Making Health Policy

Third edition

Understanding Public Health Series

Understanding Public Health is an innovative series published by Open University Press in collaboration with the London School of Hygiene and Tropical Medicine, where it is used as a key learning resource for postgraduate programmes. It provides self-directed learning covering the major issues in public health across the globe.

This is one of a series of books that provides a foundation for those wishing to join in and contribute to the twenty-first-century regeneration of public health, helping to put the concerns and perspectives of public health at the heart of policy making and service provision. While each book stands alone, together they provide a comprehensive account of the three main aims of public health: protecting the public from environmental hazards, improving the health of the public and ensuring high-quality health services are available to all. Some of the books focus on methods, others on key topics. They have been written by staff at the London School of Hygiene & Tropical Medicine with considerable experience of teaching public health to students from low-, middle- and high-income countries. Much of the material has been developed and tested with postgraduate students both in face-to-face teaching and through distance learning.

The books are designed for self-directed learning. Each chapter has explicit learning objectives, key terms are highlighted, and the text contains many activities to enable the reader to test their own understanding of the ideas and material covered. Written in a clear and accessible style, the series is essential reading for students taking postgraduate courses in public health and will also be of interest to public health practitioners and policy makers.

Titles in the series

Analytical Models for Decision-Making: Colin Sanderson, Reinhold Gruen
Applied Communicable Disease Control: Liza Cragg, Will Nutland, James Rudge (eds)
Conflict and Health: Natasha Howard, Egbert Sondorp, Annemarie Ter Veen (eds)
Economic Analysis for Management and Policy: Steven Jan, Kara Hanson, Lilani Kumarayanake, Jenny
    Roberts, Kate Archibald (eds)
Economic evaluation: Julia Fox-Rushby and John Cairns (eds)
Environmental Epidemiology: Paul Wilkinson (ed.)
Environmental Health Policy: Megan Landon, Tony Fletcher
Environment, Health and Sustainable Development, Second Edition: Emma Hutchinson, Sari Kovats (eds)
Financial Management in Health Services: Reinhold Gruen, Ann Howarth
Globalization and Global Health, Third Edition: Critical Issues and Policy: Carolyn Stephens, Benjamin
    Hawkins, Marco Liverani (eds)
Health Care Evaluation, Second Edition: Carmen Tsang, David Cromwell (eds)
Health Promotion Theory, Second Edition: Liza Cragg, Maggie Davies, Wendy Macdowall (eds)
Health Promotion Practice, Second Edition: Will Nutland, Liza Cragg (eds)
Introduction to Epidemiology, Third Edition: Ilona Carneiro
Introduction to Health Economics, Second Edition: Lorna Guinness, Virginia Wiseman (eds)
Making Health Policy, Third Edition: Kent Buse, Nicholas Mays, Manuela Colombini, Alec Fraser,
    Mishal Khan, and Helen Walls (eds)
Managing Health Services: Nick Goodwin, Reinhold Gruen, Valerie Iles
Medical Anthropology: Robert Pool, Wenzel Geissler
Principles of Social Research, Second Edition: Mary Alison Durand, Tracey Chantler (eds)
Public Health in History: Virginia Berridge, Martin Gorsky, Alex Mold (eds)
Sexual Health: A Public Health Perspective: Kaye Wellings, Kirstin Mitchell, Martine Collumbien (eds)
Understanding Health Services, Second Edition: Ipek Gurol-Urganci, Fiona Campbell, Nick Black

Forthcoming titles

Conflict and Health, Second Edition: Catherine McGowan, Bhargavi Rao, Rachael Cummings, Jerry
    Mbasha (eds)

Making Health Policy

Third edition

Kent Buse, Nicholas Mays,
Manuela Colombini, Alec Fraser,
Mishal Khan and Helen Walls

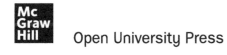
Open University Press

Open University Press
McGraw Hill
Unit 4
Foundation Park
Roxborough Way
Maidenhead
SL6 3UD

email: emea_uk_ireland@mheducation.com
world wide web: www.mheducation.co.uk

Senior Portfolio Manager: Sam Crowe
Editorial Assistant: Hannah Jones
Content Product Manager: Ali Davis

A catalogue record of this book is available from the British Library

ISBN-13: 978-0-3352-5168-1
ISBN-10: 0335251684
eISBN: 978-0-3352-5169-8

Library of Congress Cataloging-in-Publication Data
CIP data applied for

Typeset by Transforma Pvt. Ltd., Chennai, India
Printed and bound by CPI Group (UK) Ltd, Croydon, CR0 4YY

Praise page

"This third edition to 'Making Health Policy' is a welcome update. It continues to be an accessible, comprehensive yet compact introduction to the key politics and processes of health policy. It is an excellent resource for both undergraduate and graduate students who are new to this subject, as it walks them through the key debates and challenges. The broad range of examples and exercises help to bring the issues the book discusses to life. A key improvement is how the issues of colonisation and decolonisation are thoughtfully addressed throughout the book, rather than merely treated as an afterthought."
Juan Baeza, Senior lecturer in Health Policy, King's College London, UK

"Buse et al provides a remarkably succinct synthesis of a massive amount of public policy literature and offers clear applications across the health field. The third edition updates not only the literature but also reflects how the health policy field has been evolving – particularly in relation to global health. This is the ONE book not only for students but for all the policy practitioners who stumbled into the field and need to make sense of what's going on around them."
Professor Vivian Lin, Executive Associate Dean (Strategy and Operations), Professor of Public Health Practice, The University of Hong Kong

"This much-thumbed text has had a facelift! Recognising decolonial perspectives, adding new chapters on values and local-national-regional-global relationships, and updating other elements. Yet retaining the central elements that have made this text a 'must have' on your policy shelf. Educators will welcome the refresh. Generations of students will continue to appreciate the book as a true eye-opener. It's a guide to the importance of power and politics in understanding health policy – and every public health and social change activist and scholar needs to understand that!"
Prof Lucy Gilson, Professor and Head, Health Policy and Systems Division, School of Public Health University of Cape Town, South Africa

"This latest edition of an outstanding introduction to the politics of health policy making is enhanced by inclusion of critical perspectives and a new chapter on values in policymaking. The book is essential reading for anyone wanting guidance on managing the politics of the health policy process."
Prof Jeremy Shiffman, Bloomberg Distinguished Professor of Global Health Policy, Johns Hopkins University, USA

"This is the best textbook on health policy."
Prof Uta Lehmann, Director, School of Public Health, University of Western Cape, South Africa

Contents

List of figures

List of tables

List of abbreviations

ABC	abstain, be faithful and use a condom
ABPI	Association of the British Pharmaceutical Industry
ACF	Advocacy Coalition Framework
ACT UP	AIDS Coalition to Unleash Power
AIDS	acquired immune deficiency syndrome
AISP	agricultural input subsidy programme
AMR	antimicrobial resistance
ASH	Action on Smoking and Health
BIO	biotechnology innovation organization
BP	Bloomberg Philanthropies
BRICS	Brazil, Russia, India, China and South Africa
CIPRB	Centre for Injury Prevention Bangladesh
COVID-19	coronavirus disease
CVD	cardiovascular disease
EBM	evidence-based medicine
EBP	evidence-based policy
ECOSOC	United Nations Economic and Social Council
EWEC	Every Woman Every Child
EU	European Union
FAO	Food and Agricultural Organization of the United Nations
FCTC	Framework Convention on Tobacco Control
FDA	United States' Food and Drug Administration
FISP	Farm Input Subsidy Programme (Malawi)
GATT	General Agreement on Tariffs and Trade
GAVI	The Global Vaccine Alliance
GBV	gender-based violence
GIPA	principle of greater involvement of people living with AIDS
GHPs	global public–private health partnerships
GP	general (medical) practitioner
HIC	high-income country
HIV	human immunodeficiency virus
HPA	health policy analysis
ICC	International Chamber of Commerce
IHR	International Health Regulations
ILO	International Labour Organization
ILS	International Life Saving Federation
IMF	International Monetary Fund
IPC	Intellectual Property Committee

IPR	intellectual property rights
ISDS	investor-state dispute settlement
LIC	low-income country
LMICs	low- and middle-income countries
MDG	Millennium Development Goals
MIC	middle-income country
MoH	ministry of health
MMR	mumps, measles and rubella
MRVD	Maatschappij tot Redding van Drenkelingen
MSF	Médecins Sans Frontières
NCDs	non-communicable diseases
NGOs	non-governmental organizations
NHS	UK National Health Service
NICE	National Institute for Health and Care Excellence
Norad	Norwegian Agency for Development Cooperation
NPM	New Public Management
NPT	Normalization Process Theory
NRA	National Rifle Association
OECD	Organisation for Economic Co-operation and Development
PAD	Pandemic Antiviral Discovery
PbR	payment by results
PEPFAR	US President's Emergency Plan for AIDS Relief
PhRMA	Pharmaceutical Research and Manufacturers of America
PPE	personal protective equipment
PrEP	pre-exposure prophylactic
RCT	randomized controlled trial
RLSS	Royal Life Saving Society
RNLI	Royal National Lifeboat Institution
SARS	severe acute respiratory syndrome
SDGs	Sustainable Development Goals
SDG3 GAP	Global Action Plan for Healthy Lives and Wellbeing for All
Sida	Swedish International Development Agency
SMS	short message service
STI	sexually transmitted infection
SWAPs	sector-wide approaches
TAC	Treatment Action Campaign
TASC	The Alliance for Safe Children
TB	tuberculosis
TNCs	transnational corporations
TRIPS	Agreement on Trade Related Intellectual Property Rights
UK	United Kingdom
UN	United Nations
UNAIDS	United Nations Joint Programme on HIV/AIDS
UNDP	United Nations Development Programme
UNFPA	United Nations Fund for Population

UNICEF	formerly known as the United Nations Children's Emergency Fund
UNODC	UN Office on Drugs and Crime
UNOPS	United Nations Office for Project Services
US	United States of America
USA	United States of America
USAID	United States Agency for International Development
VAW	violence against women
vCJD	Variant Creutzfeldt–Jakob Disease
WCDP	World Conference on Drowning Prevention
WFP	World Food Programme
WHA	World Health Assembly
WHO	World Health Organization
WTO	World Trade Organization
XR	Extinction Rebellion

Author biographies

Kent Buse is Director of the Healthier Societies Program of the George Institute of Global Health and is Visiting Professor at Imperial College London. He served for over a decade as chief of strategy, policy and research at UNAIDS. A political-economist, Kent has been on the faculty of the Yale School of Public Health and the London School of Hygiene and Tropical Medicine.

Nicholas Mays is Professor of Health Policy at the London School of Hygiene and Tropical Medicine and a senior associate at the Nuffield Trust, a health policy and management think tank in London. His work currently focuses on health and care policy evaluation.

Manuela Colombini is an associate professor in the Faculty of Public Health and Policy at the London School of Hygiene and Tropical Medicine. A health systems and policy researcher, she specializes in health policy agenda setting and policy implementation, and systems integration.

Alec Fraser is a lecturer at King's College London and an honorary assistant professor in public policy and management at the London School of Hygiene and Tropical Medicine. His research focuses on evidence use, financial incentives and public management reform in the UK and EU countries.

Mishal Khan is an associate professor of health policy and systems at the London School of Hygiene and Tropical Medicine, visiting faculty at the Aga Khan University in Pakistan and an associate fellow at the Chatham House Global Health Programme. A social epidemiologist who has led research programmes in Asia for over 15 years, her work focuses on addressing health inequities and improving governance.

Helen Walls is an associate professor at the London School of Hygiene and Tropical Medicine. She is a public health and policy researcher whose work focuses on addressing the structural determinants of population health, particularly the political economy of food systems and nutrition.

Overview of the book

Introduction

This book provides a comprehensive introduction to the study of health policy, its political nature and its processes. Much of what is written and debated deals with the content of health policy – the 'what' of policy. This literature may use medicine, epidemiology, organizational theory or economics to provide evidence for, or evaluation of, health policy. Legions of doctors, epidemiologists, health economists and organizational theorists develop technically sound solutions to problems of public health importance. Yet, surprisingly little guidance is available to public health students, practitioners and advocates who wish to understand how issues make their way onto policy agendas (and how to frame these issues so that they are better received), how policy makers treat evidence (and how to form better relationships with decision makers) and why some policy initiatives are implemented while others languish. These political dimensions of the health policy process are rarely taught in schools of medicine or public health – but are profoundly important in determining public health outcomes.

Why study health policy?

This book integrates important concepts such as power into the study of health policy processes. Who makes and implements policy decisions (those with power) and how decisions are made (process) largely determine the content of health policy and, thereby, ultimately people's health. To illustrate this point, take the case of developing HIV policy in a country facing a tight budget constraint. Were health economists primarily involved in advising the health minister, it is likely that prevention would be emphasized (as preventive interventions tend to be more cost-effective than curative ones). If, however, the minister also consulted representatives of people living with HIV, as well as the pharmaceutical industry, it is likely that greater emphasis would be placed on treatment and care. And if powerful feminist organizations had the ear of the minister, they might lobby for interventions to empower women to protect themselves from unwanted and unprotected sex. The reconciliation of different views and the resulting policy depend on the power of various actors in the policy arena as well as the process of policy making (e.g. how widely and which groups are consulted and involved). Whether or not behavioural, curative or structural

HIV interventions are given priority will impact on the trajectory of an HIV epidemic.

All activity that takes place in society is subject to politics. For example, research into public health problems requires funding. In many universities, bench scientists and social scientists compete with each other for funds to support their research. Politics will determine the allocation of public funds to different research areas and academic disciplines, and private firms will invest in those researchers and endeavours that are most likely to lead to the highest rates of return. Politics does not end with funding, as politics is likely to govern access to study populations and even publication. Unfavourable findings can be blocked or distorted by project sponsors, and they can be disputed or ignored by decision makers or others who find them inconvenient. Politics is omnipresent. For this reason, understanding the politics of the policy process is arguably as important as understanding how health services and public health interventions improve health. Stated differently, while other academic disciplines may provide necessary evidence to improve health, in the absence of a robust understanding of the policy process, technical solutions will likely be insufficient to change practice in the real world.

This book is for those who wish to understand the policy process so that they are better equipped to influence it in their working lives. It is intended as a guide for students and professionals who wish to improve their skills in navigating and managing the health policy process – irrespective of the health issue or setting.

Evolution of the book

The first edition of this book, published in 2005, was co-authored by Kent Buse, Nicholas Mays and Gill Walt. Its starting point was the second edition of Gill Walt's earlier book, *Health Policy: An Introduction to Process and Power* (1994). The second starting point was and remains the framework for health policy analysis developed by Gill Walt and Lucy Gilson (1994). The framework attempts to simplify what are in practice highly complex relationships by visualizing them in terms of a 'policy triangle'. The framework draws attention to the 'context' within which policy is situated, the 'processes' associated with developing and implementing policy and the content of the policy. The 'actors', whose ideas and interests drive much of the policy action, are placed at the centre of the triangle. The framework can be applied in any country, to any policy, and at any policy level. A diverse range of theories and disciplinary approaches, particularly from political science, international relations, economics, sociology and organizational theory, are drawn upon throughout the book to support this simple analytical framework and provide explanations of the policy process.

For this third edition, we have updated the text, particularly with new examples where appropriate, and revised parts of the previous text in response to comments and suggestions from students and colleagues received since the second edition was published in 2012. Since that edition, there have been significant changes in the political and intellectual environment surrounding health policy analysis, especially in the field of what is currently known as, probably misleadingly, 'global health', formerly referred to as 'international health'. The most prominent is the movement to 'decolonize' and broaden the practice of global health and its related scholarship. This movement has a number of critical strands relevant to a health policy textbook, in particular: advocacy of inclusion of a wider range of theory and empirical studies by researchers originating outside North America and Europe; and challenges to the use of terminology and categories that reinforce colonial and racist assumptions about countries and peoples, especially hierarchical dichotomies such as 'developed versus developing', 'advanced versus emerging', 'resource rich versus resource poor' and so on. These challenges also relate to how people with different backgrounds are referred to and the connotations of these group labels. For example, the use of 'white' as the reference population while simultaneously relegating other people to a single grouping such as Black or even the widely used term People of Colour has been increasingly criticized for normalizing whiteness and failing to acknowledge the diversity of populations' cultures, histories and experiences (Khan et al. 2022).

We have tried to respond to these challenges in the revised text. For example, we have tried to be specific when referring to different countries and regions of the world and to avoid coarse dichotomies of countries or groups of people that risk perpetuating notions of superiority and inferiority. However, we do, from time to time, refer to broad groups of countries in terms of their income and wealth, particularly because the wealthiest countries not only have more resources to devote to improving health but also have far greater ability to determine their destinies than poorer countries. We have also incorporated additional theoretical perspectives and empirical studies from researchers who originate and work outside North America and Europe. Sometimes, we have been hampered by our collective ignorance or the preponderance of research led from North America and Europe. The process of globalizing the understanding of health policy is still in its early stages.

Structure of the book

The eleven chapters of the third edition are organized partly according to the broad contours of the health policy 'triangle' and partly according to the device of breaking the policy process into 'stages'. Chapter 1 introduces the importance and meaning of 'policy', and describes the 'policy triangle' and the 'Kaleidoscope' frameworks for health policy analysis. The latter has been informed by the increasing amount of research on the health policy process rooted in a diverse range of countries. The chapter demonstrates how both frameworks can be used to understand policy change. Chapter 2 builds on these frameworks to describe a number of theories which help explain the relationship between power and policy making, including those which deal with how power is exercised by different groups, how power is distributed and how power affects decision-making processes. The revised chapter includes a wider range of theories of the nature of power as well as perspectives on the experience of power.

Chapter 3 introduces the role of the state and, within it, the role of the government or administration in power within a country. It traces their changing roles and importance for domestic health policy making. Chapter 4 focuses on interest groups outside government and the state, principally, the private sector and the civil society (often referred to as the Third Sector in contrast to the state and the private (market) sector). These interest groups in the health sector are compared in terms of their resources, tactics and success in shaping the policy process.

Chapter 5 looks at how policy issues get onto both national and global policy agendas using three theories. It shows how the way a problem is 'framed' or presented affects whether it gets taken seriously in policy terms and also looks at the role of mass and social media in this process. Chapter 6 continues the analysis of the policy process by exploring policy implementation. It contrasts and reconciles 'top-down' and 'bottom-up' approaches to explaining implementation (or often lack thereof). Chapter 7 looks at policy evaluation and explores the different ways in which evidence enters and contributes to health policy.

Chapter 8 is a new chapter on the place of values in policy making. We think it is especially relevant because of the widespread tendency in health to view the solutions to health problems in purely technical, empirical terms, neglecting the importance for policy making of judgements about sound processes and the priority given to different goals such as equity and efficiency, which, in turn, relate to views about what a 'good society' should look like.

Chapters 9 and 10 shift attention to health policy making beyond the boundaries of individual countries to the global level. Chapter 9 looks at the actors involved in global health policy and the limits of policy making at the supra-national level. Chapter 10, also a new chapter, explores the inter-relationship between policies determined and enacted at local, country, regional and global levels.

The final chapter is devoted to doing policy analysis. It sets out in more detail the political approach to policy analysis that has guided the entire book. It reviews the main techniques for gathering, organizing and analysing data for health policy analysis. The chapter aims to assist you to analyse policy processes and to develop politically informed strategies to bring about health policy change in your professional life.

Each chapter comprises an overview, learning objectives, definition of key terms, activities, feedback on the activities, and a brief summary, further reading and list of references at the end. A number of the activities ask you to reflect on various aspects of a specific health policy, which you can select based on what you already know from previous experience or what you can find out from websites, government policy statements, independent reports, blogs, social media posts or articles in the mass media. The further readings, including websites, where relevant, at the end of each chapter have been chosen for a range of reasons: some enable you to go into greater depth; some are particularly illuminating case studies; and others offer a different perspective on the subject matter of the chapter.

Acknowledgements

We are grateful to the many colleagues and students who have commented both favourably and with constructive criticisms on the previous edition of the book. We are especially grateful to Neil Spicer for his initial thoughts on how to revise the previous edition and for taking the time to read and comment on the manuscript of the third edition and to Justin-Paul Scarr for contributing the case study on drowning prevention.

References

Khan, T., Abimbola, S., Kyobutungi, C. and Pai, M. (2022) How we classify countries and people – and why it matters, *BMJ Global Health,* 7:e009704. https://doi.org/10.1136/bmjgh-2022-009704
Walt, G. (1994) *Health Policy: An Introduction to Process and Power*, 2nd edn. London: Zed Books.
Walt, G. and Gilson, L. (1994) Reforming the health sector in developing countries: the central role of policy analysis, *Health Policy and Planning*, 9: 353–70.

Frameworks for health policy analysis

1

This chapter introduces you to what health policy is and why it is important. You will then go on to consider a simple analytical framework that incorporates the notions of context, process and actors, to demonstrate how they can help explain how and why policies do or do not change over time. Several additional frameworks will also be introduced which present complementary ways of explaining changes in health policy processes.

Learning objectives

After working through this chapter, you will be better able to:

- understand several frameworks for analysing health policy
- define the following key concepts:
  - policy
  - policy content
  - context
  - actors
  - process
- describe how health policies are made through the inter-relationship of context, process and actors
- understand a related way of looking at policy making that sees it as occurring through the ongoing interaction among interests, ideas and institutions.

Key terms

Actor Shorthand term used to denote any participant in the policy process that affects or has an interest in a policy, including individuals, organizations, groups, governments and international bodies.

Content Substance of a particular policy which details its constituent parts (e.g. its specific objectives).

Context Systemic factors – political, economic, social or cultural, local, national and international – which may affect health policy.

Decolonization The process of undoing colonial dispossession and destruction; e.g. through practices that reduce emphasis on hitherto dominant Eurocentric knowledge, and emphasize, promote and nurture indigenous and/or local knowledge production.

Epistemic community Policy community marked by shared political values, and a shared understanding of a problem and its causes.

Ideas The values, evidence, anecdote and argument that shape policy, including the way a policy problem or solution is presented or framed.

Institutions In political science, the 'rules of the game' determining how organizations, such as governments, operate. These can be formal structures and procedures, but also informal norms of behaviour that may not be written down. Confusingly, the term is also in more general use to refer to 'organizations'.

Interest What an actor or group stands to gain or lose from a policy change.

Policy Broad statement of goals, objectives and means that create the framework for activity leading to implementation with varying degrees of completeness. It often takes the form of explicit written documents, but may also be implicit or unwritten.

Policy elite Specific group of policy makers who hold senior positions in a policy system, and often have privileged access to other top members of the same, and other, organizations.

Policy makers Those who influence or make policies in organizations such as central or local government, multinational companies or local businesses, clinics or hospitals.

Policy process The way in which problems rise to policy makers' attention and policies are initiated, formulated, negotiated, adopted, communicated, implemented and evaluated.

Positionality The stance or positioning of the policy maker or policy researcher, related to their particular identity, in the social, economic and political context of a policy issue. It is thought to shape how they think about and tackle the issue.

Why is health policy important?

Health and well-being matter to most people, and often more so than income or education. Without health, as the saying goes, you have nothing. Governments also typically care about health, perhaps not as much as many people would like them to, but governments have a large stake in health – not least because the health sector is a major part of the economy as well as a major source of public and private expenditure. Some see the health sector as a sponge – absorbing large amounts of national resources to pay for the many health workers employed. Others see it as a driver of the economy, through innovation and investment in bio-medical technologies or production and sales of pharmaceuticals, or through ensuring a healthy and economically productive population. The advent of the coronavirus disease (COVID-19) pandemic in 2020 underlined how important health is to the functioning of both society and the economy as well as the policies and processes governments can and arguably should put in place to ensure public health (Loewenson et al. 2020).

Poverty, the physical environment and working conditions all have an impact on health status and health equity, and hence policies across many sectors, such as education, food, transport and urban planning directly impact on health and disease. For example, economic policies, such as taxes on sugar or alcohol are designed to influence corporate action and limit access to harmful products and encourage people to make healthier choices.

Most people come into contact with the health sector as patients or clients, through using hospitals, clinics or pharmacies, or as health professionals such as nurses, doctors, medical auxiliaries, pharmacists or managers. But it is their everyday environments – in work and leisure – that determine whether they are healthy or sick. Because the nature of decision making in relation to health often involves matters of life and death, health is often accorded a special position in comparison to other social issues.

Understanding the relationship between health policy and health, and the impact that policies in a range of sectors have on health, is important because it should help to tackle some of the major health problems of our time – such as rising obesity or heat-induced kidney disease or heart attacks. Health policy guides choices about which health technologies to develop and use, how to organize and finance health services, which drugs will be freely available or opportunities available to collaborate with non-health sectors for co-benefits (such as active transport). To understand these relationships, it is necessary to better define what is meant by health policy.

What is health policy?

In this book you will often come across the terms policy, public policy and health policy.

Policy is often thought of as the product of the decisions taken by those with responsibility for a given policy area – it may be in health or the environment, in education or in trade. The people who contribute to, influence, or are directly involved in making policies are referred to as *policy makers*. Policy may be made at many levels – in central or local government, in a multinational company or local business, in a school or hospital. While a range of individuals and groups are typically involved in policy making (and hence are policy makers), some of them can be thought of as members of a *policy elite* – a specific group of decision makers who have particularly strong influence – they may have senior positions in an organization, and often privileged access to other top members of the same, and other, organizations. For example, policy elites in government include the members of the prime minister's cabinet, all of whom would be able to contact and meet the top executives of a multinational company or of an international agency, such as the World Health Organization (WHO).

Policies are made in the private for-profit sector, the voluntary or not for profit sector, and public sector. In the private sector, multinational conglomerates may establish policies for all their companies around the world on some issues, whilst allowing local companies to decide their own policies on others, such as conditions of service. For example, corporations such as Anglo-American and Heineken introduced anti-retroviral therapy for their African employees living with HIV in the early 2000s before many governments did so. However, private sector corporations have to ensure that their policies are made within the confines of public law, made by governments.

Public policy refers to government policy or the policies of government agencies. For example, Thomas Dye (2001) says that public policy is whatever governments choose to do or not to do. He argues that failure to decide or act on a particular issue also constitutes policy. Such omissions are often not formally expressed and written down. For example, many countries have taken no legislative action requiring the use of child seats for young children in vehicles while others have regarded it as a priority for action.

The voluntary sector also makes health-related policy. Oxfam, a leading global organization in the fight against inequality, poverty and injustice, for example, has several policies on access to medicines and has led global efforts for a People's Vaccine for COVID-19.

When looking for examples of public policy, you might wish to look first for statements or formal positions issued by a government, or a government agency, as these might be the easiest to locate. These may be couched in terms that suggest the accomplishment of a particular purpose or goal (e.g. the introduction of needle exchange programmes to reduce harm among people who inject drugs) or to resolve a specific problem (e.g. charges on car journeys to reduce traffic congestion and improve air quality in urban areas).

Policies may refer to a government's health or economic policy, where policy is used as a field of activity, or to a specific proposal – 'from next year, it will be university policy to ensure students are represented on all governing bodies'. Sometimes a policy is described as a 'programme'. For example, a government's school health programme may include a number of different policies: excluding children from starting school before they are fully immunized; providing medical examinations; subsidizing school meals; and ensuring sex education in the school curriculum. The programme is thus the embodiment of health policy for school children. In this example, it is clear that policies may not arise from a single decision but could consist of a series of decisions that accumulate to lead to a broad course of action over time. These decisions or actions may or may not be intended, defined or even recognized as policy in a formal document or statement.

As you can see, there are many ways of defining public policy. Thomas Dye's simple definition of public policy as being what governments do, or do not do, contrasts with definitions that emphasize that policy is made to achieve a particular goal or purpose.

In this book, *health policy* is assumed to embrace courses of action (and inaction) that affect the set of organizations, staff, services, funding arrangements and beneficiaries of the health and health care systems. It includes policy made in the public sector (by government) as well as policies in the private, including voluntary, sector. But because health is influenced by many determinants outside the health and health care systems, health policy analysts are also interested in the actions (and lack of actions) of organizations external to the recognized health care system which have an impact on health (for example, the ministry of transportation or the environment, or the food, tobacco or pharmaceutical industries).

Analysing health policy

Just as there are various definitions of what policy is, there are many way to analyse health policy and what to focus on: an economist may say health policy is primarily about finding the most effective and efficient allocation of scarce resources for health; a public health practitioner may see it as a way to influence the determinants of health in order to improve population health equity; and for a doctor it may be all about health care services for individuals (Walt 1994). Like any field of policy, health policy is inextricably linked with politics and its analysis deals explicitly with who influences policy making, and how they exercise that influence under different conditions.

Politics cannot be divorced from health policy. If you are applying epidemiology, economics, biology or any other professional or technical knowledge to everyday life, politics will affect you. No one is unaffected by the influence of politics. For example, scientists may have to focus their research on the issues funders are interested in, rather than the questions they themselves want to explore; in prescribing drugs, health professionals may have to take into consideration potentially conflicting demands of hospital managers, government regulations and people's ability to pay. They may also be visited by drug company representatives who want to persuade them to prescribe particular drugs, and who may be permitted by government to use incentives to encourage them to do so.

Devising a framework for incorporating politics into health policy needs to go beyond the point at which many health policy analysts stop: the *content* of policy. Much health policy analysis is evaluative in that it focuses on a particular policy, describing what it purports to do, the measures proposed to achieve its goals, and whether it achieved them. For example, there has been a long-term interest in how to organize the finance and provision of health services since the 1980s, with analysts asking questions such as:

- Which would be a better policy to raise funds for services – the introduction of user fees or a social insurance system?
- Which public health services should be contracted out to the private sector – cleaning services in hospitals or blood banks or others?
- Which policy instruments are needed to undertake major changes such as these – legislation, regulation or incentives?

At other times, additional questions come to the fore. During the COVID-19 pandemic, for example, these included questions such as the optimal length of quarantine, the number of people it was safe to meet with outside, the conditions under which a mask ought to be worn, the workers who were deemed to be essential, etc. With growing concern about planetary health, policy makers are increasingly raising questions about issues such as the impact of extreme heat on specific health conditions, the best ways to decarbonize clinical trials and hospital supply chains, prevent childhood drowning or secure national food supplies within planetary boundaries.

The above-mentioned questions are the 'what' or *content* questions of health policy. But they cannot be divorced from the 'who', 'how' and 'why' questions. Who makes the decisions? Who implements them? Under what conditions will they be introduced and executed, or ignored, and why? What is the best way to generate incentives for inter-ministerial collaboration on the social determinants of health? In other words, the content is not separate from the *politics* and process of policy making. For example, in Uganda, when the President saw evidence that use of health services had fallen dramatically after the introduction of charges for health services, he overturned the earlier policy of his Ministry of Health (MoH). To understand why he made that decision, you need to know something about the political *context* (an election coming up and the desire to win votes); the *power* of the President to introduce change; and the role of *evidence* and *values* in influencing the decision, among other things. These are factors explored by Moat and Abelson (2011).

Activity 1.1

Without looking at the text below, provide a short definition of the following terms:

- policy
- public policy
- health policy.

Think of an example from your own country for each.

Feedback

- Policy refers to the decisions taken or not taken by those with responsibility for a particular policy area.
- Public policy refers to policies made by the state or the government and/or by those in the public sector (e.g. in agencies of government).
- Health policy covers courses of action (and inaction) that affect the set of organizations, staff, services, funding arrangements and beneficiaries of the health and health care system (both public and private).

You may have found it tricky to define these terms. This is because 'policy' is not a precise or self-evident term. For example, Anderson (1975) says policy is 'a purposive course of action followed by an *actor* or set of actors in dealing with a problem or matter of concern'. But this appears to make policy an 'intended' course of action, whereas many would argue that policies are sometimes the unintended result of many different decisions made over time, including decisions not to do anything. Policies may be expressed in a whole series of instruments: practices, statements, regulations and laws. They may be implicit or explicit, discretionary or statutory. Also, the word 'policy' does not always translate well: in English a distinction is often made between policy and politics, but in many languages the word for policy is the same as the word for politics.

The 'health policy triangle'

The approach to policy analysis in this book acknowledges the importance of looking not only at the *content* of policy, but also the *processes* of policy making, including how power is used in a particular health policy context. This means exploring the role of *actors* such as the nation state, international organizations and the groups making up national and global civil society, as well as the private sector, to understand how they interact

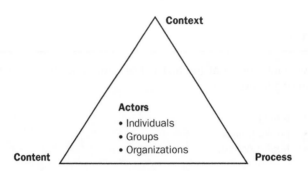

Figure 1.1: Policy analysis triangle
Source: Walt and Gilson (1994)

and influence health policy. It also means understanding the processes
through which such influence is played out (e.g. in formulating policy) and
the *context* in which these different actors and processes interact. A framework for analysing health policy that brings these elements together was
developed by Walt and Gilson (1994) (Figure 1.1). It focuses on content,
context, process and actors. It is useful for this book because it helps
to conceptualize four domains important for systematically exploring the
political nature of health policy and it can be applied in a range of contexts
including in high-, middle- and low-income countries. It provides a starting
point for health policy analysis but other factors shaping policy such as
the distribution of power, the role of values and the contribution of evidence
need to be taken into account. These and other influences on policy are
discussed in the chapters that follow.

The health policy triangle is clearly a highly simplified representation of
a complex set of inter-relationships, and may give the impression that the
four factors can be considered separately. This is not so! In reality, actors
are influenced (as individuals or members of groups or organizations) by the
context within which they live and work, including, for example, the prevailing ideology and culture, their disciplinary training, and the process of policy
making. And the processes of policy making – for example, how issues get
on to policy agendas, and how they fare once there – are affected by actors,
their position in power structures, and their own values and expectations.
The content of policy will likely reflect some or all of these factors. So, while
the policy triangle is useful for helping us to think systematically about all
the different factors that might affect policy, it is like a map that shows the
main roads but lacks contours, rivers, forests, paths and dwellings.

The actors who make or influence policy

As you can see from Figure 1.1, Walt and Gilson place actors at the centre
of the health policy framework. The term actor may be used to denote individuals (e.g. a particular statesperson), organizations such as the World

Bank or multinational companies such as Shell, or the state or government. It is important, however, to recognize that this is a simplification. Individuals cannot be separated from the organizations within which they work, and any organization or group is made up of many different people, not all of whom speak with one voice and whose values, beliefs and interests may differ on policy issues.

In the chapters that follow you will look at many different actors and ways of differentiating between them in order to analyse who has influence in the policy process. For example, there are many ways of describing groups that are outside the realm of the state. In international relations it has been customary to talk about non-state actors (actors outside government). Political scientists talk about interest or pressure groups. In the development literature, these groups are usually referred to as civil society organizations or non-governmental organizations (NGOs) (organizations which fall between the state and the individual or household). What differentiates all these actors from government or state actors and political parties is that they do not seek formal political power for themselves, although they do want to influence those with formal political power.

Sometimes many different groups get together to demonstrate strong feelings about particular issues – these are called social movements or popular movements. For example, the early twenty-first century has been marked by the activities of a global social movement loosely united under the anti-globalization banner. It organized major protests against what was perceived as the unfair and unregulated power and greed of multinational corporations and banks. Over the past decade disruptive eco-justice and planetary health movements have emerged as people seek to ensure stronger government action and accountability on the global climate crisis.

Actors may try to influence the policy process at the local, national, regional or international level. Often, they become parts of networks to consult and decide on policy at all of these levels. At the local level, for example, community health workers may interact with environmental health officers, teachers in local schools, or local businesses in the implementation of health policy. At the international level, actors may be linked with others across state borders. For example, they may be members of inter-governmental networks (i.e. government officials in one department of government in one country, learning lessons about policy alternatives from government officials from another country); or they may be part of policy or *epistemic communities* – networks of collaborating professionals with recognized expertise and relevant knowledge in a specific field of policy. Others may form issue networks – coming together to act on a particular issue. In Chapter 4 you will learn more about the differences between these groups and their roles in the policy process.

To understand the variation between actors in how much they influence the policy process means understanding the concept of power, and how it is exercised. Actors may seek to influence policy, but the extent to which they will be able to do so will depend, among other things, on their perceived and actual power. Power may be characterized by a mixture of individual wealth, personality (charisma), level of or access to knowledge, or authority, but it is strongly tied up with the organizations and structures (including networks and 'social contracts' such as patriarchy or white supremacy) within which the individual actor works and lives as well as the position or office that the individual holds. Sociologists and political scientists talk about the interplay between 'agency' and 'structure'. 'Agency' refers to the power or capacity of actors to act independently and to make their own free choices. 'Structure', by contrast, denotes the arrangements which limit the choices and opportunities available to specific actors. In practice, the power of actors (agents) is intertwined with the structures (organizations) to which they belong. In this book it is assumed that power is the result of the interaction between agency and structure, about which you will learn more in Chapter 2.

Activity 1.2

Make a list of the different actors who might be involved in making policy on HIV and/or AIDS in your own country. Place the actors into wider groups.

Feedback

You might have grouped actors in different ways and in each country the list will differ and will change over time. The examples below may or may not apply to your country but they give an idea of the sorts of categories and actors you might have thought of. Where you do not know them, do not worry as we discuss these actors in the following chapters:

- government (e.g. ministries of health, education, interior);
- international NGOs (e.g. Médecins Sans Frontières);
- national NGOs (e.g. of people living with HIV, faith-based organizations);
- pressure/interest groups (e.g. the Treatment Action Campaign);
- international organizations (e.g. WHO, UNAIDS, the World Bank);
- bilateral agencies (e.g. Norad, Sida);
- funding organizations (e.g. the Global Fund, PEPFAR);
- private sector companies (e.g. Anglo-American, Heineken, Merck & Co);
- researchers (e.g. from universities, think tanks).

Contextual factors that affect policy

Context refers to systemic factors – political, economic and social, present at local, regional, national and international levels – which may have an effect on health policy. There are many ways of categorizing such factors, but one useful way is provided by Leichter (1979):

- *Situational factors* are the more or less transient or idiosyncratic conditions which may influence policy (e.g. wars, droughts). These are sometimes called 'focusing events' (see Chapter 5). These may be a one-off occurrence, such as an earthquake which leads to changes in hospital building regulations. They may also be associated with a longer, delayed and diffused public recognition of a problem. For example, the advent of the HIV epidemic (which took time to be acknowledged as an epidemic on a world scale) gradually produced new treatment and control policies for tuberculosis (TB) because of the inter-relationship of the two diseases – people living with HIV are more susceptible to diseases, and latent tuberculosis may be triggered by HIV. The health impacts of the global climate crisis may not be transient per se but provide a succession of focusing events that contribute to increasing research attention that over time informs subsequent policy action.
- *Structural factors* are the relatively unchanging elements of the society. They may include the political system, and extent to which it is open or closed; that is, whether or not there are opportunities for civil society to participate in policy discussions and decisions; structural factors may also include the type of economy and the employment base. For example, where wages for nurses are low, or where workloads are unrealistically high, countries may suffer migration of these professionals to other societies where there is a shortage or better working conditions. Other structural factors that will affect a country's health policy will include demographic features or technological advances. For example, long-term care costs rise for countries with ageing populations, as their care needs increase with age. Technological change has increased the number of women giving birth by caesarean section in many countries. Among the reasons given are increasing professional reliance on monitoring technology that has led to reluctance among some doctors and midwives to take any risks, and a fear of litigation. And, of course, a country's national wealth will have a strong effect on which health services can be afforded. A country's energy sources may be considered a structural factor that has implications for how quickly the health sector can decarbonize or the priority placed on mass and active transport, for example.
- *Cultural factors* may also affect health policy. In societies where formal hierarchies are important, it may be difficult to question senior officials or elder statespersons. The position of ethnic minorities or

linguistic differences may lead to certain groups being poorly informed about their rights, or receiving services that do not meet their particular needs. In some countries where women cannot easily access health services (e.g. because they have to be accompanied by their husbands) or where there is considerable stigma about a particular disease or services, some authorities have developed systems of home visits or 'door-step' delivery (e.g. PrEP for HIV). As a result of COVID-19, online services, for example for mental health, have also become more common. Religious factors can also strongly affect policy, as evidenced by the so-called 'gag rule' adopted by successive Republican administrations in the United States, which seeks among other things to curb the availability of safe abortion services. The 'expanded' global gag rule adopted under the Presidency of Trump and Pence blocked global health assistance to non-American organizations using their own, non-American funds to provide information, referrals or services for legal abortion or to advocate for access to abortion services in their own countries. This impacted millions of people around the world as reproductive health services offered by NGOs were heavily curtailed for fear of the failure to comply with American right-wing cultural mores on sexual health (see Chapter 8 on values in health policy).

- *International or exogenous factors* leading to greater inter-dependence between states and influencing sovereignty and international co-operation in health may also affect health policy (see Chapters 9 and 10). Although many health problems are dealt with by national governments, some demand co-operation between national, regional or multilateral organizations. For example, the nearly complete eradication of polio has taken place in many parts of the world through national and regional action, sometimes with the assistance from international organizations such as the WHO. However, even if one state manages to immunize all its children against polio and to sustain coverage, the polio virus can be imported by people who have not been immunized crossing the border from a neighbouring country.

These contextual factors are complex, and unique in both time and setting. In recent years, scholars have emphasized the 'active' role of context. With this emphasis, context is not something in the background – but rather in the foreground shaping policy development, helping understand the 'when' and 'why' of change. It is worth considering both the 'outer context' – the elements highlighted by Leichter above – and the 'inner context' of organizations which include organizational cultural factors crucial to policy implementation (see Chapter 6). Some contexts may be more or less receptive to policy change – this helps explain why some policies are implemented in some places more quickly or fully than others (Robert and Fulop 2014).

The implementation of specialist stroke units in England provides an example of how context shapes policy making (Langhorne 2021). There was early evidence from Northern Ireland in the 1950s that stroke patients had better outcomes if treated on specialist wards. From the late 1970s, stroke units were implemented in Norway and Sweden. Large clinical trials in the 1990s in the United States of America (US) highlighted the benefits of thrombolytic drugs and the logic of centralizing and specializing stroke care. European clinicians came together to call for Stroke Unit care across the continent in 2000, and the WHO offered further support through the Helsingborg Declaration in 2006. Despite international recognition of the value of more specialized centres, adoption in England remained patchy until the government committed to large-scale stroke care improvements in 2007 through a National Stroke Care Strategy. Until this point, the context had not been receptive to changing stroke care. Stroke was seen as a low clinical and political priority because stroke patients tended to be elderly and there was seemingly little effective treatment. However, during the early 2000s, the context had been gradually changing – technological and medical advances meant that stroke patients could receive much more effective care. Stroke as a medical specialism gained higher status, and stroke patients and their families established support groups and campaigning organizations to demand better care. In addition, as England's population was ageing, stroke was becoming more of an economic burden, so it made more sense for the government to prioritize stroke care (alongside heart disease and cancer care). Finally, the development of clinical audit and international comparisons of outcomes highlighted the costs of inaction and prompted a political response.

To understand how health policies change, or do not, implies an ability to analyse the context in which they are made, and an attempt to assess how far any, or some, of these sorts of factors may influence policy outcomes.

✎ Activity 1.3

Consider urban air pollution linked to petrol and diesel transport policy in your own country. Identify some contextual factors that might have influenced the way policy has (or has not) developed. Bear in mind the way context was divided into four different factors in the description above.

Feedback

Each setting is unique, but the sorts of contextual factors you may have identified are summarized below.

Situational

- A new prime minister/president or regional mayor coming to power and making air pollution policy a priority.
- The high-profile death of a person acknowledged publicly to be linked to air pollution.
- New research findings on the impact of air pollution on specific population groups.

Structural

- The role of individual campaigners, the media or NGOs in publicizing, or not, air pollution – relating to the extent to which the political system is open or closed.
- Evidence of growing mortality and morbidity linked to air pollution made public – perhaps among a particular group such as children and the elderly.
- Wider transport and industrial policies and implications of change, including availability of resources for public transport, impacts upon jobs and the influence of pro-car lobbyists.

Cultural

- The actions and beliefs of individual actors in relation to travelling by car as opposed to public transport.
- Prevailing norms equating driving with freedom conflicting with views about the rights of citizens to clean air.
- Scandals highlighting dishonesty and illegality on the part of car manufacturers in 'cheating' emissions regulations.

International

- The role of international fossil fuel and car manufacturing corporations.
- Technical norms and standards on air pollution promoted by international agencies, for example by the European Union.

The processes of policy making

Process refers to the way in which policies are initiated, developed or formulated, negotiated, communicated, implemented and evaluated. The most common approach to understanding policy processes is to use what is called the 'stages heuristic' (Sabatier and Jenkins-Smith 1993). This is an approach that breaks the policy process into a series of easily under-standable steps, but it is acknowledged that this does not represent what happens in the real world. Nevertheless, it can be helpful to analyse policy making in terms of these different stages:

- *Problem identification and issue recognition*: explores how some issues get on to the policy agenda, while others do not even get discussed. In Chapter 5 you will go into this stage in more detail.
- *Policy formulation*: explores who is involved in formulating policy, how policies are arrived at, agreed upon, and how they are communi-cated. Berlan et al. (2014) is a useful analysis of the process of policy formulation.
- *Policy implementation*: this was traditionally the most neglected phase of policy making and is sometimes seen as quite divorced from the first two stages. However, this is arguably the most important phase of policy making because if policies are not implemented, or are diverted or changed during implementation, then something may be going wrong from the point of view of the policy originator – and the policy outcomes may not be those which were sought. These issues are discussed in Chapter 6.
- *Policy evaluation*: identifies what happens once a policy is put into effect – how it is monitored, whether it achieves its objectives and whether it has unintended consequences. This may be the stage at which policies are changed or terminated and new policies introduced. This aspect of the policy process is covered in Chapter 7.

There are caveats to using this useful but simple framework. First, it makes it look as if the policy process is linear – in other words, proceeding smoothly from one stage to another, from problem recognition to imple-mentation and evaluation. However, it is seldom so clear or obvious a process. It may be at the stage of implementation that more sophisticated problem recognition occurs or policies may be formulated but never reach implementation. In other words, policy making is seldom a neat or fully *rational* process – it is iterative and affected by interests – i.e. actors. Others have noted that there are numerous interacting cycles taking place simultaneously which defy efforts to delineate and represent the policy process in a simple and singular cycle. Hence, analysts tend to agree with Lindblom (1959) that the policy process is one which policy makers 'muddle through' as they negotiate with competing interest groups and hold imper-fect information.

Nevertheless, the 'stages heuristic' continues to be a useful device. It can be used for exploring national as well as regional and international policies in order to try to understand how policies are transferred around the world.

While the policy triangle (see Figure 1.1) and the stages heuristic are both helpful frameworks for simplifying the extremely complex, dynamic and inter-active nature of policy making, some feel that both pay too little explicit attention to other factors that explain why and how policies change. John (1998) and Howlett et al. (2009), for example, refer to the importance of the interaction of ideas, institutions (meaning how policy processes are typically organized) and interests (or actors) in changing policy. The notion of *ideas* provides a useful lens for looking at how issues and their related policies are framed and presented, because as ideas change, or issues are re-defined and re-packaged (for instance in light of new evidence), so policy may be affected – making it more or less palatable to different interest groups.

When you get to Activity 1.4 on drowning prevention, you will see how the framing and packaging of the issue as one connected to development rather than to recreational swimming changed prevailing ideas about the feasibility of addressing this pressing but neglected global challenge which, in turn, led to policy action. Alcohol provides a different example, where the alcohol industry favours the idea of harm reduction through encouraging individual responsibility, and the public health community promotes ideas of collective action that promote taxation, and restrictions on sales and marketing. These different policy ideas reflect the competing values of individual versus collective responsibility – as well as underlying interests – profits made from selling alcohol versus an obligation to protect health – which affect how evidence of the effectiveness of different interventions is interpreted.

We use the term *institutions* in the field of policy analysis to mean the 'rules of the game' or 'how things are done' in a particular setting – in other words, the patterns of formal and informal rules and norms governing how policy-making processes are shaped. This is a little confusing since the word 'institution' is used more commonly to mean an organization, especially an enclosed one like a prison. As already discussed, *interests* refer to actors who may be individuals or groups, organized or informal and who want to see policy that furthers their goals or at least does not threaten their attainment.

Other analysts have stressed other concepts useful to understanding policy change. Shiffman and Smith's (2007) framework builds on the policy triangle's notions of actors and context (although they use the term 'environment' for context), but gives greater space for consideration of ideas (the ways in which those involved with the issue understand and portray it), following John (1998) and Howlett et al. (2009), and issue characteristics. In their framework, institutions are perceived as part of actor power. The policy triangle reminds us more about processes – and how useful it is to understand the cycle of policy making from agenda-setting to implementation and evaluation, but its broad approach can be enhanced by adding ideas and actor power (when thinking about how different actors influence policy), in thinking about the rules and norms of organizations when they make policy, and in considering issue characteristics when considering the content of a particular problem and how actors are likely to respond to it.

A further framework, developed as a practical guide for assessing when and where investments in policy reforms are most feasible in any given context, builds on the above theoretical understandings of the policy process as well as a review of a series of examples of policy change in Zambia (Resnick et al. 2018). The framework, called the 'kaleidoscope model' (see Figure 1.2), emerged as an attempt to identify a 'core' set of variables from the proliferation of those proposed in disparate disciplinary literatures over

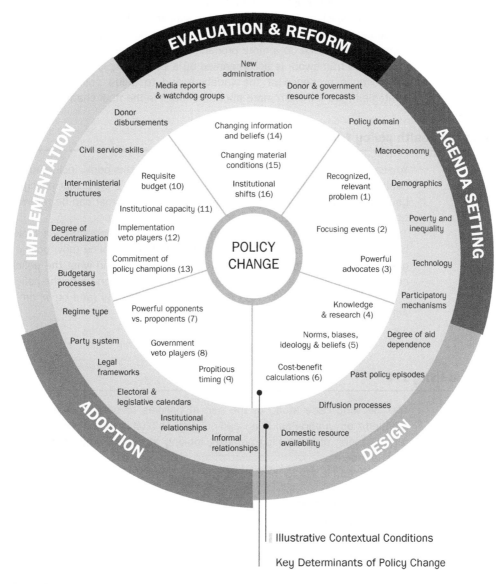

Figure 1.2: Kaleidoscope model of policy change

Source: Resnick et al. (2018)

the preceding decades. The resultant 16 core variables were repeatedly observed during episodes of policy change across diverse contexts. In the model, these variables are then loosely mapped to the stages heuristic as some variables are more strongly affiliated to a particular stage of the policy process than to other stages. The authors describe the model as kaleidoscopic 'because just as shifting a kaleidoscope refracts light in a new pattern, so does focusing on a particular stage of the policy process reveal a different constellation of key variables that are important for driving change' (Resnick et al, 2018). And hence similar to a kaleidoscope, many of the contextual factors might remain static, but as policy processes proceed, some variables take on a more pronounced role in shaping the policy than others. The framework is accompanied by a set of simple tools to assess the absence/presence of the variables and to guide policy-influencing strategies (you will learn more about the latter in the final chapter).

Using the health policy triangle

You can use many of the frameworks introduced in this book, including the health policy triangle, to help analyse or understand a particular policy or you can apply them to plan a particular policy. The former can be referred to as analysis *of* policy, the latter as analysis *for* policy.

Analysis *of* policy is generally retrospective and explanatory – it looks back to explore factors such as the determination of policy (how policies got on to the agenda, were initiated and formulated) and what the policy consisted of (content). It also includes evaluating and monitoring the policy – did it achieve its goals? Was it considered successful (and by whom)? Activity 1.4 focuses on this type of policy analysis.

✎ Activity 1.4

The following case study of the rise of policies to prevent drowning, adapted from Justin-Paul Scarr and colleagues (2022), describes the different stages of the policy process, looking at context and actors as well as process.

As you read it, apply the health policy triangle by:

1. identifying the actors;
2. identifying the policy processes;
3. describing the context;
4. assessing how content contributed to determining the eventual policy;
5. identifying any examples of interests, ideas, institutions or issue characteristics that enhance understanding of the policy process in this case.

Getting drowning prevention on the policy agenda and formulating the UN Resolution on Global Drowning Prevention

Eighteenth to twentieth centuries: maritime safety, swimming and lifesaving

Drowning prevention today can be traced to two historical periods. First, eighteenth-century maritime accidents increased the focus on safety, and resulted in innovations including lifeboats, lifejackets and rescue stations. Maritime safety charities soon followed. One such charity, the Maatschappij tot Redding van Drenkelingen (MRVD), formed for the rescue of drowning victims in Amsterdam in 1767. Another, the Royal National Lifeboat Institution (RNLI), was established in England in 1824.

Around the same time the growing popularity of swimming prompted the development of lifesaving techniques and organizations to protect swimmers from drowning. For example, the Swimmers' Lifesaving Society formed in London in 1894. Known today as the Royal Life Saving Society (RLSS), it initially focused on water safety education. Water safety, education and rescue were central to drowning prevention policy for the century that followed.

1980s: the child survival and development revolution

In the 1980s, UNICEF launched the 'Child Survival and Development Revolution' aiming to save the lives of millions of children each year through low-cost measures. In 1970, all-cause under-five mortality rates in Bangladesh were approximately 206 per 1,000 live births, but by 2005 that had reduced to 65 per 1,000. This success revealed less appreciated causes of child death, including drowning.

2000s: contestation on problems and solutions

In 2002, MRVD under leadership of Professor Joost Bierens, a resuscitation specialist, gathered experts at the World Congress on Drowning in Amsterdam. Although high-income country actors and contexts dominated debate, and a new medical definition for drowning resulted, a small group gathered to discuss the issue in other parts of the world. UNICEF and WHO convened similar meetings throughout the 2000s at which research using community surveys, not hospital data, was presented showing that drowning was a much bigger problem than previously understood but there were no obvious solutions.

In 2005, UNICEF and The Alliance for Safe Children (TASC) formed the Centre for Injury Prevention Bangladesh (CIPRB) to assess solutions to drowning in rural areas. Two emerged: day-care for under-fives and swimming lessons for school-aged children. The latter faced scepticism from scientists who pointed to a lack of robust evidence and concerns that teaching swimming skills could increase risk taking among children.

Two advocates, Douglas 'Pete' Peterson, a former US Ambassador to Vietnam, and CIPRB Director Dr Aminur Rahman, railed against complacency, challenged prevailing approaches to data collection and called on global actors to reach consensus. The policy debate was dominated by high-income country (HIC) interests and lacked appreciation of the low- and middle-income country (LMIC) contexts where different solutions were needed to address the problem of children drowning in ditches or wells, usually within metres of their homes.

2010–2015: building a global platform to reduce drowning

Global experts again gathered, this time in Danang, Vietnam for the International Life Saving Federation's (ILS) World Conference on Drowning Prevention 2011 ('WCDP 2011'). Convened by RLSS-Australia, the event was reframed from 'World Water Safety' to 'Drowning Prevention', to the consternation of some HIC interests. Scholarships were awarded to 150 LMIC actors, and participants cycled into rural villages to experience first-hand the challenges of preventing drowning in everyday life. The closing declaration 'Building a global platform to reduce drowning' (ILS 2014) outlined a call for high-level action.

At a similar time, Michael Bloomberg's charitable foundation, Bloomberg Philanthropies (BP), convened a workshop to scope drowning prevention. BP decided to fund the first WHO Global Report on Drowning in 2014 (World Health Organization 2014). At the launch, WHO Director General, Margaret Chan, described drowning as a public health challenge never targeted by a global strategic prevention effort. Experts welcomed increasing consensus, but technical disagreements and posturing among actors detracted from global policy maker attention. Nonetheless a small group clung to the idea of building a global platform for drowning prevention.

2015–2022: achieving a historic first UN Resolution on Drowning Prevention

In 2015, RNLI employed advocacy specialists who set about pitching a resolution at the World Health Assembly (WHA). Drowning was framed as a neglected public health issue, but a WHA policy agenda change gazumped the proposal. Aspirations shifted to the UN General Assembly in New York, where a UN Group of Friends for Drowning Prevention agreed to pitch a resolution in health and development terms. A secretariat worked with key UN missions to brief Member States and negotiate the resolution. A debate in the United Kingdom (UK) media that challenged RNLI's use of funds for overseas aid almost derailed the agenda. COVID-19 then forced postponement of UN policy debate until 2021.

The General Assembly passed the Resolution on Global Drowning Prevention (United Nations 2021) in April 2021. In speeches, Bangladeshi UN Ambassador, Rabab Fatima, presented Bangladesh as being in the front line in the fight against drowning, and framed drowning prevention as critical to the Sustainable Development Goals (SDGs). Irish UN Ambassador, Geraldine Byrne Nason, linked drowning to climate action and disaster risk reduction. The Resolution delegates co-ordination responsibilities to WHO and encourages Member States to strengthen their data on occupational and adolescent drowning, build plans, implement maritime safety measures and include swimming lessons in school curricula. Given the diverse issue characteristics, and non-health sector solutions that arise, advocating drowning to become part of sustainable development agendas is thought to be critical to ensuring action at global, national or community levels.

Source: Adapted from Scarr et al. (2022)

Feedback

1. You may have named the following as actors:
   (a) Professor Bierens, Dr Rahman, Michael Bloomberg, WHO Director General, Ambassadors Peterson, Fatima and Byrne Nason and the organizations within which they worked, which provided the base for their influence: MRVD, CIPRB, TASC, BP, WHO, Bangladesh and Ireland's missions to the UN.
   (b) Unnamed advocacy specialists, injury experts and scientists.
   (c) WHO, UNICEF.
   (d) Networks of drowning prevention advocates; technical and scientific experts interested in drowning resuscitation, lifesaving rescue, swimming and child health.
   (e) NGOs including RNLI, CIPRB, ILS and RLSS-Australia.
2. Processes – the story is divided into decades that suggest three eras:
   • Pre-2010 – growing awareness of the problem because of changes in scientific methods (community surveys), impact of the child survival resolution reducing child mortality and revealing previously underreported rates of drowning, and the process and

challenges of developing solutions relevant to drowning prevention in LMICs.

- 2010–2015 – building a global platform. You could have noted the
use of conferences including WCDP 2011 and workshops with
donors to build an agenda for drowning prevention, and advocate
action to policy makers.
- 2015–2021 – achieving a Resolution on Global Drowning Prevention. You might have seen the shift from technical and scientific processes to an emphasis on policy advocacy, and use
of advocacy specialists to influence policy makers at WHA and
subsequently at the UN. You could have noted the influence of
donors (e.g. Bloomberg Philanthropies) in prioritizing and funding certain activities that lead to evidence-informed policy-making processes.

3. Context – some points you might consider under context include:
- Tensions between HIC framing of the problem (i.e. recreational)
and solutions (i.e. rescue, resuscitation, swimming) and those
relevant to LIMC contexts such as barriers around wells and
waterways, or early failures to achieve consensus on problems
and solutions.
- You might have mentioned the impact of WHO bringing institutional power and legitimacy to reframe drowning as a major global
public health issue that had been relatively neglected in terms of
prevention, as well as the strengthening cohesion among the key
actors to give legitimacy to specific interventions.

4. Content
- You may have noted that the technical content for drowning prevention policy was drawn from numerous studies which were
reflected in the WHO Global Report on Drowning.
- You might have noted that solutions centred around child drowning and the need to act in LMICs.
- You might have observed technical elements of the UN Resolution
on Global Drowning Prevention, and the reframing of drowning as
relevant to SDGs, climate action and disaster risk reduction.
- You might have noted the contrast between ideas of drowning
prevention in HICs and those in LMICs, including the reframing of
ideas from water safety into drowning prevention.

These could all be described as issue characteristics.

Analysis *for* policy is usually prospective – it looks forward and tries to
anticipate what will happen if a particular policy is introduced. It feeds
into strategic thinking about how to modify policy and may lead to policy advocacy or lobbying. For example, following a multi-disciplinary study

to inform HIV prevention policy among high-risk groups in Pakistan, the government commissioned a prospective analysis of the major policy recommendations made by the researchers. This involved a survey of relevant policy elites who were asked to express their level of agreement with 15 statements concerning each recommendation where each question related to a variable associated with presumed success of the feasibility of adopting and implementing the recommendation. This survey was followed by semi-structured interviews with a range of interest groups. The results of the analysis were used by the researchers and government officials to tailor the content of the recommendations to make them more politically palatable (Buse et al. 2009). In Chapter 11, you will learn some of the methods, such as stakeholder analysis, to help in prospective analysis for policy.

An example of how analysis *of* a policy can help to identify action *for* policy was seen in a study undertaken by McKee et al. (1996) in which they compared policies across a number of HICs to prevent sudden infant deaths – sometimes called 'cot deaths'. Research had highlighted that many of these deaths were avoidable by putting infants to sleep lying on their backs. The study showed that evidence had been available from the early 1980s, but it was some years before it was acted on. The study suggested that statistical evidence seemed to have been of little importance as governments in many countries failed to recognize the steady rise in sudden infant deaths, even though the evidence was available to them. Instead focusing events, such as television programmes which drew media attention and the activities from NGOs, were much more important. The lessons *for* policy depended to some extent on the political system: in federal forms of government, it seemed that authority was diffused, so strong central actions were difficult. This could be overcome by well-developed regional campaigning within countries, and encouraging NGOs and the media to take up the issue. In one country, it seemed that a decentralized statistical service had led to delays in pooling mortality data, so recognition of the problem took longer. The authors concluded that many countries needed to review their arrangements to respond to evidence of challenges to public health.

Health policy analysis and the field of 'global health'

All policy analysis is a product of the analyst(s)' prevailing values and ideas and as well as the theories, approaches and methods they use. It is similarly the product of the organizations that support and publish the work. Interest groups that might stand to gain or lose from the analysis might facilitate or block access to materials that shed light on the policy issue. The material itself also reflects prevailing ideas which tend to serve dominant interests. Thus, policy analysis is subjective and is as likely to serve the status quo as to change it.

The field of public policy analysis – and health policy analysis – has been largely financed and framed by funders based in HICs, and undertaken and or led by researchers situated in organizations in those countries. This includes much analysis of health policy and health systems in LMICs that often goes under the misleading term of 'global health'. The authors of this textbook all have affiliations with prestigious universities in London, UK which are part of this tradition. Particular forms of quantitative and experimental research knowledge tend to be privileged by HIC health organizations, such as universities and policy agencies, and, at the same time, much of the general policy-making theory used for health policy analysis is derived from studies of HICs.

Despite this, the global health agenda itself, and in particular the question of who has the power to set the agenda, has come under increasing scrutiny in recent years. The origins of the enterprise that is today thought of as the 'global health system' have been characterized as marked by 'unequal power relationships, including colonialism, imperialism, post-World War II governance structures, and patriarchal systems and practices' (Global Health 50/50 2020). These forces of inequality have resulted in a global health system where decision-making power remains vested in an unrepresentative group – the leadership of a sample of 201 global health organizations, for example, is predominantly male (70 per cent), from HICs (80 per cent) and educated in HICs (90 per cent). The same analysis found that women from low-income countries (LICs) account for just 1 per cent of board seats (Global Health 50/50 2022). Thus, not only is there inequality in terms of who the leadership is, but also a lack of diversity in the systems of knowledge and understanding about what counts as 'evidence' within the decision-making processes (Loewenson et al. 2021).

Over the past decades, the injustice of a global health agenda, set largely in Western capitals to be implemented by governments elsewhere in the world, has been increasingly highlighted. Calls for gender equality across the system, for *decolonizing* the global health system and for a system that is more representative and fairer have been heard from people in social movements (Women in Global Health 2022), health practitioners in LMICs (Oti and Ncayiyana 2021) and academics across a range of settings advocating research partnerships led by analysts from LMICs (Abimbola and Pai 2020; Mogaka et al. 2021). We have yet to see similar movements in global health based on other aspects of inequality such as class, caste, migration status, etc., but health policy making and policy analysis that is truly inclusive will encompass and address these by asking where power lies and how the existing distribution can be changed.

An increasing number of health policy analyses are being published by authors from organizations in LMICs (see the special issue of *International Journal of Health Policy and Management* on 'Analysing the Politics of Health Policy Change in Low- and Middle-Income Countries: The HPA Fellowship Programme 2017–2019' edited by Gilson et al. (2021)). This is part of a wider movement to decolonize global health and global health policy analysis. Though there is no settled definition of what this entails in practical, day-to-day terms, Khan et al. (2021: 1) define it as:

> a movement that fights against ingrained systems of dominance and power in the work to improve the health of populations, whether this occurs between countries, including between previously colonizing and plundered nations, and within countries, for example the privileging of ... research-based knowledge formation over the lived experience of people themselves.

The goal is for new frameworks and tools to be developed to help answer a different set of questions that reflect different values, interests and experiences, as well as a greater diversity of perspectives on priority problems, and related feasible and acceptable solutions.

Among other things, decolonizing health policy analysis involves attending to *positionality*. This refers to understanding and confronting how the stance or positioning of the researcher in the social and political context of the study affects how they think about and tackle the topic of the study.

Positionality matters because a researcher's beliefs, biases, preferences and relative privilege and power influence their research. In the same way that we encourage students to think critically about who is involved in policy processes, whose interest they represent and whose priorities they reflect, policy analysts should reflect on how their own values, identities, including characteristics such as gender and ethnicity, their institutional base, their perceived power, legitimacy and interests as well their prior involvement in policy communities influence their analyses. Chapters 2 and 11 will help you better understand positionality so that you can incorporate a more reflexive approach in your analysis.

Summary

In this chapter you have been introduced to definitions of policy and health policy and several analytical frameworks that bring together domains such as context, process and actors to help you make sense of the policy-making process and its political nature. You have learned that these frameworks can be used both retrospectively – to analyse past policy – and prospectively – to help shape future policy. You have also been introduced to current debates relating to decolonizing the conduct both of global health policy making and policy analysis. In part, this involves confronting the privileged position and world view enjoyed by those who currently dominate the field. Many of the concepts you have been introduced to will be expanded and illustrated in the chapters that follow. A useful online resource covering concepts associated with the politics of public policy can be found at Paul Cairney's website (https://paulcairney.wordpress.com/), while Lucy Gilson and colleagues have developed a helpful health policy analysis reader (Gilson et al. 2018).

Further reading

Affun-Adegbulu, C. and Adegbulu, O. (2020) Decolonising global (public) health: from Western universalism to global pluriversalities, *BMJ Global Health*, 1; 5(8): e002947.

Berlan, D., Buse, K., Shiffman, J. and Tanaka, S. (2014) The bit in the middle: a synthesis of global health literature on policy formulation and adoption, *Health Policy and Planning*, 29(suppl 3): iii23–34. https://doi.org/10.1093/heapol/czu060

Gilson, L., Agyepong, I.A. and Shiffman, J. (2018) Part A Health policy analysis: starting points, in *A Health Policy Analysis Reader: The Politics of Policy Change in Low- and Middle-Income Countries*. Geneva: Alliance for Health Policy and Systems Research, pp. 10–30.

Resnick, D., Haggblade, S., Babu, S. et al. (2018) The Kaleidoscope Model of policy change: applications to food security policy in Zambia, *World Development*, 109: 101–20.

Walt, G. and Gilson, L. (1994) Reforming the health sector in developing countries: the central role of policy analysis, *Health Policy and Planning*, 9: 353–70.

Website

Paul Cairney: Politics and Public Policy, https://paulcairney.wordpress.com

References

Abimbola, S. and Pai, M. (2020) Will global health survive its decolonisation?, *The Lancet*, 396(10263): 1627–8.

Anderson, J. (1975) *Public Policy Making*. London: Nelson.

Berlan, D., Buse, K., Shiffman, J. and Tanaka, S. (2014) The bit in the middle: a synthesis of global health literature on policy formulation and adoption, *Health Policy and Planning*, 29(suppl 3): iii23–34. https://doi.org/10.1093/heapol/czu060

Buse, K., Lalji, N., Mohamad, I., Mayhew, S.H. and Hawkes, S. (2009) Political feasibility of scaling-up five evidence informed HIV policies: in search of deeper and wider policy commitment, *Sexually Transmitted Infections*, 85(suppl 2): ii37–42.

Dye, T. (2001) *Top Down Policymaking*. London: Chatham House Publishers.

Gilson, L., Orgill, M. and Shroff, Z. (2018) *A Health Policy Analysis Reader: The Politics of Policy Change in Low- and Middle-Income Countries*. Geneva: WHO.

Gilson, L., Shroff, Z.C. and Shung-King, M. (2021) Introduction to the Special Issue on 'Analysing the Politics of Health Policy Change in Low- and Middle-Income Countries: The HPA Fellowship Programme 2017–2019', *International Journal of Health Policy and Management*, 10(7):360–3. https://doi.org/10.34172/ijhpm.2021.43

Global Health 50/50 (2020) *Power, Privilege and Priorities*. Available at: https://globalhealth5050.org/2020report/ (accessed 3 October 2022).

Global Health 50/50 (2022) *Boards for All? A Review of Power, Policy and People on the Boards of Organisations Active in Global Health*. Available at https://globalhealth5050.org/2022-report/ (accessed 3 October 2022).

Howlett, M., Ramesh, M. and Perl, A. (2009) *Studying Public Policy*. Oxford: Oxford University Press.

International Life Saving Federation (2014) Building a global platform to reduce drowning. ILS. Available at: www.royallifesaving.com.au/__data/assets/pdf_file/0020/43715/WCDP2011_Conference-Declaration-Building-a-global-platform-to-reduce-drowning-LR.pdf (accessed 3 October 2022).

John, P. (1998) *Analysing Public Policy*. London: Bloomsbury Publishing.

Khan, M., Abimbola, S., Aloudat, T. et al. (2021) Decolonising global health in 2021: a roadmap to move from rhetoric to reform, *BMJ Global Health*, 6: e005604. https://doi.org/10.1136/bmjgh-2021-005604

Langhorne, P. (2021) The stroke unit story: where have we been and where are we going? *Cerebrovascular Diseases*, 50: 636–43.

Leichter, H. (1979) *A Comparative Approach to Policy Analysis: Health Care Policy in Four Nations*. Cambridge: Cambridge University Press.

Lindblom, C.E. (1959) The science of muddling through, *Public Administrative Review*, 19: 79–88.

Loewenson, R., Accoe, K., Bajpai, N. et al. (2020) Reclaiming comprehensive public health, *BMJ Global Health*, 5: e003886.

Loewenson, R., Villar, E., Baru, R. et al. (2021) Engaging globally with how to achieve healthy societies: insights from India, Latin America and East and Southern Africa, *BMJ Global Health*, 6: e005257.

McKee, M., Fulop, N., Bouvier, P. et al. (1996) Preventing sudden infant deaths – the slow diffusion of an idea, *Health Policy*, 37: 117–35.

Moat, K.A. and Abelson, J. (2011) Analyzing the influence of institutions on health policy development in Uganda: a case study of the decision to abolish user fees, *African Health Sciences*, 11(4): 578–86.

Mogaka, O.F., Stewart, J. and Bukusi, E. (2021) Why and for whom are we decolonising global health?, *Lancet Global Health*, 9(10): E1359–60.

Oti, S.O. and Ncayiyana, J. (2021) Decolonising global health: where are the Southern voices?, *BMJ Global Health*, 6: e006576.

Resnick, D., Haggblade, S., Babu, S. et al. (2018) The Kaleidoscope Model of policy change: applications to food security policy in Zambia, *World Development*, 109: 101–20. https://doi.org/10.1016/j.worlddev.2018.04.004

Robert, G. and Fulop, N. (2014) The role of context in successful improvement. *Perspectives on Context*. London: Health Foundation, 31.

Sabatier, P. and Jenkins-Smith, H. (1993) *Policy Change and Learning*. Boulder, CO: Westview Press.

Scarr, J.P., Buse, K., Norton, R. et al. (2022) Tracing the emergence of drowning prevention on the global health and development agenda: a policy analysis, *The Lancet Global Health*, 10(7): e1058–66.

Shiffman, J. and Smith, S. (2007) Generation of political priority for global health initiatives: a framework and case study of maternal mortality, *The Lancet*, 370: 1370–9.

United Nations (2021) *Global Drowning Prevention*, A/RES/75/273. Seventy-fifth session of UNGA. New York, USA.

Walt, G. (1994) *Health Policy: An Introduction to Process and Power*. London: Zed Books.

Walt, G. and Gilson, L. (1994) Reforming the health sector in developing countries: the central role of policy analysis, *Health Policy and Planning*, 9: 353–70.

Women in Global Health (2022) *About Women in Global Health*. Available at https://womeningh.org/about/ (accessed 3 October 2022).

World Health Organization (2014) *Global Report on Drowning: Preventing a Leading Killer*, Geneva: World Health Organization.

2   Power

In this chapter you will learn why understanding power is fundamental to policy analysis and be introduced to a number of theories which will help you understand the role of power in policy making. These include explanations of the sources of power, its distribution in society and frameworks for undertaking power analyses. These theoretical insights help to explain why decision making is not simply a rational process but more likely the result of struggles between competing groups of actors.

Learning objectives

After working through this chapter, you will be better able to:

- differentiate between the 'three faces of power' described by Lukes and apply each to health policy making
- contrast theories that account differently for the distribution of power in society and understand their implications for who is thought to determine health policy
- reflect on these theories in terms of who developed them (reflecting power in society), and the implications of this for health policy analysis
- use these theories to understand key health policy issues of our time.

Key terms

Agency The capacity of individuals to act independently and to make their own free choices.

Authority Whereas power concerns the ability to influence others, authority is the right to do so.

Colonization The action or process of settling among and establishing control over the indigenous people of an area.

Decolonization The process of undoing colonial dispossession and destruction; for example, through practices that reduce emphasis on Eurocentric knowledge production, and emphasize, promote and nurture other including indigenous knowledge production.

Elitism   The theory that power is concentrated in a small minority in society.

Feminism   A range of socio-political movements, ideologies and scholarly theories that aim to define and establish the political, economic, personal and social equality of the sexes.

Marxism   A political theory named after Karl Marx. It asserts that the owners of capital and means of production inevitably exploit those who only have their labour to offer in the capitalist system. It examines the consequences of this for the position of labour, capitalist productivity and economic development.

Pluralism   The theory that power is widely distributed in society.

Power   The ability to control resources and influence people, leading them to do things that they otherwise may not do.

Public choice (theory)   The theory that explains government decision making as a result of the actions of self-interested and rational public actors.

Racism   The belief that different human groups possess distinct and inherited characteristics, abilities or qualities with some of these groups superior to others as a result.

Social contract   A theory that concerns the legitimacy of the state's authority over the individual, or of those that rule over those that are ruled. It is based on the idea that individuals have consented, either explicitly or tacitly, to surrender some of their freedoms and submit to the authority of the state or ruler.

Social structure   The recurrent patterned arrangements which influence or limit the choices and opportunities available to people in society.

White supremacy   The belief that white people constitute a superior race and should dominate societies, to the exclusion or detriment of other racial and ethnic groups.

Introduction

This chapter introduces you to the concept of *power* in policy making. The exercise of power is central to every policy process, and understanding it is essential to identifying how to bring about the policy change necessary to improve health and health equity. Health policy decision making is typically characterized as involving multiple actors with competing interests, beliefs, values, resources and influence, as well as *authority*, over the policy-making process. Many health policy issues are highly contested, and there can be large differences of view between the individuals and groups with an interest in a policy issue (see Chapter 8 for more on this). Actors with great power and influence – whether they are larger rich countries, multinational corporations, or some other actor with relative advantage – can have considerable influence over the policy-making process. This power and influence can also be exercised in a variety of ways, some observable and some concealed. Therefore, understanding policy making requires an appreciation of the nature of power, how it is distributed and the manner through which it is exercised.

First, the meaning of power is explained and several conceptualizations of power presented, then the chapter presents theories relating to how power is exercised and distributed. Importantly, you will also have the opportunity to consider how your positionality – your identity in any social and political context – shapes the way you may understand and view power and the theories presented, as all are somewhat dependent on particular views of the world.

This chapter deepens understanding of the relationships between the 'process', 'content', 'context' and 'actors' elements in the 'policy triangle' (Walt and Gilson 1994) introduced in Chapter 1. It provides the basis for a more in-depth analysis of the influence of different policy actors on policy making, and the processes of agenda setting and policy formulation, implementation and evaluation in later chapters.

What is power?

What is 'power' in regard to policy making? How is it defined? Power can be considered as the ability to influence people, and in particular to control resources. However, there is considerable debate over the meaning of power, including, for example, whether power is best understood as 'power over' in a relational sense, describing the ability to influence others, or 'power to' in terms of the ability to achieve particular goals. Power is multi-dimensional and is generated from, and constrained by, the broader historical, social, political, cultural and organizational context of policy decision making (Gilson et al. 2018).

Different theories try to explain where power lies. Some of these theories focus on 'structure', arguing that power lies in the structure of relationships and institutions, including the structure of language (Levi-Strauss 1968). Other theories focus more on 'agency', arguing that an actor's ability to achieve influence and further their own goals is independent of the constraints of *social structure* (Campbell 2009). Yet other theories integrate both structure- and agency-based power, arguing that power can both be voluntarily exercised by actors via agency and expressed through the social structures actors are embedded within (Giddens 1984). From this third perspective, the structure of social systems has the power to constrain and enable social (inter)action but is, at the same time, produced and reproduced through social (inter)action over time. In contrast, a further group of scholars focus less on agency and structural forms of power. Foucault, for example, instead claimed that 'power is everywhere' (Foucault 1998). He argued that power is embedded within accepted forms of knowledge, scientific understanding and 'truth' that are produced under different forms of constraints and determine the limits of acceptable discourse and behaviour in society (Gaventa 2003).

Understanding power can help understand many of the 'big' issues of our time, and throughout history. These include global and national economic and material inequalities linked to exploitative capitalist practices, including colonial, post-colonial and corporate influence in policy making with implications for issues such as malnutrition, climate change and vaccine equity. Indeed, the way we are taught about and understand power is itself a manifestation of power.

Many of the theories of power that dominate traditional academic approaches to policy analysis have been developed by white male scholars from the Anglophone and Francophone Global North. It is increasingly recognized that these theories have limitations and that a wider set of perspectives are both available and would improve our understanding of how power dynamics shape the critical challenges of our times. Going beyond dominant theories and approaches to engage with a wider range of perspectives can support identification of new and even transformative solutions for global health (Stoeva 2022). A number of newer voices and ways of thinking have emerged or been given greater recognition in recent years, some of which we profile in this chapter. Table 2.1 presents some important theories and frameworks in regard to the conceptualization of power. These include classic general work published in the twentieth century alongside some more recent work from this century, some of which focuses on health policy explicitly, and the use of theories and frameworks in LMICs.

Table 2.1 Key theories and frameworks on the conceptualization of power

Author, year of publication	Key features
Weber, 1948	Political authority as legitimate domination, distinct from coercion/force. Three sources of political authority: traditional (derived from established customs and social structures), charismatic (derived from individual leader characteristics) and rational-legal authority (derived from the formal rules and laws of the state) (Weber 1948).

(Continued)

Table 2.1 (Continued)

Author, year of publication	Key features
Foucault, 1978	Concept of 'power/knowledge' holds that rather than being an instrument of power, knowledge is constitutive of power and inseparable from it. Discourses and institutions (in regard to the way that decisions are organized), create systems of disciplinary power (Foucault 1978).
Pateman, 1988	Describes the social contract that establishes modern patriarchy, which continues to aid oppression of women and girls (Pateman 1988).
Bourdieu, 1990	Combines agency and structure to produce different forms of 'capital'. A person has and can develop different forms of capital – or power. Actors use forms of capital (economic, cultural, social or symbolic) to advance their self-interest and preferences (Bourdieu 1990).
Mills, 1997	Describes the social contract that establishes white supremacy over all other groups of people (Mills 1997).
Veneklasen and Miller, 2002	A framework of four expressions of power: power over (authority over others), power to (individual powers to act on something), power with (to act with others or collaborations) and power within (the ability of a person to recognize their self-knowledge, abilities or a sense of self-worth) (Veneklasen and Miller 2002).
Barnett and Duvall, 2005	A framework for conceptualizing types of power produced through different social relations in the international sphere: compulsory, institutional, structural and productive power (Barnett and Duvall 2005).
Farnsworth and Holden, 2006	Theory on corporate structural and agency-based (political engagement, institutional participation and provision/production) power in social policy (Farnsworth and Holden 2006).
Moon, 2019	A (global health) systems approach to the conceptualization of power. Eight types of power: physical, economic, structural, institutional, moral, discursive, expert and network (Moon 2019).

 Activity 2.1

In Chapter 1 we describe the importance of a person's positionality in relation to understanding health policy processes. This is particularly the case with understanding an issue such as power. Consider how your positionality shapes your own power and privilege, and how this may influence your understanding of power and your interpretation of the theories of power to be discussed in this chapter.

Feedback

Considering your identity and its association with power and privilege can be complex. We all have a range of characteristics relating to our age, race and ethnicity, gender, sexuality and socio-economic position, as well as our nationality, disability status and whether or not we are from an HIC, MIC or LIC. The combined effect of these characteristics on a person's position and power in society is referred to as 'intersectionality'– a term coined by the American race theorist Kimberlé Crenshaw (1991). You may think of the impact of other characteristics as well – for example, whether or not you are a refugee or asylum seeker. Some of the combinations of these characteristics are associated with greater power and privilege, others with less. Some of the characteristics change over time. For some characteristics, their association with power and privilege changes depending on the social setting. However, there are also often some fairly stable associations.

What comes to mind to you when you hear the word 'power'? Are your connotations positive or negative? Do you think of opportunity and perhaps excitement, or instead oppression and struggle? This may depend on your personal experience of the exercise of power.

People's identities are usually multi-faceted. However, if your identity is largely one associated with power and privilege, you may understand power quite differently to someone whose identity is largely not. Someone whose identity is not associated with power and privilege may be particularly aware of the structural aspects of power, while someone whose identity is associated with power and privilege may be more likely to highlight their 'agency' or ability to act. If your identity is one of less power and privilege, you may feel particular resonance with concepts such as 'cultural hegemony, 'mental domination' and the 'disciplinary' nature of social institutions. Others may be able to relate more closely to perspectives on power that highlight actor expertise and resources and the concept of power as 'capital'.

Not surprisingly, some of the most evocative writing on power comes from the self-described black lesbian poet Audre Lorde. For Lorde, speaking and writing as a black woman was very important in a world that takes the white man as a 'mythical norm'. As the feminist writer Sara Ahmed commented, Lorde wrote of what she faced – 'the brutalising and devastating structures of racism, sexism, classism, ageism and heterosexism' (Ahmed, quoted in Lorde 2017).

For further reading on some of these ideas, you may also wish to explore the writing of the English feminist and political theorist Carole Pateman and the Jamaican-American philosopher Charles W. Mills (Pateman 1988, Mills 1997). They theorize how society is built on the oppression of women and people of colour, respectively, in order to uphold systems of patriarchy and white supremacy (see below for more on feminism and white supremacy).

Stigma and oppression shapes people's 'being' in the world in many ways as articulated by the British writer Matthew Todd in regard to LGBT identities (Todd 2018), who describes how it manifests as low self-worth rendering it all the more difficult to challenge those in power. Of particular relevance to this chapter, Mills describes how white philosophers take their white privilege for granted, so that they fail to recognize that white supremacy is a political system and that this shapes their theorizing (Mills 1997).

How is power expressed?

In much theorizing on policy making, power is typically thought of in a relational sense as having 'power over' others – the ability to achieve a desired outcome, to 'do' something. Thus, power is said to be exercised when A has B do something that B would not have otherwise done.

A can achieve this end over B in a number of ways, which have been characterized as the three 'faces' or 'dimensions' of power:

- First face: power as decision making.
- Second face: power as non-decision making.
- Third face: power as thought control.

Table 2.2 summarizes the evolution of social-science thinking about power that contributed to the identification of the three 'faces' of power eventually described by Steven Lukes (1974). The three dimensions have been very influential, informing, for example, later conceptualizations such as Gaventa's 'power cube', for analysing the levels, spaces and forms of power and their interrelationship (Gaventa 2006, Gaventa et al. 2011), and Fuchs and Lederer's theory on the power of corporations (Fuchs and Lederer 2007).

Marxism is a political theory developed by Karl Marx, a German philosopher of the nineteenth century. It asserts that the owners of capital and means of production inevitably exploit those who only have their labour to offer in the capitalist system. It examines the consequences of this for the position of labour, capitalist productivity and economic development (Marx 1867).

Lukes' third face of power, described below, stems from Marxist thinking that working class subordination is secured via the socialization and indoctrination of the working class to accept ruling-class ideology and values

Table 2.2 Key theories leading to the three 'faces' of power

Author, year of publication	Key features
Marx, 1867	Theory focused on the struggle between capitalists and workers, with these power relationships considered inherently exploitative and inevitably leading to class conflict. Power is held by a ruling capitalist class which controls the state (Marx 1867).
Gramsci, 1971 (written 1929–1935)	Concept of cultural 'hegemony', by which the state and the ruling classes use ideology, rather than violence, force or economic modalities, to control and maintain capitalist power (Gramsci 1971).
Dahl, 1957	Theory of power as decision making (also described as the first dimension of power) (Dahl 1957).
Bachrach and Baratz, 1962	Theory of power as decision making and agenda setting (also described as the first and second dimensions of power) (Bachrach and Baratz 1962).
Lukes, 1974, 2005	Theory of power as decision making, agenda setting and preference shaping (the three dimensions of power) (Lukes 1974, 2005).

through key institutions that generate a 'false consciousness' within the working class (Marx 1976). These ruling-class ideologies and values and their permeation in society relate to today's economic system of capitalism supported by neoliberal thinking. Many scholars are now identifying the way in which ruling-class ideology considerably weakens societal capacities to respond to important issues of our time, including infectious disease pandemics, high levels of non-communicable disease, the climate crisis, and growing economic and social inequities (Navarro 2007, 2020, Fremsted and Paul 2022, Milsom et al. 2022).

Building on these ideas, and also relating to the third face of power described below, the Marxist intellectual Antonio Gramsci developed the concept of 'cultural hegemony' to explain how the state and the ruling classes use ideology, rather than violence, force or economic modalities, to control and maintain capitalist power (Gramsci 1971).

The first face of power – power as decision making

The first dimension of power – power as decision making – was first proposed by the American political scientist Robert Dahl writing about municipal politics in the US in the 1950s. Dahl saw power as a 'relation among people', being about the ability of a person to achieve compliance from others who change how they behave as a result of power being exerted over them where 'A has power over B to the extent that he can get B to do something that B would not otherwise do' (Dahl 2005 [1961]; Robinson 2006). The first face of power is often observable or overt, and it is how power was traditionally described as operating. It relates directly to the way that decisions are made, for instance, through counting votes in a formal political arena – the party or parties that can summon the most votes will be able to pass their legislation. Compared to other forms of the exercise of power, it is possible simply to identify the winners and losers of policy disputes. It is also associated with visible conflict.

Examples of the first dimension of power in regard to the exercise of power over HIV policy include the decision of the South African government in 1999 to make AIDS a notifiable disease (Baleta 1999), or the more recent policy outlined by the government of the UK in an HIV action plan, backed by £23 million of government funding, to reduce new infections by 80 per cent between 2022 and 2025 in England (Department of Health and Social Care (UK) 2021).

The second face of power – power as non-decision making

The second face of power identifies who has the power to set the political agenda (and keep particular issues off the agenda). It was identified in the 1970s, again in US politics by Bachrach and Baratz in response to Dahl's analysis of the first dimension of power. This second dimension or 'face' of power is a less visible form of power and is sometimes described as 'covert', or power in inaction. With this second dimension of power, power is exercised 'when A devotes their energies to creating or reinforcing social and political values and institutional practices that limit the scope of the political process to public consideration of only those issues which are comparatively innocuous to A' (Bachrach and Baratz 1962). Consequently, power as agenda setting highlights the way in which powerful groups control the agenda to keep threatening issues off the policy radar screen. Expressed differently, power as 'non-decision making' involves 'the practice of limiting the scope of actual decision making to safe issues by manipulating the dominant community values, myths and political institutions and procedures' (Bachrach and Baratz 1963). In this dimension of power, some issues remain latent and fail to enter the policy arena. With this dimension, we cannot count votes because the issue does not make it into the legislative chamber to be voted upon. Instead, we would need to observe the 'corridors of power' – including the 'lobby' (see below) and the interactions between politicians and other actors which decide what gets onto the agenda or not (see Chapter 5 on agenda setting).

An example of the second dimension of power is the food industry partnering with public health organizations to influence agenda setting – with the aim of warding off tough regulatory measures such as nutrition labelling. With alcohol policy, for example, Hawkins et al. (2021) examined how a 'Drink Free Days' campaign (2018–2019) was run by Public Health England, an executive agency of the UK government, in partnership with Drinkaware, an industry-funded 'alcohol education charity' to encourage middle-aged drinkers to abstain from drinking on some days (Hawkins et al. 2021). Such partnerships with government by industry-associated bodies such as Drinkaware have been identified as key components of industry strategy to influence policy and regulatory agenda – particularly, to keep strong regulatory measures that might harm industry profits off the political agenda. In doing so, such partnerships are an example of industry's use of the second face of power.

The third dimension of power – power as thought control

The American political and social theorist Steven Lukes built on Dahl and Bachrach and Baratz by adding a 'third dimension of power' to explain how the powerful secure the willing, unreflective compliance of those they dominate. This dimension is conceptualized as 'power as thought control'. In other words, power is a function of the ability to influence others by shaping their preferences. In this dimension, 'A exercises power over B when A affects B in a manner contrary to B's interests' (Lukes 1974). Lukes argues that thought control is achieved through the control of information, mass media and socialization (Lukes 1974). With parallels to the work of Ngũgĩ wa Thiong'o, a Kenyan scholar, in regard to the role of language in shaping the 'mental universe' of the colonized (wa Thiong'o 2011), Lukes argues that power is exercised by shaping people's perceptions and interests without their own awareness – with A thus gaining B's compliance through subtle means. This form of power includes the ability to shape meanings and perceptions of reality of which advertising is the most obvious example. However, this dimension also relates more broadly to the way that society is structured, and how this influences our thinking. To help identify the behind-the-scenes use of this third dimension of power, questions to ask yourself include: what assumptions and worldviews do we take for granted and whose interest is it for these to be propagated?

Lukes finds the third dimension of power the 'the supreme and most insidious' form as it dissuades people from having objections by:

> shaping their perceptions, cognitions and preferences in such a way that they accept their role in the existing order of things, either because they can see or imagine no alternative to it, or because they see it as natural and unchangeable, or because they value it as divinely ordained and beneficial. (Lukes 1974: 28)

The 2016 referendum in the UK on European Union (EU) membership provides an example of this face of power. Many areas of England and Wales voted to leave the EU (Brexit) despite the fact that it would make them poorer (Pollards 2021). The role of the anti-EU British press over the previous 30 years was integral to the development of a Euro-sceptic discourse that erroneously equated domestic UK policy failings with those of the EU and an out-of-touch political elite.

Another example is the influence of free market fundamentalism in English-speaking countries since the 1980s, specifically the taken for granted, widely held view, propagated by the dominant mass media corporations that: the state must reduce its interventions in economic and social activities, and labour and financial markets must be deregulated to grow the economy and raise living standards. The ideology behind this is neoliberalism – the political economic paradigm of our time (Schrecker 2019).

The third face of power is not merely harnessed by the state or commercial sector, but also by a wide array of other actors and their networks – and included here are social and mass media. The rise of social media platforms in recent decades has contributed to populist views of both the left and right, such as those demonstrated by the Tea Party movement in the US, the international Occupy movement of 2011, and the election of leaders such as Donald Trump and Jair Bolsonaro. It has also contributed to a rise in discontent at odds with public health evidence, for example with anti-vaccination campaigns locally and globally as dangerously powerful disinformation is rapidly circulated through unregulated new technologies (Perera et al. 2019). Of course, this is just one view. At the same time, those actively opposed to vaccination (the 'anti-vaxxers') might say that the mass media has contributed to people being systematically misinformed about vaccination so that Big Pharma can continue to profit. They might see their efforts as contributing to pulling back the curtain of illusion put in place by experts' use of the third face of power.

You will see that the third face of power is complex and often less straightforward to apply than the first and the second dimensions of power. This is because the third dimension of power can be mobilized in very subtle ways, and it often operates over a long timeframe. This makes it difficult for the researcher or policy analyst to identify it, and once identified its meaning requires interpretation, which means it may be open to contestation from others. Some of these interpretive issues have been exacerbated by what has been termed a shift to 'post-truth' politics in recent years whereby certain populist politicians have been seen to perpetuate falsehoods and use poorly regulated social media sites.

Due to their considerable resources, in all capitalist countries corporate actors wield considerable power over health policy making. They deploy all three 'faces' of power in pursuit of their interests. The term 'commercial determinants of health', first coined by the researchers West and Marteau (2013), is used by the public health community to describe this influence and its often detrimental impacts for health policy and health outcomes (Mialon 2020). Take the example of multi-national motor car manufacturers. Motor cars are problematic from a public health perspective. They contribute to many millions of road traffic accidents globally each year leading to death and disability. They promote and contribute to increasingly sedentary lifestyles across the world. They are highly polluting – both making air hazardous to breathe in urban areas and leading to premature deaths and respiratory illnesses, and of course, petrol and diesel cars are very significant contributors to global carbon dioxide emissions thus the climate crisis. Recent scandals have also shown that many of these corporations have been involved in largescale malpractice to 'cheat' emissions regulations in many jurisdictions (Jung and Sharon 2019). At the same time, national and local governments in most countries are keen to facilitate motor car manufacturing and welcome investment from multinational motor car manufacturers as there are large economic benefits related to motor car manufacturing – the industry provides many high-skilled, well-paid jobs, as well as many further political, economic and lifestyle benefits for governments and individuals.

The issue can be examined using the three faces of power, for example:

- In terms of the first dimension of power, we can observe votes at the national and local level to welcome investment from multinational motor car corporations to set up enabling legislation for the establishment of new car production plants.
- In terms of the second dimension of power, we can speculate about and devise research studies to examine how some multinational motor car corporations were able to manipulate and undermine effective regulation for many years in relation to carbon emissions.
- In terms of the third dimension of power, we can observe the influence of motor car advertising around the world in promoting car ownership as something aspirational, aligned with notions of freedom and excitement: in essence, maximizing the 'positive' elements of cars and minimizing the 'negative' ones.

Over recent decades, public health researchers have exposed multiple strategies used by corporations to prevent regulation of health-harmful commodities. These corporations cover a wide range of industries, including the alcohol, tobacco and highly processed food and beverage industries, as well as fossil fuels. The strategies of the tobacco industry have been particularly well documented, but similar tactics are increasingly being identified in relation to other health-harming industries.

Public–private partnerships are another oft-used tactic to keep certain issues (especially government regulation of the industry) off political agendas. We previously described this in relation to the Drink Free Days (DFD) campaign in England (Hawkins et al. 2021). Such tactics are an example of the second face of power.

Industry also frames health issues in ways that resonate with and amplify the neoliberal ideology that supports the current capitalist political economic system. Such processes may reinforce the notion that health and disease are the responsibility of the individual rather than a wider set of actors processes, restrict conceivable policy solutions and perpetuate

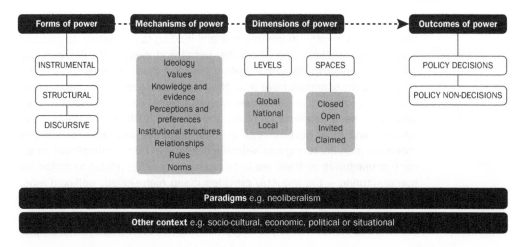

Figure 2.1: Milsom et al.'s framework for analysing power in public health policy making

Source: Milsom et al. 2020, Reproduced under the Attribution 4.0 International (CC BY 4.0) License https://creativecommons.org/licenses/by/4.0/

policy-making norms that privilege certain interests (e.g. economic or trade interests) over health (Milsom et al. 2020).

Milsom and colleagues developed a framework (see Figure 2.1) to analyse the different forms and mechanisms of power operating in trade and health policy that enable corporate actors to prevent government regulation. It is useful for analysing power in public health policy making including how powerful actors such as corporations achieve a policy decision or promote *non-decision making* (e.g. policy inertia).

✎ Activity 2.2

The following describes a classic study of air pollution in the United States of America (USA). As you read it consider:

1. Which dimension of power is described?
2. Does the study indicate that power as thought control may also have been in play?

Air pollution in the USA

In the 1960s, the political scientist Matthew Crenson sought to explain why air pollution remained a 'non-issue' in many American cities. In particular, he attempted to identify relationships between the neglect of air pollution and characteristics of political leaders and institutions (the way that decision-making processes are organized).

Crenson's approach, examining why things do not happen, contrasted with Robert Dahl's study which looked at why they do (2005 [1961]). Crenson adopted this strategy to test whether the study of political inactivity (or non-decision making, sometimes described as policy inertia) would shed new light on ways of thinking about power. He also wondered if this different approach would support the claims made by Dahl that the policy-making process was open to many groups in society.

Crenson began by demonstrating that action or inaction on pollution in US cities could not be attributed to differences in actual pollution level or to differences in social attributes of the populations in different cities. The study involved two neighbouring cities in Indiana which were both equally polluted and had similar demographic profiles. One of the cities, East Chicago, had taken action to deal with air pollution in 1949, while the other, Gary, did nothing until 1962. Crenson argues that the difference arose because Gary was a single-employer town dominated by US Steel, with a strong political party organization, while Chicago was home to a number of steel companies and had no strong party organization when it passed air pollution legislation. In Gary, anticipated negative reactions from the company were thought to have prevented activists and city leaders from placing the issue on the agenda. Crenson also interviewed political leaders from 51 American cities. These suggested that 'the air pollution issue tends not to flourish in cities where industry enjoys a reputation for power'.

Crenson's major findings were that, first, power may consist of the ability to prevent some items from becoming issues; second, that power does not need to be exercised for it to be effective: the mere reputation for power can restrict the scope of decision making; third, those affected by political power, 'the victims', may remain invisible, because the power or reputation of the powerful may deter the less powerful from entering the policy-making arena. He concluded that 'non-issues are not politically random oversights but instances of politically enforced neglect'.

Feedback

1. Crenson's study describes and provides an empirical basis for power as non-decision making, i.e. the second face of power.
2. Given that people would probably prefer not to be poisoned by air pollution, the case suggests that people will not necessarily act on their preferences and interests. This is presumably due to some form of manipulation or indoctrination, policy making by thought control. Milsom et al.'s (2020) framework is useful to identify and explain policy inertia.

From what you have learned so far, drawing particularly on the three faces of power, provide three simple examples of how the relationship between A and B reveals that A is exercising power over B.

Feedback

A can get B to do what B may not have otherwise done. A can keep issues that are of interest to B off the policy agenda. A can manipulate B in a way that B fails to understand their true interests.

So far, you have learned that power is the ability to achieve a desired result, with a variety of means to achieve this. It concerns the ability to get an actor to do what they would not have otherwise done. Common to the different perspectives on how to achieve the desired results is the notion that the policy process involves the exercise of power by competing actors to control scarce resources. The manner in which these struggles are resolved depends in large part on who has power in society.

How widely is power distributed and who can use it?

Power is often described in relational terms and there are different perspectives on its possible distribution. With health policy, the distribution of influence will depend on the specific policy content and context – and on the position/positionality of those involved. Consider a country where tobacco constitutes a considerable proportion of the gross domestic product and is a valuable source of government revenue. In this country, which is likely to have more influence over tobacco control policy: the tobacco industry, the MoH or public health and consumer interest groups? The answer is, probably, the tobacco industry. Yet, in the same country, industry may have less influence over policy to screen for cancer than, for example, the MoH, the medical profession and patient groups.

Despite the differences that policy content and context exert over the distribution of power in a given policy process, attempts have been made to arrive at general theories. These theories relate to the nature of society and the state. While some theories locate power in society as opposed to the state, all are concerned with the role of the state and the interests which the state is thought to represent in the policy process. The focus is on the state because of the dominant role that it often plays in policy processes (see Chapter 3). Theorists differ, however, in two important and related respects: first, in their assessment of whether the state is independent of society or a reflection of the distribution of power in society; second, in their view of the state serving the common good or the interests of a privileged group. You will now learn about how the theories differ and consider the implication of these differences for health policy.

We will start by discussing *pluralism*, *elitism* and *public choice* theory. There are a number of elitist frameworks which locate power in specific groups in society. These include professional power (described as part of elitism) and Marxism (described earlier in the chapter), and also feminism and white supremacy, which we discuss below.

Pluralism

The pluralist view on power, held by Dahl and others, asserts that there are multiple possible sources of power (e.g. legal authority, skills, knowledge, prestige, money, charisma) and that while decision-making power is located primarily within the framework of government and the state, other groups can also exert influence and have power.

Pluralism represents the dominant school of thought on theories of the distribution of power in liberal democracies. In its classical form, pluralism views power as dispersed throughout society – with no individual group holding absolute power and the state arbitrating among competing interests in the development of policy. Elite pluralism, a sub-category of pluralism, considers that some groups have more power than others (Dahl 1957).

Key characteristics supporting pluralism in society include:

- open electoral competition among a number of political parties;
- ability of individuals to organize themselves into pressure groups and political parties;
- ability of pressure groups to air their views freely;
- openness of the state to lobbying on the part of all pressure groups;
- the state acting as a neutral referee adjudicating between competing demands;
- although society has elite groups, no elite group dominates consistently.

For pluralists, health policy emerges as the result of conflict and bargaining among large numbers of groups organized to protect the specific interests of their members. The state selects from initiatives and proposals put forward by interest groups according to what is best for society.

Pluralism has been subject to considerable criticism for its portrayal of the state as a neutral arbiter in the distribution of power and for downplaying the existence of privileged groups that appear consistently to prevail. Most contemporary pluralists would now acknowledge that the policy-making playing field is not level. For example, they note the privileged position of organized business, and the role that the media and socialization play in most political systems.

Elitism

Elitist theorists contend that policy is dominated by and reflects the values and interests of a privileged minority – business, political and military elites (Mills 1956) – not 'the people' or wider population as claimed by pluralists. Modern elitists question the extent to which modern democratic political systems live up to the democratic ideals suggested by the pluralists. For example, in the UK during the early stages of the COVID-19 pandemic, the government awarded contracts worth hundreds of millions of pounds to suppliers of personal protective equipment (PPE) with whom they had personal links. A High Court judge later ruled that it was unlawful for these companies to be given this preferential treatment. Furthermore, many of the masks and other PPE supplied by two of the companies were not suitable for use, resulting in a monumental waste of taxpayer's money (Dyer 2022). In contrast, groups representing small business, labour and consumer interests are only able to exert influence at the margins of the policy process.

As far as health policy is concerned, does elitist theory overstate the capacities of the elite to wield power? Some may argue that most health policy is of relatively marginal importance on political agendas and that, consequently, it may be that elitist theories are less useful in accounting for power in health policy. Such marginal issues are sometimes referred to as 'low politics' on the grounds that they focus on technical issues of expert opinion. An example might relate to the work done by the National Institute for Health and Care Excellence (NICE) in the UK in relation to recommending a specific drug or health technology for use in the National Health Service (NHS). Nonetheless, you will see many examples in this book which suggest that an elite wields considerable influence in health policy making. Furthermore, if accounting for the upstream influences (macro-level influences on health, such as social, economic and environmental factors) on health outcomes, including for example the activities of fossil fuel companies and wars involving the military, health policy is a much broader field including many aspects of 'high politics'.

The various groups making up the 'elite' have been described as including:

> *members of the government and of the high administration, military leaders, and, in some cases, politically influential families . . . and leaders of powerful economic enterprises, and the political class, comprising the political elite but also leaders of political parties in opposition, trade union leaders, businessmen [sic] and politically active intellectuals.* (Bottomore 1966: 14–15)

Other members of the social elite may be those of professions such as law and medicine. Professional power draws attention to the power of specific professional groups and the way they wield influence over the policy process (Abbott 1988). Sociologists have highlighted both inter- and intra-professional power dynamics. Eliot Freidson (1970) suggested the 'professional dominance' of medics in the US in the middle of the twenti-eth century came under increasing challenge as the century wore on. The story in the UK is similar, where government reforms since the 1980s have increased the powers of managers in health care, and also furthered the responsibilities and rights of nursing and allied health professionals – lead-ing some to claim that the power of doctors has been reduced (Harrison and Ahmad 2000). Whilst the autonomy of the medical profession of 30 or 40 years ago has reduced, doctors – both individually and collectively – remain powerful actors in health care with considerable influence over health poli-cy-making processes (see Chapter 4 for further discussion of this).

It can be inferred from this that, for elite theorists, power is drawn from a variety of resources: wealth, family connections, technical expertise, pro-fessional identity or office. Yet what is also important is that the power of any one member of the elite is unlikely to depend on a single source.

According to elite theorists:

- society is comprised of the few with power and the many without, with only the few who have power making public policy;
- those who govern are unlike those who do not, with, in particular, the elite coming from the higher socio-economic strata;
- non-elites may be inducted into the governing circles if they accept the basic consensus of the existing elite;
- public policy reflects the values of the elite, although this may not imply a conflict with the values of the masses; indeed, as Lukes (1974) argued, the elite can manipulate the values of the masses to reflect their own interests;
- interest groups exist but they are not all equally powerful and do not have equal access to the policy-making process;
- the values of the elite are conservative and consequently any policy change is likely to be incremental.

Elitist theory could be considered relevant to many countries where politi-cians, senior bureaucrats, business people, professionals and the military make up tight policy circles that become a dominant or ruling class. In some places, the elite may be so few in number that they can be recog-nized by their family name.

The notion that not all interest groups are equally influential may reso-nate with you. Corporate actors in certain industries (for example, tobacco, alcohol and pharmaceuticals) have increasing concentrations of power (Wood et al. 2021) – and often have greater leverage over health policy than public health groups They also pay lobbyists to increase the odds that their views will be heard and acted on by governments. The following section highlights the results of a study by Russ and colleagues examin-ing business expenditure devoted to lobbying the US federal government to shape US policy toward WHO, including the funding of WHO (Russ et al. 2022).

Corporate lobbying in the United States towards the World Health Organization

The term 'lobby' as a noun relates to the areas in parliament buildings where citizens can meet and make demands on legislators. The term is also used as a verb, meaning to make direct representation to a policy maker. Lobbyists and interest groups are similar in that they both attempt to influence policy makers but lobbyists are hired by interest groups to represent their interests.

Russ and colleagues report that between 2006 and 2015 expenditure on lobbying of US federal government officials focused on the WHO or the WHA averaged US$12.5 million annually. Numerous industries were involved in this lobbying, including food processing, chemicals, agricultural product, alcohol and pharmaceuticals. There was also evidence of considerable cross-industry co-ordination. The lobbying covered the following topics: WHO health policies and guidelines related to the products of the corporate actors; specific internal WHO processes and operations that conflict with commercial interests; US engagement with WHO; and US funding for WHO in 2018.

The greater the amount of funding, the more likely it is that interest groups are able to influence legislators. The authors expressed the concern that 'our data demonstrate a pre-existing, coordinated effort by the corporate sector not only to influence global health policy, but also to sow doubt in the integrity of the WHO' (Russ et al. 2022). During the period of study, WHO-related lobbying expenditure also increased – to US$46 million in 2020, which the authors describe as approximately 15 per cent of average total annual US planned (pre-pandemic) contributions to WHO for 2020–2021' (Russ et al. 2022). The researchers also found an intensification of effort to influence US appropriations for the WHO starting around 2016 – and that this was associated with specific demands for greater private sector involvement in WHO policy making. This highlights the increasing financial commitment given to lobbying by the corporate sector to influence US engagement with WHO and health policy outside the US.

Public choice

Public choice is a theory of the power of the state derived from free market economics. Public choice theorists dispute the idea that the state acts neutrally on behalf of all societal interests. Instead, they assert that the state is itself an interest group which wields power over the policy process since elected public officials (politicians) and civil servants wish to pursue their own interests, often at the expense of the good of society as a whole. For example, to remain in power, elected officials consciously seek to reward particular groups with public expenditure, goods, services and favourable regulation in the expectation that these groups will keep them in power. Similarly, public servants use their offices and proximity to political decision makers to increase the importance (and budgets) of their own offices and staff over time. As a result, public servants strive to expand their bureaucratic empires as this will lead to bigger salaries and more opportunities for promotion, power, patronage and prestige. The state is, therefore, said to have an inbuilt dynamic which leads it to grow and increase in power, thereby squeezing out more efficient ways of governing and delivering public services.

Public choice theorists argue that the self-interested behaviour of state officials may lead to policy that is captured by narrow interest groups outside the state. As a result, policies are likely to be distorted in economically inefficient ways, and not in the public's interest. From this perspective, for example, health policies which involve rolling back the state will be resisted by bureaucrats, not because of their technical merits or demerits, but because bureaucrats will favour policies that entrench their positions and influence. In Bangladesh, MoH and Family Welfare officials resisted proposals to contract out public sector management and service delivery to the private sector. Public choice adherents would explain this resistance on the basis of fear of staff redundancies, diminished opportunities for rent-seeking and patronage, and concerns about the diminution of statutory responsibilities. This view would assert that politicians would try to use their position to reward past and potential future supporters at the expense of the rest of the population. Critics suggest that public choice theory both overstates the power of the bureaucracy in the policy process and is largely fuelled by ideological opposition to 'big government'.

✎ Activity 2.4

Consider how it is possible for scholars to arrive at such different conclusions as to the distribution of power in a country like the US. As you may recall, Dahl (1957) and others argued that many groups can influence the policy process, while other theorists argued that the power resides with a ruling class or elite, consisting of the captains of business, political executive and the military establishment.

Feedback

The answer lies in what the scholars have observed and studied. Dahl and other pluralists focused on actual conflicts among different groups over municipal politics. Elitist theorists emphasized that those with a reputation for power are effective at keeping controversial issues off the policy agenda (indicative of the second dimension of power), which are, therefore, beyond the purview of the conflicts studied by Dahl (who focused on the first dimension of power). You may also want to reflect on how the positionality/identity of the different theorists may have shaped their understanding of the distribution of power in societies. For example, it is possible that theorists from privileged backgrounds tend to assume that power is widely distributed because they have little experience of having their actions dictated by other more powerful groups.

Feminism

Feminism is about the achievement of political, economic and social equality of the sexes and highlights the adverse impact of patriarchy on women's lives. It focuses on the systematic, pervasive and institutionalized power that men wield over women in the domestic/familial and public spheres, and the organized activity to address these gender-based injustices. In patriarchal societies, it is most often men who define societal problems and their solutions, and men who decide which issues are policy-worthy and which are not. In line with the third face of power as thought control (1974), women are socialized to accept their lower status within this schema. In the most patriarchal societies, women are expected to remain in the domestic domain (as mothers and wives) while public affairs, such as the economy and the state, are run by and for men. As many of these gender-based injustices are institutionalized in the laws and policies of our societies, feminist efforts have often targeted public law and public policy (Pateman 1988; Hawkesworth 1994).

In Japan for example, the number of female policy makers and law makers is much lower than the global average – which is already reflective of the fact that most societies are patriarchal. For example, women constitute only 10 per cent of members in Japan's House of Representatives and 20 per cent in the House of Councillors. According to the World Economic Forum, the gender gap index ranks Japan 120th out of 156 countries in the world, and for women's political empowerment Japan ranks 147th (Akimoto 2021). In such a situation, it is hardly surprising to find that three decades after more than 70 countries had made emergency contraception available to women without them having to seek their partners' consent, this was still a subject of debate in 2022 in Japan. Activists in Japan have said that this situation 'reflects the low priority the country's male-dominated parliament and medical community give to women's health' (McCurry 2022). Japan is, however, just a more extreme example of how a patriarchal system plays out in countries globally.

Theories of policy making are usually presented without any regard for gender. This raises issues of policy (analysis) goals and values – discussed in Chapter 8. You may wish to read the work of feminist scholars such as the American feminist social worker Beverly McPhail, who describes key issues for consideration in feminist policy frameworks including the importance of acknowledging the multiple forms of feminism. McPhail presents a feminist policy analysis framework that examines policy through a gendered lens by posing a series of questions, relating to areas such as values (e.g. Do feminist values undergird the policy? Which feminism, which values?), multiple identities (e.g. Are white, middle-class, heterosexual women the assumed standard for all women?) and gender neutrality (Does presumed gender neutrality hide the reality of the gendered nature of the problem or solution?) (McPhail 2003). Whilst directly addressing issues of power, such a framework may help to augment understanding of all aspects of the policy process including in regard to the conceptualizations and frameworks presented in the other chapters of this textbook.

White supremacy

White supremacy is the belief that white people are superior to those of other races or ethnicities. It has imposed and thereby maintains domination – social, political, historical and institutional – by white people over non-white people (however defined, as this has changed over time and place). This ideology was institutionalized in legal structures such as the Atlantic slave trade, Jim Crow laws in the US (the state and local laws that enforced racial segregation in southern parts of the country), White Australia policies from the 1890s to mid-1970s, and apartheid in South Africa. However, it remains institutionalized throughout many countries in many other areas of life – both formally and in less obvious ways. An example for a prominent global health institution is the findings of the independent review to address discrimination and advance anti-racism at the London School of Hygiene and Tropical Medicine (Nous Group 2021). Such findings at this institution and elsewhere have been the result of and further catalysed moves to '*decolonize*' global health. White supremacy also describes a social system in which white people have structural advantages (privileges) over other groups, despite legal equality. White people normalize and thus fail to see, and take for granted, these privileges. This is similar to the feminist critique of the assumptions and unreflective behaviour of men in a wide range of societies. In both cases, the concept of power as thought control and as something that profoundly shapes our worldviews can help with understanding how this institutionalization is maintained.

Some scholars have argued that white supremacy is itself a political system. The philosopher Charles Mills, introduced previously, has drawn on *social contract* theory, which addresses how people live together in society, to describe the social contracts which establish white supremacy and the associated power differentials – which he describes as the racial contract (Mills 1997).

Related to these issues of oppression and discrimination and their institutionalization is the concept of structural violence, a term coined by the Norwegian sociologist Johan Galtung (Galtung 1969). Structural violence is a form of violence relating to the characteristics of social structures and social institutions and how they harm (some) people from meeting their basic needs, including protecting their health. For example, in research on physical violence as a leading cause of injury and death amongst Black youth in the US, Wendel et al. (2021) describe how physical violence is shaped by structural violence. They define structural violence as the 'ideologies, systems, institutions, and policies that utilize power to create and perpetuate social, political and economic environments that harm some groups of people while empowering or privileging others' (Wendel et al. 2021).

As with patriarchal values and misogyny, white supremacy enters and affects the health policy-making process through many ways. This includes through the evidence that is generated in regard to health problems and their solutions and how (and by whom) it is interpreted; the power held by different actors in society and who (in a society that privileges white people, and particularly white men) is most likely to be represented in actor groups with greatest power; and the values, assumptions and interests of different actors including those with greatest power and influence.

Summary

This chapter has introduced you to a range of different theories and perspectives relating to the sources and distribution of power in societies with particular reference to health policy making, including some that are less commonly discussed in public policy textbooks such as the power relations inherent in the pervasive assumption of white supremacy.

Critically, we have also asked you to consider how your own power and privilege ('positionality') may shape your understanding of power. Such reflection is important for cultivating a deeper understanding of the policy process and the role of power in influencing that process.

The differences between the theories presented are sometimes quite stark, particularly between those which consider power as widely dispersed in societies and those which consider it as accumulating disproportionately in particular groups, whether they are large corporations, government officials, high-status professionals such as doctors, men over women, or white people over others. Some of the differences relate to the focus of attention, such as political conflict and formal decision making as against non-decision making. Some have been softened over time, such as pluralists' recognition of consistent power imbalances in society. In other cases, there is a need to integrate theory, for example, to enable issues of

---

patriarchy and white supremacy to be incorporated in theories which focus on capital (business) versus labour (employee) dynamics.

It is perhaps surprising that there is reasonable empirical evidence in support of many of the competing theories. How can this be? To return to a point you read at the start of this chapter, the nature and distribution of power depends on the specific policy context and the nature (content) of the policy issue. Technical issues such as the decision of which drug to fund by a national health service are often decided by a small group of experts. Many issues of high politics such as whether to go to war are made by a political elite (perhaps endorsed by a parliament), but some are highly debated and influenced by a range of interest groups – an example here being the UK's Brexit, ultimately decided by referendum. What is ultimately useful about the theories is that they provide different ways of trying to understand power in policy issues in different settings.

Further reading

Lukes, S. (2005) *Power: A Radical View*, 2nd edn. New York: Palgrave Macmillan.

Petticrew, M., Maani, N., Pettigrew, L. et al. (2020) Dark nudges and sludge in big alcohol: behavioral economics, cognitive biases, and alcohol industry corporate social responsibility, *The Milbank Quarterly*, 98(4): 1290–328.

Sriram, V., Topp, S.M., Schaaf, M. et al. (2018) 10 best resources on power in health policy and systems in low-and middle-income countries, *Health Policy and Planning*, 33(4): 611–21.

Topp, S.M., Schaaf, M., Sriram, V. et al. (2021) Power analysis in health policy and systems research: a guide to research conceptualisation, *BMJ Global Health*, 6(11): e007268.

wa Thiong'o, N. (2011) *Decolonising the Mind: The Politics of Language in African Literature*. Martlesham: James Curry.

References

Abbott, A. (1988) *The System of Professions: An Essay on the Division of Expert Labour*. Chicago, IL: University of Chicago Press.

Akimoto, D. (2021) Can Japan fix the gender gap in its politics?, *The Diplomat*, June.

Bachrach, P. and Baratz, M. (1962) The two faces of power, *American Political Science Review*, 56: 941–52.

Baleta, A. (1999) Zuma defends decision to make AIDS a notifiable disease, *The Lancet*, 353(9164): P1599.

Barnett, M. and Duvall, R. (2005) Power in international politics, *International Organisations*, 59: 39–75.

Bottomore, T.B. (1966) Elites and Society, Penguin, New York

Bourdieu, P. (1990) *The Logic of Practice*. Stanford, CA: Stanford University Press.

Campbell, C. (2009) Distinguishing the power of agency from agentic power: a note on Weber and the 'black box' of personal agency, *Sociological Theory*, 27(4): 407–18.

Crenshaw, K. (1991) Mapping the margins: intersectionality, identity politics, and violence against women of color, *Stanford Law Review*, 43(6): 1241–99.

Dahl, R.A. (1957) The concept of power, *Behavioral Science*, 2: 201–15.

Dahl, R.A. (2005 [1961]) *Who Governs? Democracy and Power in an American City*. New Haven, CT: Yale University Press.

Department of Health and Social Care (UK) (2021) Over £23 million investment to end new HIV infections by 2030. Available at: www.gov.uk/government/news/over-23-million-investment-to-end-new-hiv-infections-by-2030 (accessed 30 October 2022).

Dyer, C. (2022) Covid-19: government's use of VIP lane for awarding PPE contracts was unlawful, says judge, *British Medical Journal*, 376: o96.

Farnsworth, K. and Holden, C. (2006) The business-social policy nexus: corporate power and corporate inputs into social policy, *Journal of Social Policy*, 35(3): 473–94.

Foucault, M. (1978) *The History of Sexuality*. New York: Random House.

Foucault, M. (1998) *The History of Sexuality: The Will to Knowledge*. London: Penguin.

Freidson, E. (1970) *Profession of Medicine: A Study of the Sociology of Applied Knowledge*. New York: Harper & Row.

Fremsted, A. and Paul, M. (2022) Neoliberalism and climate change: how the free-market myth has prevented climate action, *Ecological Economics*, 197: 107353.

Fuchs, D. and Lederer, M. (2007) The power of business, *Business Power and Global Governance*, 9(3): 1–17. https://doi.org/10.2202/1469-3569.1214

Galtung, J. (1969) Violence, peace and peace research, *Journal of Peace Research*, 6(3): 167–91.

Gaventa, J. (2003) *Power after Lukes: A Review of the Literature*. Brighton: Institute of Development Studies.

Gaventa, J. (2006) Finding the spaces for change: a power analysis, *IDS Bulletin-Institute of Development Studies*, 37.

Gaventa, J., Pettit, J. and Cornish, L. (2011) *Power Pack, Understanding Power for Social Change*. Brighton: Institute for Developmental Studies.

Giddens, A. (1984) *The Constitution of Society: Outline of the Theory of Structuration*. Cambridge: Polity Press.

Gilson, L., Orgill, M. and Shroff, Z.C. (2018) *A Health Policy Analysis Reader: The Politics of Policy Change in Low- and Middle-Income Countries*. Geneva: World Health Organization.

Gramsci, A. (1971) *Selections From the Prison Notebooks of Antonio Gramsci*. New York: International Publishers.

Harrison, S. and Ahmad, W. (2000) Medical autonomy and the UK state 1975 to 2025, *Sociology*, 34(1): 129–46.

Hawkesworth, M. (1994) Policy studies within a feminist frame, *Policy Studies*, 27: 97–118.

Hawkins, B., Durrance-Bagale, A. and Walls H. (2021) Co-regulation and alcohol industry political strategy: a case study of the Public Health England-Drinkaware Drink Free Days Campaign, *Social Science & Medicine*, 285: 114175.

Jung, J. and Sharon, E. (2019) The Volkswagen emissions scandal and its aftermath, *Global Business and Organizational Excellence*, 38(4): 6–15.

Levi-Strauss, C. (1968) *Structural Anthropology*. New York: Allen Lane, The Penguin Press.

Lorde, A. (2017) *Your Silence Will Not Protect You*. London: Silver Press.

Lukes, S. (1974) *Power: A Radical View*. London, Macmillan.

Lukes, S. (2005) *Power: A Radical View*, 2nd edn. New York, Palgrave Macmillan.

Marx, K. (1867) *Capital: Critique of Political Economy*. Moscow: Progress Publishers.

Marx, K. (1976) *Capital*. Harmondsworth: Penguin.

McCurry, J. (2022) Japan to approve abortion pill – but partner's consent will be required, *The Guardian*, 31 May.

McPhail, B. (2003) A feminist policy analysis framework: through a gendered lens, *Social Policy Journal*, 2: 39–61.

Mialon, M. (2020) An overview of the commercial determinants of health, *Globalization and Health*, 16: 74.

Mills, C. W. (1956) *The Power Elite*. New York: Oxford University Press.

Mills, C. W. (1997) *The Racial Contract*. Ithaca, NY: Cornell University Press.

Milsom, P., Smith, R., Baker, P. and Walls, H. (2020) Corporate power and the international trade regime preventing progressive policy action on non-communicable diseases: a realist review, *Health Policy and Planning*, 36(4): 498–508.

Milsom, P., Smith, R. and Walls, H. (2022) Expanding public health policy analysis for transformative change: the importance of power and ideas. Comment on 'What generates attention to health in trade policy-making? Lessons from success in tobacco control and access to medicines: a qualitative study of Australia and the (Comprehensive and Progressive) Trans-Pacific Partnership', *International Journal of Health Policy and Management*, 11(4).

Moon, S. (2019) Power in global governance: an expanded typology from global health, *Globalization and Health*, 15(1): 74.

Navarro, V. (2007) Neoliberalism as a class ideology; or, the political causes of the growth of inequalities, *International Journal of Health Services*, 37(1): 47–62.

Navarro, V. (2020) The consequences of neoliberalism in the current pandemic, *International Journal of Health Services*, 50(3): 271–5.

Nous Group (2021) *Independent Review to Address Discrimination and Advance Anti-racism*. London School of Hygiene and Tropical Medicine, Nous Group. Available at: www.lshtm.ac.uk/media/56316 (accessed 15 April 2023).

Pateman, C. (1988) *The Sexual Contract*. Stanford, CA: Stanford University Press.

Perera, K., Timms, H. and Heimans, J. (2019) New power versus old: to beat antivaccination campaigners we need to learn from them – an essay by Kathryn Perera, Henry Timms, and Jeremy Heimans, *British Medical Journal*, 367: l6447.

Pollards, J. (2021) Brexit and the wider UK economy, *Geoforum*, 125: 197–8.

Robinson, N. (2006) *Learning from Lukes? The Three Faces of Power and the European Union*. ECPR Research Session. Nicosia.

Russ, K., Baker, P., Kang, M. and McCoy, D. (2022) Corporate lobbying on US positions towards the World Health Organization: evidence of intensification and cross-industry coordination, *Global Health Governance*, 27(1): 37–83.

Schrecker, T. (2019) Globalization and health: political grand challenges, *Review of International Political Economy*, 27(1): 26–47.

Stoeva, P. (2022) How can engagement with political science and international relations for health be improved? *The Lancet*, 399: 1977–1990.

Todd, M. (2018) *Straight Jacket: Overcoming Society's Legacy of Gay Shame*. London: Transworld Digital.

Veneklasen, L. and Miller, V. (2002) *A New Weave of Power, People & Politics: The Action Guide for Advocacy and Citizen Participation*. Oklahoma City, OK: World Neighbors.

wa Thiong'o, N. (2011) *Decolonising the Mind: The Politics of Language in African Literature*. Martlesham: James Curry.

Walt, G. and Gilson, L. (1994) Reforming the health sector in developing countries: the central role of policy analysis, *Health Policy and Planning*, 9: 353–70.

Weber, M. (1948) The meaning of discipline, in H.H. Gerth and C. Wright Mills (eds.) *From Max Weber: Essays in Sociology*. London: Routledge.

Wendel, M., Nation, W., Williams, W. et al. (2021) The structural violence of white supremacy: addressing root causes to prevent youth violence, *Archives of Psychiatric Nursing*, 35: 127–8.

West, R. and Marteau, T. (2013) Commentary on Casswell (2013): the commercial determinants of health, *Addiction*, 108(4): 686–87.

Wood, B., Williams, O., Baker, P. et al. (2021) The influence of corporate market power on health: exploring the structure-conduct-performance model from a public health perspective, *Globalization and Health*, 14: 41.

3   Government and the state

This chapter focuses on the roles of the government and the wider state (or public sector) in the formulation of policy, and the extent of their influence in the policy process. While policy formulation usually involves taking account of a wide variety of interests, albeit driven by the ideological assumptions of the government in power, the way this happens is dependent on the type of government and state institutions of a country. Thus the state is typically a central focus of policy and policy analysis. This is in part the result of its omnipresence and its role in implementing the decisions of the government of the day, despite recognition of the limits on nation states in the context of global inter-dependency and the influence of powerful interest groups, particularly multinational corporations (see Chapter 4 for the role of the private sector).

Learning objectives

After working through this chapter, you will be better able to:

- describe the main state bodies involved in policy making – legislature, executive, bureaucracy and judiciary – and their roles
- understand how these bodies relate to one another differently in different types of political system and how these relationships shape how policy is made
- understand how different parts of government (e.g. ministries of health, finance, business, employment, housing, social security, etc.) and different levels (e.g. national, regional and local) require active co-ordination if policies are to be successful
- describe and account for the changing role of the state in the past few decades, and what this has implied for the state's role in health policy
- describe the formal organizational structure of the health system of your country and be aware that the official chart of its organization may not reflect the true pattern of power and influence in the system and, by extension, in health policy making.

Key terms

Bureaucracy   This term can refer to: (1) institutions through which government policy is pursued; (2) public officials, often known as civil servants, whose job it is to advise ministers (the executive) on how best to take forward their policy goals and then to manage the process of policy implementation; and (3) a hierarchical and rule-based approach to public administration.

Decentralization   The transfer of authority and responsibilities from central government to local levels.

Executive   Leadership of a country (i.e. the president and/or prime minister and other ministers). The prime minister/president and senior ministers are often referred to as the cabinet.

Federal system   A government system in which the sub-national (i.e. state or provincial) level of government is not subordinate to the national government but has substantial powers of its own which the national government cannot take away without changing the constitution.

Government   That part of the state comprising the executive ('the government of the day') and the bureaucracy (civil or public service and ministries).

Institutions   In political science, the 'rules of the game' determining how organizations, such as governments, operate. These can be formal structures and procedures, but also informal norms of behaviour that may not be written down. Confusingly, the term is also in more general use to refer to 'organizations'.

Judiciary   Judges and courts responsible for ensuring that the government of the day (the executive) acts according to the laws passed by the legislature and/or in line with the constitution.

Legislature   Body that enacts the laws that govern a country and oversees the executive. It is normally democratically elected in order to represent the people of the country and commonly referred to as the parliament or assembly. Many countries have two chambers or 'houses' of parliament.

Majoritarian   A government system in which election results are determined by a simple numerical majority of the votes cast and/or the parliamentary seats won, sometimes referred to as 'first past the post'.

Parliamentary system   A system of government in which the members of the executive (the cabinet) are also members of the legislature and are chosen from the members of the legislature who represent political parties that have a majority in the legislature.

Path dependency The phenomenon in which decisions taken in one period influence the scope and direction of later policy by reinforcing the position of particular interest groups or putting in place specific ways of working that restrict future action.

Populism An approach to politics that is difficult to define since it is not intellectually coherent but usually includes leaders and potential leaders who define themselves as the champions of ordinary people, purport to be anti-elitist and who brand opponents as disloyal to the country. Populism particularly appeals to those who are concerned to protect the security and cultural integrity of their country against outsiders ('others') but who are also sceptical of the ability of democratically elected government to do so.

Presidential system A system of government in which the president (i.e. the head of the government of the day – the executive) is not a member of the legislature but elected separately. Presidential systems vary in the extent to which the president has directive powers that do not depend on the will of the legislature.

Proportional representation Voting system which is designed to ensure as far as possible that the proportion of votes received by each political party equates to their share of the seats in the legislature.

Regulation The rules and standards made and maintained by an authority – often by government (e.g. in a private market for goods and services to prevent anti-competitive behaviour or false claims).

State A set of public bodies that enjoy legal sovereignty over a fixed territorial area and extends beyond the government of the day, comprising the executive, legislature, bureaucracy, judiciary, courts and military as well as other public bodies, including the specialized agencies that regulate aspects of the health and health care system.

Stewardship The role of governments in directing and overseeing the health system, improving its performance and ensuring that it is maintained in good order for future generations (e.g. by ensuring a future supply of trained health workers).

Unitary system A system of government in which the lower levels of government are constitutionally subordinate to the national government and derive their authority entirely from central government.

Introduction

Policy decisions of *governments* and the wider *state* extend deeply into people's personal lives from the relatively trivial to the life changing. In recent decades, states have, for example:

- regulated the number of children people can have (China);
- prohibited private medical practice (Cuba);
- prohibited commercial sex work (about a third of countries);
- determined the age at which gender reassignment procedures are allowed (ages vary between countries);
- determined whether or not emergency contraception is available without a medical prescription (countries' policies vary widely).

For much of the twentieth century the state played a dominant role in the economies of most countries: airlines were owned and operated by the state as were other utilities such as railways, water, electricity and telephones. Many governments presided over 'command and control' economies in the context of five-year development plans. In many newly independent post-colonial countries, the government also became the major employer. For example, in Tanzania the government's workforce grew from 27 per cent of those formally employed in 1962 to over 66 per cent in 1974 (Perkins and Roemer 1991). By the 1980s things began to change; states were 'rolled back' and the private sector was encouraged to enter fields that were once the preserve of the state – including health care. This shift has been maintained and has had implications both for the content of health policy as well as the actors participating in the health policy process.

This chapter explores government policy making and the role of the wider state mainly focusing on democracies; that is, settings where there are periodic opportunities for the people to change their leaders. The chapter looks first at the role of the parts of the state most frequently assumed to be directly involved in shaping and carrying out policies: the legislature, the executive, the bureaucracy and the judiciary. The chapter continues by looking at the involvement of the wider state or public sector in health and presents arguments which justify its prominent role.

In terms of the two generic frameworks for policy analysis introduced in Chapter 1, the focus in this chapter is on a particular set of official 'actors' within the policy process and their relationships. In terms of the 'policy stages' model also discussed in Chapter 1, the main focus is on policy formulation with some reference to policy implementation.

Government and public policy

Chapter 2 introduced a range of different ways of understanding public policy based on underlying notions of the distribution of power in society. An alternative approach is to seek to explain the formulation and implementation of public policies by reference to the characteristics of the government and wider state system (see Figure 3.1). This approach sees individual politicians and bureaucrats as actors driven by their ideas and their self-interest, but also sees the organization of government and the public sector as a set of structures and rules that shape the policy process (Evans et al. 1985). The latter are referred to by political scientists as *institutions* – that is, the norms and procedures of government such as the electoral system, the body with the right to initiate legislation, the relations between the legislature and judiciary (see below), the rules governing lobbying of political representatives by agents of interest groups, the way in which specific interest groups are consulted by government, the norms of transparency and so on. A focus on institutions tends to draw attention to the obstacles and limits on policy change since structures and procedures, particularly constitutions, tend to change less frequently than, for example, the distribution of support between political parties. A focus on institutions also tends to emphasize how institutional arrangements, both formal and informal, constrain policy development processes and thinking – keeping them to well-worn paths so that decisions in the past limit the room for manoeuvre in the future. This phenomenon is known as *path dependency*. It has been used extensively to explain the very prolonged process in the US to extend health insurance coverage despite much popular support and why the Affordable Care Act (known as 'Obamacare') is incomplete compared with the systems of universal public insurance in Western European countries (Steinmo and Watts 1995).

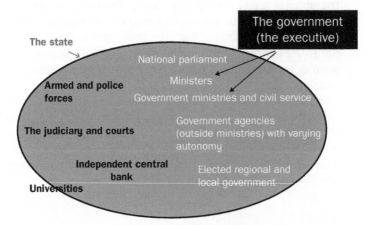

Figure 3.1: The distinction between the wider state and the government in a parliamentary system

Characterizing government systems

Two features of government systems have a major effect on the ability of governments to make and implement policy: autonomy and capacity (Howlett et al. 2009). In this context, *autonomy* means the ability of the government to resist being captured by self-interested groups and to act fairly as an arbiter of social conflicts. The government system may not be neutral in a political sense (after all, it serves governments of different ideological complexions), but, if it is truly autonomous, it strives to operate as far as possible with objective regard to improving the welfare of the whole country not just advancing the interests of the sections of the community who support the government of the day. The rise and consolidation of populist authoritarian regimes in countries such as Brazil and Hungary in the early twenty-first century has shown that governments can also act very differently, maintaining their power base by dividing society, labelling opponents as 'enemies of the state' and favouring their supporters. Similarly, government agencies can become 'captured' by the interests they seek to regulate, as in the case of the US Food and Drug Administration (FDA), which failed to protect the public from the harm caused by Purdue Pharma's opioid, OxyContin.

Capacity refers to the ability of the government system to make and implement policy. It springs from the expertise, resources and coherence of the machinery of government. For example, it is essential that a government is able to pay its civil servants on time and keep corruption in check. It also improves policy making if individual ministries respect the fact that their decisions and behaviour can have major implications for other arms of government and refrain from self-interested actions. More positively, this would mean an MoH that supported other ministries to pursue policies beyond health that were health promoting and protecting (so-called 'health in all policies') (De Leeuw et al. 2021). The different forms of government system have implications for the autonomy and capacity of government policy making.

Federal versus unitary systems

All governments operate at a variety of levels between the national and the local (e.g. publicly funded health systems frequently have national and regional levels of administration). However, there is an important, basic distinction between *unitary* and *federal* systems which cannot be overlooked when thinking about policy change in health systems. In the former, there is a clear chain of command linking the different levels of government so that lower levels are strictly subordinate to higher levels. In France, for example, the national government has potentially all the decision-making powers. It can delegate these powers to lower levels of government, but can also take these powers back relatively easily. China,

Japan and New Zealand are similar. The UK has a largely unitary system in which local government derives its powers from central government, but Scotland, Wales and Northern Ireland were granted their own powers over most of their domestic affairs, including health, under legislation passed by the national parliament in London in 1999 (see 'Devolution of the UK's National Health Service (NHS) to Scotland, Wales and Northern Ireland' in Chapter 10, page 266). Thus, the UK sits uneasily somewhere between a unitary and federal state.

In fully federal systems, the sub-national level of government is not subordinate to the national level but enjoys a high level of freedom over those matters under its jurisdiction. Central government cannot remove these freedoms without consent of the sub-national tier which normally means rewriting the constitution of the country. For example, Australia, Brazil, Canada, India, Nigeria and the US are all federal countries. In Canada, for instance, the health system is a responsibility of the provinces, not the federal government, though the latter contributes some of the funding for health services. This leads to lengthy negotiations and disputes between the two levels of government about who pays for what and what decision rights each level of government has and should have.

Indeed, federalism is widely regarded as a major reason for the relative inability of governments in these countries to bring about major, nation-wide policy changes in the health sector except when circumstances are highly favourable. A further complication is that federal and sub-national governments may be controlled by different political parties with different values and goals. Moreover, elections at one or the other level rarely coincide, so policy development processes that require lengthy negotiations between the affected interests can be disrupted by a change of government at either level. Typically, unitary government systems are associated with far more rapid policy change and less need to compromise when formulating policy. However, this does not necessarily mean that policies developed in this way will be implemented as intended (see Chapter 6). Even in unitary systems with relatively few constitutional obstacles to legislative change, the underlying conditions for fundamental system reform rarely occur. These are typically a combination of a government with a high level of authority (e.g. a strong parliamentary majority), the political will to incur the risks of major change (i.e. reform must be sufficiently central to its policy agenda) and strong capacity (Tuohy 2004).

Role of political parties

In democracies, people are free to set up political parties and put themselves forward for election on behalf of those parties without executive and judicial interference. Parties produce manifestos on which they campaign at elections and devise strategies to promote their goals and marginalize their opponents. Voters are normally invited to support a broad package of measures designed to maximize the party's appeal. The detail of which policies reach the government agenda and how they are developed subsequently is outside the direct control of the party and the voters (see Chapter 5). Of course, a government in office has to be careful not to move too far away from what it promised its party members, supporters, funders (e.g. from business or trade unions) and the voters at the election, even if circumstances change, otherwise it will jeopardize its future support. In office, politicians may find that turning manifesto promises into coherent policy is far more difficult technically and politically than they had envisaged while in opposition.

The evidence suggests that political parties have a modest direct effect on policy – their greatest contribution being at the early stages of policy identification – but a larger indirect effect through influencing the staffing of the legislature and executive (and sometimes the judiciary).

In single or dominant party systems, one political party formulates all or most policies and it becomes the task of the government to find the best ways of implementing them. On the whole, elections in single-party systems do not provide voters with any real choices or policy alternatives, and criticism of the ruling party and its government are often muted or stifled. For example, opposition parties and independent media organizations had already effectively been stifled before the 2022 Hungarian general election when the self-styled 'illiberal democrat', authoritarian *populist* prime minister, Viktor Orbán was re-elected president for the fourth time. Orbán had skilfully used seemingly innocuous media ownership laws to enable his supporters to take over media organizations without explicit political control (Geva 2021). In single-party regimes, the party can also intervene directly in policy. There is no clear-cut or simple separation between the party and the executive or legislature. Both the latter can be criticized by the party to the extent that ministers and members of parliament can be removed for not responding with sufficient zeal to the party's views.

By contrast, in liberal democracies, once a political party wins power at an election, the government is in charge. Ministers can adapt party policy in the light of the political pressures placed upon them and the changing nature of the policy environment.

Majoritarian versus proportional electoral systems

Another basic distinction between government systems relates to the rules governing parliamentary elections. In *majoritarian* systems, typically candidates from different political parties compete for votes within electoral districts, sometimes known as constituencies. The candidate with the most votes represents the district in parliament and political parties aim to win as many such contests as possible so as to have the most seats in parliament and thus be best placed to form the executive or government of the day. Under *proportional representation*, the number of seats gained by each party is related to its share of the national vote (though different systems do this to differing degrees) and the aim of political parties is to maximize total votes. This difference can affect the policies promoted by parties to the electorate. Under proportional representation, the goal is to appeal to a wide range of potential voters whereas under the majoritarian 'first past the post' system, parties may tailor their policies to the issues affecting particular constituencies within the country.

Roles and inter-relationships of the legislature, the executive and the judiciary

Another feature of each country's government system affecting how public policy is formulated concerns the relations between the legislature or parliament, the executive and the judiciary. The *legislature* is the body which represents the people, enacts the laws that govern the people and oversees the *executive* which is the leadership of the country (i.e. the president and/or prime minister and other ministers, commonly referred to in democracies as 'the government of the day' or the cabinet). Typically, in *parliamentary* systems, the executive (the administration, or 'government of the day') is chosen by the legislature from among its members (i.e. ministers are members of the parliament and are generally from the party or parties that can command a majority in the parliament). The executive remains in office as long as it has majority support among the legislators. Typically, in *presidential* systems, such as Brazil or the US, the executive (the president and their team) are detached from the legislature, with the president elected separately by the public. Thus, the president does not require the support of the majority of members of the legislature to win office but is hampered in governing effectively if the majority of the legislature is from an opposing political party.

In presidential systems, the executive can propose policy but the approval of the legislature is required for the policy to become law. As a result, the US president, for example, frequently has to offer concessions to the legislature in one area of policy in return for support in another since in the US system, the president has to rely on the legislature (the House of Representatives) to initiate legislation. In addition, members of the legislature can play an active part in designing and amending policies. This means that the policy development process is more consultative than in parliamentary systems and there are more obvious attempts by interest groups to exert influence, and for complex bargaining to occur between interests and political representatives. This is particularly the case for large-scale business interest groups which also provide party political funding.

In parliamentary systems, while there may be some dispute and bargaining over policies within the governing political party or coalition, this usually takes place behind the scenes and the executive can normally rely on its majority in the legislature to obtain support for the measures it wishes to enact. Where the executive does not have an outright majority in the legislature, as happens more often in countries with systems of proportional representation where there may be a larger number of political parties and coalition governments are more common, it has to compromise in order to get policies through the legislature. This makes the policy process slower and more complex, but not as difficult as policy making in presidential systems. Policy making is still ultimately centralized in the executive in all types of parliamentary systems.

🖊 Activity 3.1

As well as the separation of powers between the executive (the president and their staff) and the legislature (the two Houses of Congress), which other parts of the governmental system make major policy change (e.g. a wholesale reform of the financing of the health care system) more difficult in the US than in many other countries?

Feedback

The US system is federal so the individual states will have to be persuaded to support any major change in domestic policy. By contrast, the states have no role in foreign and defence policy. This explains why presidents of the US tend to spend quite a lot of time and energy on defence and foreign policy where their power is less restricted and they can act on behalf of the entire nation.

The position of the judiciary also affects the government policy process. In *federal systems* and/or those based on a written constitution, there is typically an autonomous judiciary, usually in the form of a supreme court charged with adjudicating in the case of disputes between the different tiers of government and with ensuring that the laws and actions of the government are consistent with the principles of the constitution. For example, the US Supreme Court has frequently challenged the laws of individual states: in the 1950s, it enforced the civil liberties of black people by overturning legislation in the southern states which would have segregated schools between black and white. In 2022, it did the reverse by challenging women's constitutional rights to abortion, thereby opening the way for states to enact legislation to limit or ban abortion. In countries like Britain without a written constitution, though independent of government, the courts are more limited in what they can do to constrain the executive in the protection of the rights and liberties of individual citizens and executive policy making is easier.

Real-world government systems are built of combinations of the features discussed above so that the effects of one may be mitigated by another. Thus, a country such as New Zealand has a unitary, parliamentary system with only one parliamentary chamber (see below). This arrangement tends to concentrate power in the single parliamentary chamber. Nonetheless, members of parliament are elected by proportional representation, thereby giving a wider range of political opinion a say in who is elected and reducing the odds of sharp changes in policy between successive governments, since governments are generally coalitions of political parties. This system also produces a stronger representation of the interests of minority groups such as the indigenous Maori population.

✎ Activity 3.2

Imagine that you are a national minister of health wishing to introduce a major change into a health care system, such as user fees for patients to use public hospitals. List the different considerations you would have to take into account if you were trying to introduce such legislation in a federal, presidential system versus a unitary, parliamentary system. Make two lists of factors.

Feedback

Your notes might look something like those presented in Table 3.1.

You will immediately see the larger number and greater complexity of the considerations which the minister of health in a federal, presidential system will have to take into account compared with his counterpart in the unitary, parliamentary system. Thus, US President Barrack Obama faced many formal and informal *institutional* obstacles in his quest to widen health care insurance coverage and lower its cost. As a result, the original reform bill included many concessions to opponents of reform and further concessions had to be made throughout the legislative process, most notably to circumvent the filibustering tactics of opponents in the upper house, the Senate (Hacker 2010). Filibustering is also known as 'talking out' and is an anti-majoritarian barrier to change in which a member(s) of a parliament speaks for as long as possible in debate to prevent a piece of legislation being voted on and passed. It is now a taken for granted Senate rule that any legislation of more than trivial significance requires at least 60 out of approximately 100 Senators to vote to end a debate and overcome a filibuster rather than a simple majority. By contrast, the Australian parliament has strict rules on how long members can speak, thereby largely preventing filibusters.

Table 3.1 Federal, presidential and unitary, parliamentary systems compared

Federal, presidential system	Unitary, parliamentary system
Which level of government is responsible for which aspects of health policy? Is this change within the jurisdiction of national government?	Has the intended reform been discussed in the governing political party or parties? Is it in the election manifesto or coalition agreement? What does the governing political party or parties think about the intended reform? Are they broadly supportive? If not, are the majority of members of the legislature from the government party or parties likely to be in support?
Does national government control the aspects of health policy most relevant to the proposed changes? For example, does national government control all the necessary resources to bring about the change?	Has the government got a majority in the legislature (parliament) to enact the changes? If not, can the government get sufficient votes from other parties?
Is the national legislature likely to support the changes? If not, what concessions might be made either in health or in other areas of policy to win the necessary support? Are these concessions worth making for this reform?	What concessions, if any, will be needed to get a majority in support of the reforms?
What are the odds of the proposed legislation passing through the national legislature without substantial amendment?	
If the government will be dependent on the support of states or provinces to bring about the changes, what are the likely reactions of states or provinces to the reform? Which states or provinces have governments of the same political persuasion as the national government?	
What concessions to the states/provinces could the government make in health or other areas of policy without undermining its position with its supporters in order to obtain sufficient support for the health reforms, particularly from states/provinces governed by opposition parties? For example, will national government have to fund the changes in their entirety to have any chance of getting them accepted?	
What view are the courts likely to take of the reforms?	

The role of the legislature

In the overwhelming majority of countries, the constitution states that the decisions of the legislature are the expression of the will of the people (i.e. there is popular sovereignty) and that the legislature is the highest decision-making body. Most have three formal functions: to represent the people; to enact legislation (the most formal manifestation of policy intent); and to oversee the executive (the prime minister or president and ministers). Legislatures in democracies are generally composed exclusively of elected members (known as deputies, senators or members of parliament). Three-fifths of the countries in the world have unicameral or single-chamber legislatures; the rest have bicameral arrangements with two chambers or houses that are typically elected and composed differently. Generally, the job of the upper house is to review and refine draft legislation that has started out in the lower house and thereby contribute to better policy and law making. In presidential systems, as we saw earlier, the legislature has autonomy from the executive and, on occasions, can make policy. In parliamentary systems, the task of the legislature is primarily to hold the government to account on behalf of the public for its performance rather than to initiate policy. Legislators can identify problems in draft legislation and request changes but the executive generally holds the advantage backed by its parliamentary majority.

In a range of different government systems, legislatures are increasingly regarded as bodies that rubber-stamp decisions taken elsewhere, struggle to hold the executive to account and fail to protect basic population rights. For example, the human rights monitoring platform, Civicus (2021), reported that freedom of expression, peaceful assembly and association continued to deteriorate globally. Civicus reported that almost 90 per cent of the world's population now lived in countries which significantly restricted these rights. Authoritarian governments, in particular, but not exclusively, had taken advantage of the COVID-19 pandemic to pass laws to restrict popular dissent, to limit the ability of opposition political parties to criticize them or mobilize public opinion and to entrench their electoral position, for instance, by extending governmental term limits. Laws passed during a public health emergency tended not to be repealed.

Efforts have been made in a number of countries to strengthen the role and influence of the legislature, principally by ensuring that members of parliament have the powers, staff and other resources to investigate and critique the activities of the executive and to develop alternatives to government policies. Civil society also appears to be more active in some countries, attempting to put issues on the agenda of the government of the day (the executive) and holding it to account (see Chapters 4 and 5).

✎ **Activity 3.3**

What obstacles do national legislatures (i.e. parliaments and assemblies) typically face in influencing government policy making and in holding the executive to account?

Feedback

Five main reasons are usually given for the difficulties faced by legislatures in fulfilling their functions. The relative importance of each depends on the country in question, but most are related directly or indirectly to the rising power of the executive:

- increasingly strong political party discipline, controlling the activities of members and reducing criticism of the executive;
- the ability of the executive to use its powers of patronage (i.e. the ability to offer or withhold opportunities for promotion into ministerial and other positions) to control potentially dissident members of the legislature;
- the shift of much political and policy debate from the parliamentary debating chamber to the mass media (e.g. to the set-piece television interview or debate between party leaders) and particularly to social media, thereby bypassing the legislature;
- the expansion of government activities and their delegation to a range of specialized state agencies so that many decisions can be taken by bureaucrats and special advisers far from parliament without the need for new laws or legislative debate;
- the increasing influence of supra-national bodies such as the EU, the International Monetary Fund (IMF) or the World Trade Organization (WTO) that limit or remove issues from domestic legislative politics (see Chapters 9 and 10).

Although some legislatures rarely propose new laws and others struggle to fulfil their three main functions, they survive because they have great symbolic value, upholding the ideal of democratic representation of the public. Also, particularly in presidential systems, they can block some of the proposals of the executive by right. In parliamentary systems, legislators can scrutinize and delay legislation, but where an executive has a parliamentary majority and reasonable party discipline, it will prevail over the views of members of parliament. Only where there is no clear majority and the government is dependent on several smaller parties do individual legislators have opportunities to shape policies directly. This is one of the arguments in favour of an electoral system of proportional representation.

The role of the executive

As you have seen, in most countries with multi-party systems and even more in one-party states, most of the power to initiate and make policy lies with the executive – the elected politicians who become prime minister or president and their ministers or immediate advisers. This group is usually called the 'cabinet'. The executive is generally more powerful in parliamentary than presidential systems, though this depends on the constitution of the country in question. The elected and appointed members of the executive are supported by bureaucrats (civil servants) who both advise ministers and take direction from them. There is debate about the relative influence on policy of elected officials and bureaucrats. It depends strongly on the country and the period studied as well as the nature of the policy issue at stake. In some countries, the senior level(s) of the *bureaucracy* are political appointees liable to change as the government changes, thereby blurring the distinction between political and bureaucratic influence on policy, while in others the civil service is permanent, politically neutral and separate from elected politicians. In the latter systems, there has been a trend towards ministers appointing their own political advisers in addition to the ministry civil servants to give political, presentational and policy advice to ministers, including helping write political speeches.

Compared with the legislature, the executive or cabinet has far greater informational, financial and personnel resources. The cabinet has the authority to govern the country and usually has the ultimate authority to initiate policies. Crucially, it can generally choose when to introduce draft laws to the legislature, though not in all presidential systems. In parliamentary systems, as long as the government has majority support in the legislature, there can be few limits on the power of the executive. In presidential systems, the executive has to convince the legislature to approve its proposed measures where these involve legislation. However, there are still wide areas of policy where the executive has discretion, particularly in relation to defence, national security and foreign policy where legislation is rarely needed for action. Frequently, once the budget has been approved by the legislature, the executive has a great deal of control over the detail of how public resources are used.

Traditionally, minister of health was not seen as a very prestigious cabinet post and rarely a route to the most senior ministerial positions such as minister of finance. However, as the economic importance of a healthy population has become more apparent and spending on health services has risen as a share of national incomes, the post has grown in prominence along with the profile of the MoH (see below).

The role of the chief executive

If the executive is very powerful, does this power emanate from the collective decision making of the cabinet, or from the strength of the prime minister or president who occupies a position similar to the chief executive of a private corporation? In countries where constitutional checks on the executive are weak, most major policy decisions will be in the hands of the chief executive and their most politically trusted or strategically important ministers. The minister of finance is usually in the latter group of core ministers.

Thus, individual political leadership does matter, even in the complex and inter-connected contemporary world which constrains national governments in many ways (as you will see in Chapters 9 and 10). One of the most striking examples of the impact of contrasting leadership decisions concerned government policy on AIDS in South Africa and Uganda in the late 1990s and early 2000s. Both countries had a high prevalence of HIV. In South Africa, President Thabo Mbeki denied the link between HIV and AIDS as part of a national political struggle over the control of information and resistance to Western dominance of science (Schneider 2002). His government refused to support the purchase of anti-retroviral drugs for the treatment of people living with AIDS. In Uganda, President Yoweri Museveni was widely credited with a quite different policy of openly discussing AIDS and inviting all groups to help develop a national response to the epidemic. Although the wider political environment in Uganda particularly favoured such a stance (e.g. there was no major tourist industry to be harmed by openness), the President himself contributed decisively to the direction of policy (Parkhurst 2001).

Similarly, during the COVID-19 pandemic, there were big differences in behaviour and decision making between political leaders, all of whom struggled to know how best to respond. Some so-called '*populist*' leaders at the time in countries such as Brazil, India and the United States were heavily criticized by some observers for initially denying the severity of the virus, undermining the efforts of public health agencies, or delaying the response in the name of protecting the ordinary population and the economy against an out-of-touch technocratic elite (McKee et al. 2020).

The role of the bureaucracy

The appointed officials who administer the system of government are referred to as civil or public servants. Although referred to as 'servants' of the politicians, their role extends beyond this to managing policy processes in many areas of policy. There are far too many functions for the executive to discharge more than a fraction of the highest profile ones, delegating many to bureaucrats to carry out in their name. Civil servants can also have influence because of their expertise and experience. While ministers and governments may come and go, most of the bureaucrats remain to maintain the system of government. Even in countries such as the US and most of Latin America, where top civil servants change when the ruling government changes, most other public servants' jobs are unaffected.

Countries generally try to strike a balance between a self-interested civil service unresponsive to political leadership and an excessively politicized civil service which serves the interests of the ruling parties rather than the national interest. There are subtle forms of politicization even in merit-based, politically neutral civil service systems. For example, in Australia and Canada, the prime minister has considerable freedom to appoint the most senior civil servants without reference to ability or open competition.

New governments and new ministers are clearly more dependent on their officials for information, if only until they are familiar with what is happening in their field of responsibility and with the detail of how the system of government works, but they may also be suspicious of officials who until recently had served a government led by their opponents and less likely to accept their views on policy options. In such situations, they tend to rely on their own political advisers who play increasingly important roles as the eyes and ears of the minister, and an extension of their reach.

The power of the bureaucracy vis-à-vis politicians differs from country to country, over time and from sector to sector. In France, India, Japan, South Korea and Singapore the civil service traditionally has high status, a neutral professional ethos and a clear mandate to provide independent advice to politicians. After a long period of training, civil servants form a homogeneous, well-informed group and pursue a life-long career in government.

Looking around the world, it becomes apparent that countries like South Korea with strong bureaucracies are exceptional. In many countries, particularly poorer, post-colonial ones, bureaucracies often do not have sufficient capability and capacity to deal with the problems the country faces. In such settings, there is a perennial risk that the executive and its political supporters will try to use the government machinery and policy to pursue their own interests, at the expense of the needs and well-being of the majority of the population. In other words, the state lacks the twin features of *autonomy* and *capacity* introduced earlier in the chapter – often linked to ongoing neo-colonial dependencies and foreign or global capitalist interests which perpetuate exploitative government practices, wealth extraction and corruption.

Even in countries with a much better equipped civil service, the power of the bureaucracy depends on its internal organization within a particular sector. Thus, if in the health sector there are a small number of agencies and a small number of officials in each body who have some decision-making power independent of politicians, bureaucrats will tend to be influential in certain health policy processes. By contrast, if there are a large number of agencies each with some authority, no one group of officials is likely to be influential on a specific issue and politicians will most likely have more direct influence over a wider range of policy areas.

Similarly, the influence of the civil service on policy formation also depends on the extent to which it has a monopoly over advice reaching ministers. Thus, in Australia, New Zealand and UK, where traditionally the professional, politically neutral civil service was the main source of advice to ministers, governments have acted in the last 40 years to widen the range of sources of advice to ministers, for example, by developing policy and strategy units within government staffed by a mixture of political advisers, secondees from business and handpicked civil servants, and by opening up civil service posts to outside applicants. One approach is to recruit successful entrepreneurs or consultancy firms to advise on the reform of government itself as well as its policies. In this way, the boundaries between the civil service and the political sphere together with other walks of life such as business and academia have been deliberately blurred, and political appointees have grown in number and influence within the government process.

Finally, the influence of the bureaucrats depends on the type of policy at issue. Major policies (e.g. macro-economic policy) and/or those with a high profile and ideological significance (i.e. 'high' politics) are more likely to be driven by the senior politicians and their personal advisers. The civil service role will be confined to ensuring that the wishes of the government are implemented. By contrast, on issues of 'low politics' – dealing with technical problems relating to the day-to-day working of government such as the detail of hospital reimbursement systems – civil servants tend to have much greater influence in defining the problem and providing the solution.

The role of the ministry of health

The bureaucracy is divided into departments or ministries, as well as other agencies with specific functions. Indeed, specialization is a feature of bureaucracies. Each of these organizations will have its own interests and ways of operating. The ministry of finance is generally the most powerful since it is responsible for allocating resources between different ministries in line with government priorities. Sectoral ministries, such as health, are, in turn, responsible for ensuring that the needs of their sectors are properly represented when decisions are made. Some conflict is inevitable as each ministry argues for what it regards as its proper share of the government's budget. In addition, different ministries relate to different 'policy communities' or 'policy networks' (i.e. more or less organized clusters of groups inside and outside government in a particular sector trying to influence government policy, see Chapter 4), which can vary in complexity and scale, thereby shaping the way ministries function.

Ministries are internally divided, often along functional, technical or policy lines. Thus, an MoH might have divisions relating to the main contours of the health system such as hospitals, primary health care and public health or the main diseases such as malaria, tuberculosis and HIV, as well as medical, nursing and other professional advisory departments which cut across these divisions – with each division pursuing its own interests and ideas in relation to policy prioritization, formulation and implementation. There are also likely to be regional or district levels of the ministry or separate health authorities which may not play a large part in policy identification and formulation, but are important for policy implementation, depending on the extent of *decentralization* in the government system (more on this in Chapter 6).

Ministries of health play an essential function in governing and steering health systems. This function is sometimes referred to as *stewardship* or overall system oversight, which 'encompasses the tasks of defining the vision and direction of health policy, exerting influence through *regulation* and advocacy, and collecting and using information' (World Health Organization 2000: xiv). Ministries shape and maintain the policy and regulatory framework within which health services are paid for and delivered. These frameworks, often in the form of legislation, define the respective roles, responsibilities and accountabilities of the ministry and other health system agencies.

The roles and responsibilities of ministries of health vary depending on how decentralized the health system is, but the following are usual, particularly in systems paid for from taxation (ministries generally have more regulatory and fewer planning and resource allocation roles in systems based on social or private insurance):

- advising the minister of health and the wider government on how to respond to the health problems facing the country currently and in the future;
- developing, implementing and enforcing legislation and related regulations;
- negotiating the operating and capital budgets for the public system with the ministry of finance in tax financed systems, or ensuring the financial viability of the insurance funds in social insurance systems;
- defining which services are covered by the public system and setting prices for goods and services (particularly in social insurance systems);
- allocating resources (money, staff, equipment, facilities) to different parts of the country and/or services through strategies and plans;
- planning the future workforce and subsidizing training;
- setting standards and regulating the quality of care at organizational and individual professional levels;
- monitoring health and health system performance according to goals of equity, efficiency, acceptability, responsiveness, etc.;
- providing infrastructural services such as for information technology, payment of physicians, etc.;
- co-ordinating action with other ministries and agencies that have roles to play in protecting health (e.g. in transport, agriculture and food);
- generating appropriate information and research evidence to support all the above activities;
- engaging in international co-operation to improve health policy and outcomes – for example through the World Health Assembly (see Chapter 9).

✎ **Activity 3.4**

Ministries have differing status. The political importance of health ministries to governments has been rising in relative terms. Where do you think the MoH and health policy sits in the hierarchy of status and attention in your country? Why do you think this is the case?

Feedback

Explanations for a low status include the possibility that the country faces very pressing economic problems, the solutions to which are generally seen as lying in reforming and stimulating the economy rather than investing in people's health. The economists in dominant ministries of finance frequently regard spending on health as 'consumption' (i.e. current spending which produces only current benefits) and tend not to see it as 'investment' (i.e. spending now to produce a stream of benefits into the future) to which they would give higher priority. Their approach traditionally has been to try to restrict consumption as far as possible in favour of investment in fields such as infrastructure (roads, harbours, drainage schemes) with a view to making longer term economic gains. However, it is increasingly being recognized that wisely targeted spending on health improvement (e.g. HIV prevention, reducing the incidence of type 2 diabetes) can be a worthwhile investment, and should be seen as integral to economic policy since a healthier workforce is highly likely to be more productive.

Despite these insights, it is still true to say that health issues tend to come to the attention of the cabinet most forcibly at times of crisis (see Chapter 5). Although there may be crises driven by epidemics, such as cholera, malaria, TB, AIDS or COVID-19, economic crises are still more likely to force discussions about health issues in terms of how to pay for expensive medicines or new technologies against a background of falling government revenues. It is very common in such circumstances to see intensive discussion of proposals to introduce or increase user fees.

'Health in all policies': the relationship between health and other ministries

In all countries, the range of ministries whose policies affect health tend to be absorbed in their own sectoral policy issues rather than concerned to contribute to a government-wide set of policies that improve health. For example, ministries of environment, agriculture and education have their own goals to pursue and are accountable for meeting them. As a result, they may not give high priority to the human health implications of their decisions (e.g. subsidizing the production of unhealthy commodities). In response, countries started to establish cross-government bodies in the 1970s for the development and implementation of health policy (e.g. a national health council in Sri Lanka). More recently, many countries set up national committees or task forces to co-ordinate the response to the COVID-19 pandemic across government. Despite these continuing efforts, most policies tend to be pursued sectorally, in part because there are undoubtedly some advantages for governments in being able to call on the expertise of specialized agencies. The challenge is to align the incentives of such bodies.

De Leeuw and Clavier (2011) argue that the main cause of the failure to develop 'health in all policies' or 'healthy public policies' at national level has been the absence of the voice of the public. Without this support (i.e. popular demands), health advocates have been unable to mobilize political change across government. Health issues have continued to be debated and responded to in isolation from wider policy concerns. These authors contend that it may be easier to engage and mobilize the public in relation to cross-sectoral health issues at local level where these are more immediate and visible to communities. Another limitation may spring from the inability of the largely biomedically trained leadership in ministries of health to mobilize other ministries to give health sufficient policy priority.

✏ Activity 3.5

Can you provide three examples of government policy decisions in your country that would have been different if their health implications had been taken into account properly?

Feedback

Your answer will obviously be specific to your country and your experience. Typically, policies such as large environmental projects (e.g. dams or highways) are not thoroughly assessed for their health consequences either directly or indirectly. For example, better and faster roads, unless well engineered with a view to reducing pedestrian injuries and deaths can have major adverse consequences, especially for children. Such effects are often not well understood or not weighed in the balance against other costs and benefits. If they were, policy decisions might be different. Another example of policy that might well have been different if the health implications had been taken into account relates to government subsidies for the production of tobacco in a number of LMICs. The costs of dealing with the health outcomes of consuming locally produced tobacco can outweigh the economic gains from production and exports.

While health will not always be the predominant goal of government decisions, since there are many other objectives that contribute to the well-being of populations and to better health (e.g. higher educational attainment), it is important for the full range of consequences of major policy decisions to be taken into account as far as possible. Governments in Wales in the UK and New Zealand have been notable in promoting a more intersectoral approach and longer-term approach to government policy making focused on improving 'well-being' (including intergenerationally) rather than prioritizing economic growth above all else (Welsh Government 2015; New Zealand Government 2019). The idea is that all ministries should be required by legislation to show how they are contributing to improving the outcomes which the government values most, such as improving literacy and infant health, by the actions they take in their individual sectors. In principle, under such a system of reporting and accountability, the ministries of education and health should be more likely to take into account the inter-dependence of their activities since children's health is important for their educational attainment and vice versa. While rational, this cross-sectoral approach to policy formulation and implementation is difficult to achieve.

Activity 3.6

Now that you have read about the main elements in systems of government, prepare a description of the government system in your country. The following questions will help you organize your account:

1. How many political parties are there? How do elections work (i.e. is there a form of proportional representation or a majoritarian system)? How does this affect policy making?
2. Is the system of government unitary or federal; i.e. are there regions or provinces which have substantial freedom to organize their own affairs (e.g. in health services) or are all the main decisions taken at national level and simply carried out at lower levels?
3. How is the national legislature structured? How much influence does the legislature have compared with the executive (cabinet)? Can its members question or challenge the decisions of the president and/or prime minister?

4. Who makes up the executive? Is the executive entirely separate from the legislature or do members of the executive have to come from the legislature? How strong is the chief executive (president or prime minister) compared with other ministers in the executive?
5. What are the powers of the judiciary in relation to the actions of the executive and legislature? How independent are the judges of the governing party or parties? Is there a written constitution? Is it enforced by the courts?
6. How are public servants recruited and what is their role? How influential are civil servants on the actions of the elected government?
7. Overall, what sort of government system would you say you have in your country? Refer to the types of political regimes described in Chapter 2. How does the system shape the policy process?

Feedback

If you find that there are important gaps in your knowledge, you need to consult reference books and/or government publications to complete your description.

Activity 3.7

Now that you have an understanding of the government system in your country, it is time to sketch out the main organizations of government that relate to the health system. The following questions should help you structure your account:

1. Is there a minister of health at national level or is the portfolio shared with other areas of policy? What is the scope of the relevant minister's responsibilities? Is the post regarded as an attractive one for politicians?
2. Is there a national MoH or is health part of another ministry? What are its responsibilities? How is the ministry staffed (i.e. by generalists, specialists or a mix) and how is it organized internally? Is there a hierarchy of national, regional, district and local functions and activities in the ministry, or does the ministry just operate at national level (e.g. setting the general direction of policy)? What is the nature of the accountability of the health system to the ministry and/or minister of health?
3. Are there other national organizations relevant to health policy (e.g. official bodies responsible for training, quality improvement, information, or bodies responsible for inter-ministerial co-ordination with

a health goal, etc.)? What does each do? How do these bodies relate either to the minister or ministry of health? How are their activities co-ordinated?
4. If there are advisers or experts from international agencies involved at national level, what do they do and how do they relate to the MoH?
5. How is the health system organized below the national level? Who owns the provider organizations? Is the clinical workforce employed by these organizations or contracted privately?
6. How do you think each of the organizational features you have described above affects the way that health policy decisions are made and implemented in your country?
7. How does the wider government system which you summarized in the previous activity shape the way that the MoH and health system operate?

You will probably find it helpful to draw a diagram of how the different bodies relate to one another. This is known as an *organogram* or organizational chart. It is a convenient way of summarizing a lot of organizational information relatively simply. Typically, the chart shows lines of authority and accountability between different levels in a hierarchy. Arrows can also be used to show how resources and information flow between bodies, as well as consultative and advisory relationships. Figure 3.2 is an example of an organizational chart for the health system of Nepal.

Feedback

Your answer to these questions will depend on your country of choice. It is important to be aware that organizational charts are a highly abstract picture of the system and can be misleading. The way a system works in practice may not correspond very closely to the way it is presented formally on an organizational diagram. The organizational chart perhaps most closely reflects the idealized rational stages model of the policy process (see Chapter 1). One of the aims of this book is to show that while this may be an aspiration, it is rarely an accurate depiction of the policy process. Chapters 4 and 5 on the role of interest groups and on how issues get onto the policy agenda show that the health policy process is strongly influenced by groups outside the formal decision-making structure. In addition, the hierarchical, 'top-down' way in which systems are typically represented often fails to capture the way in which frontline staff can play a critical role in whether, and if so how, policies developed at higher levels are implemented (see Chapter 6).

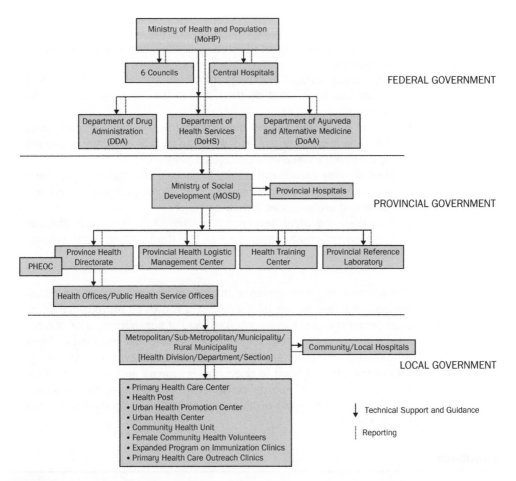

Figure 3.2: Organogram and reporting mechanism of the Nepalese health system in a federal context

Source: Public Health Update (2021)

The role of the state in health systems

In all countries, to varying degrees, government and wider state agencies make and implement policies for health and care services, but also policies that directly and indirectly shape population health in other ways. Mills and Ranson (2005) identified a wide range of regulatory mechanisms which have been applied in LMICs to assure the quality and availability of services, for example, licensing providers and facilities, or providing incentives for clinical staff to work in underserved areas.

Arguably of greater importance for population health, states have assumed a range of wider public health functions, for example, to ensure safe water and food purity, establish quarantine and border control measures to stop the spread of infectious diseases, regulate roads and workplaces to reduce the threat of injuries, legislate to reduce environmental pollution, and set standards for food labelling, air pollution, and tar and nicotine in cigarettes.

You could likely add to the above selective list which is meant to illustrate the range of state involvement in health in the early twenty-first century. This raises the question of how such growth has been justified.

Activity 3.8

The following case study reviews the rationale for the involvement of the state in health and health care. While reading through the section, make notes as to the main reasons for state involvement in the health system.

The involvement of the state in health and health care

Economists have focused on 'market failure' as the principal reason for a pronounced role for the state in health care finance and provision as well as wider public health (e.g. regulating and charging businesses for their environmental pollution). Efficient markets depend on a number of conditions. These are often not met because of specific characteristics of health and health services. First, the optimal amount of health services will not always be produced or consumed because the externalities (costs and benefits) are not taken into consideration by consumers or producers. For example, childhood immunization rates fell in many high-income countries in the 2000s because parents' decisions relate to the perceived risks and benefits of protecting their children as opposed to the benefits of protection of others by reducing the pool of susceptible children. Second, the market will fail to provide many so-called 'public goods' because of the lack of incentives to do so. Public goods are those that are 'non-rival' in consumption (consumption by one person does not affect consumption of the same good by others) and 'non-excludable' (it is not possible to prevent a consumer from benefiting by making them pay), for example, control of mosquito breeding or producing knowledge through research. Third, monopoly power may lead to overcharging. Monopolies could be established by the medical profession, the drug industry or a hospital in a given catchment area, or the privatized water sector. However, some economists argue that the lack of efficient health care markets provides relatively weak justification for state delivery of health services (except in relation to public and preventive health services) as market failure could be dealt with through regulation.

Another argument in favour of a strong state role hinges around the 'information asymmetry' between consumer and providers. Consumers are at a disadvantage, and private providers are in an unusually strong position to take advantage of this imbalance through profit seeking and over-treatment. Another characteristic of the health care market is that the need for health care is uncertain and often costly. This provides an argument in favour of insurance. However, experience suggests that private insurance markets do not work well in health. Both of these reasons provide compelling support for state involvement.

Yet it is unlikely that these economic arguments can account entirely for the prominent role of the state in health and health care. An additional powerful justification for state intervention is on grounds of equity or fairness, specifically that some individuals will be too poor to afford to pay for the health care they need themselves. From this perspective, access to health care is a right of all citizens, irrespective of their income or wealth. Furthermore, since health is so important for life chances, on equity grounds, the state has a responsibility to mitigate the unequal social and economic determinants of ill health and curb the harmful influence of the 'unhealthy commodities industries'. There is convincing evidence that the tobacco, alcohol and ultra-processed food and drink industries, especially transnational corporations, make a major contribution to the global epidemic of non-communicable disease. Another target for state intervention are the industries that are responsible for harmful climate change through the burning of fossil fuels. It is clear that state regulation and intervening in the private market are the only effective ways to prevent the health harm all these industries cause. Self-regulation (e.g. voluntary codes) has repeatedly been shown not to work to protect public health (Bryden et al. 2013). On the positive side, the state can intervene to promote physical activity by planning towns and neighbourhoods that are conducive to walking and cycling. It can also support low-environmental-impact food producers and dietary choices.

Feedback

The main justifications for state involvement are:

- market failure;
- information asymmetry between consumer and provider;
- uncertain and often costly need for care;
- to achieve equity of access to care, and protect and reduce inequalities in population health.

Summary

In this chapter you have learned about the justification for and the wide-ranging roles and responsibilities of the government and wider state (the public sector) in health policy. You have learned why the state is often the most important actor in policy making, including in health. The ideology and decisions of national governments differ, and this affects their policies and the outcomes. Decision making is shaped both by government and state institutional arrangements, and the country context. In most sectors, the executive (ministers) and the bureaucracy (civil servants) usually have the resources and position to control what gets on to the policy agenda and is formulated into policy, with the legislators in a subsidiary role, particularly in parliamentary systems. Where politicians change frequently, a permanent bureaucracy may have very significant power in policy formulation, but, in general, politicians initiate the formulation of policies in areas of major political concern.

Further reading

Colebatch, H.K. (2014) Making sense of governance, *Policy and Society*, 33: 307–16. https://doi.org/10.1016/j.polsoc.2014.10.001

Greer, S.L., Fonseca, E.M., Raj, M. and Willison, C.E. (2022) Institutions and the politics of agency in COVID-19 response: federalism, executive power, and public health policy in Brazil, India, and the US, *Journal of Social Policy*, 1–19. https://doi.org/10.1017/S0047279422000642

Greer, S.L., Wismar, M. and Figueras, J. (eds.) (2016) *Strengthening Health System Governance: Better Policies, Stronger Performance*. Maidenhead: Open University Press McGraw Hill, Chapters 1–3 and 5. Available at: https://eurohealthobservatory.who.int/publications/m/strengthening-health-system-governance-better-policies-stronger-performance (accessed 24 April 2023).

Lownes, V. and Roberts, M. (2013) *Why Institutions Matter, The New Institutionalism in Political Science*. Basingstoke: Palgrave Macmillan, especially Chapter 1.

Siddiqi, S., Masud, T.I., Nishtar, S. et al. (2008) Framework for assessing governance of the health system in developing countries: gateway to good governance, *Health Policy*, 90: 13–25. https://doi.org/10.1016/j.healthpol.2008.08.005

References

Bryden, A., Petticrew, M., Mays, N. et al. (2013) Voluntary agreements between government and business – a scoping review of the literature with specific reference to the Public Health Responsibility Deal, *Health Policy*, 110: 186–97. https://doi.org/10.1016/j.healthpol.2013.02.009

Civicus (2021) 13 countries downgraded in new ratings report as civic rights deteriorate globally. Press release, 8 December. Available at: https://findings2021.monitor.civicus.org/rating-changes.html#global-press-release (accessed 24 April 2023).

De Leeuw, E. and Clavier, C. (2011) Healthy public in all policies, *Health Promotion International*, 26(S2): ii237–44. https://doi.org/10.1093/heapro/dar071

De Leeuw, E., Harris, P., Kim, J. and Yashadhana, A. (2021) A health political science for health promotion, *Global Health Promotion*, 28(4): 17–25. https://doi.org/10.1177/17579759211034418

Evans, P.B., Rueschemeyer, D. and Skocpol, T. (eds.) (1985) *Bringing the State Back in*. Cambridge: Cambridge University Press.

Geva, D. (2021) Orban's Ordonationalism as post-neoliberal hegemony, *Theory, Culture & Society*, 38(6): 71–93. https://journals.sagepub.com/doi/pdf/10.1177/0263276421999435

Hacker, J.S. (2010) The road to somewhere: why health reform happened – or why political scientists who write about public policy shouldn't assume they know how to shape it, *Perspectives on Politics*, 8: 861–76.

Howlett, M., Ramesh, M. and Perl, A. (2009) *Studying Public Policy: Policy Cycles and Policy Subsystems*. Don Mills, Ontario: Oxford University Press.

McKee, M, Gugushvili, A., Koltai, J. and Stuckler, D. (2021) Are populist leaders creating the conditions for the spread of COVID-19? Comment on 'A Scoping Review of Populist Radical Right Parties' Influence on Welfare Policy and its Implications for Population Health in Europe', *International Journal of Health Policy and Management*, 10(8): 511–15. https://doi.org/10.34172/IJHPM.2020.124

Mills, A.J. and Ranson, M.K. (2005) The design of health systems, in M.H. Merson, R.E. Black and A.J. Mills (eds.) *International Public Health: Disease, Programs, Systems and Policies*. Sudbury, MA: Jones and Bartlett.

New Zealand Government (2019) *The Wellbeing Budget*. Wellington: New Zealand Treasury. Available at: www.treasury.govt.nz/sites/default/files/2019-05/b19-wellbeingbudget.pdf (accessed 24 April 2023).

Parkhurst, J.O. (2001) The crisis of AIDS and the politics of response: the case of Uganda, *International Relations*, 15: 69–87.

Perkins, D. and Roemer, M. (1991) *The Reform of Economic Systems in Developing Countries*. Cambridge, MA: Harvard University Press.

Public Health Update (2021) Organogram and reporting mechanism of Nepalese health system in federal context. Available at: https://publichealthupdate.com/organogram-and-reporting-mechanism-of-nepalese-health-system-in-federal-context/ (accessed 8 May 2022).

Schneider, H. (2002) On the fault-line: the politics of AIDS policy in contemporary South Africa, *African Studies*, 61: 145–67.

Steinmo, S. and Watts, J. (1995) It's the institutions stupid! Why comprehensive national health insurance always fails in America, *Journal of Health Politics, Policy and Law*, 20: 329–72.

Tuohy, C.H. (2004) Health care reform strategies in cross-national context: implications for primary care in Ontario, in R. Wilson, S.E.D. Shortt and J. Dorland (eds.) *Implementing Primary Care Reform: Barriers and Facilitators*. Montreal and Kingston: McGill-Queen's University Press, pp. 73–96.

Welsh Government (2015) *Well-being of Future Generations (Wales) Act 2015*. Available at: www.futuregenerations.wales/wp-content/uploads/2017/01/WFGAct-English.pdf (accessed 24 April 2023).

World Health Organization (2000) *World Health Report 2000. Health Systems, Improving Performance*. Geneva: WHO.

Interest groups

4

Chapter 3 focused on the role of government and the wider state and explained how government policy makers are often at the heart of the policy process. However, neither politicians nor civil servants operate in a sealed system, especially not in well-functioning democracies, even if the government does tend to be at the centre of decision making. To use the terminology of the 'policy triangle' in Chapter 1, there are many other actors in the policy process. Governments often consult external (non-governmental) *interest groups* to see what they think about issues and to obtain information, including on political support for their intended policies. Governments may also fund non-governmental groups, or treat some preferentially. In turn, interest groups outside government attempt to influence ministers and civil servants. They use a range of tactics to get their voices heard including building relationships with those in power, lobbying them, mobilizing the media, setting up formal discussions or providing the political opposition with criticisms of government policy. Some interest groups are far more influential than others: in the health field, the medical profession and industries such as pharmaceuticals, health insurance, food, alcohol and gambling exert significant influence on governments in most countries. Increasingly, governments, at least in liberal democracies, tend to operate in partnership with, and through networks of, these non-governmental actors. This is typically referred to as a shift from *government* to *governance* as governments are forced and/or choose to work with and through *civil society* and private sector organizations rather than entirely on their own terms.

Learning objectives

After working through this chapter, you will be better able to:

- explain what an interest group is
- classify the different types of interest groups
- describe the tactics used by different interest groups to get their voices heard and exert pressure on governments
- appreciate the differential resources available to different sorts of interest groups, including new interests such as large social media corporations

- identify how networks of interest groups and government actors form around particular fields of policy
- account for the increasing prominence of market-related private sector and civil society interest groups in health policy making and the need to manage resulting conflicts of interest that can arise
- understand what is meant by the shift from 'government' to 'governance'.

Key terms

Advocacy coalition   Grouping of actors within a policy sub-system distinguished by a shared set of norms, beliefs and resources. It can include politicians, civil servants, members of interest groups, journalists and academics who share ideas about policy goals and to a lesser extent about solutions.

Cause group   Civil society group whose main goal is to promote a particular issue or cause such as free speech or prison reform.

Civil society   The part of society that is outside the private sphere of the family or household, the market and the state.

Civil society group   A non-market (i.e. not for profit) interest group or organization which is also not part of the state. These groups are sometimes referred to as the Third Sector.

Conflict of interest   A set of circumstances that create a risk that an individual's ability to apply professional judgement is, or could be, or could be perceived to be, impaired or influenced by a secondary interest (such as a financial one).

Corporation   An association of stockholders (shareholders) which is regarded as a legal entity or a 'person' under most national laws. Ownership is marked by ease of transferability and the limited liability of stockholders.

Governance   The process of societal decision making where there are many policy actors involved, and where the relationship between the government of the day and these policy actors is not entirely rules-based or hierarchical.

Insider groups   Interest groups which pursue a strategy designed to win themselves the status of legitimate participants in the government policy process.

Interest group   Any group outside the state, including market-related and civil society groups, that attempts to influence government policy to achieve goals that are either directly beneficial to the group's members or advance the societal goal it seeks.

Iron triangle   Small, stable and exclusive policy community usually involving executive agencies of government, legislative committees and private market interest groups (e.g. around defence procurement).

Issue network   Loose, extensive, diverse network of policy actors who come together informally to try to draw attention to an issue, address a specific problem or promote a particular solution.

Market-related interest groups   Interest groups such as business, professional and employer associations.

Multinational   Business which operates in at least one country other than its home country.

Non-governmental organization (NGO)   Any not for-profit organization outside the state (i.e. in civil society), though the term also tends to be used more narrowly to refer to larger, structured organizations providing services rather than all of civil society.

Outsider groups   Interest groups which have either failed to attain insider status or have deliberately chosen a path of confrontation with government.

Policy community (and sub-system)   Relatively stable network of organizations (interest groups and state agencies) and individuals involved in a recognizable field of wider public policy such as health policy. Within each of these fields there will be identifiable sub-systems, such as for mental health policy, with their own policy communities.

Policy network   Generic term for inter-dependent organizations (e.g. interest groups and state agencies) involved in an area of policy that exchange resources and bargain to varying degrees to attain their specific goals.

Private sector   The part of the economy that is not under direct government control and operates primarily on a for-profit basis.

Regulation   The rules and standards made and maintained by an authority – often by government (e.g. in a private market for goods and services to prevent anti-competitive behaviour or false claims).

> **Social movement**   Loose grouping of individuals sharing certain views and attempting to influence others (e.g. through use of social media, demonstrations, etc.) but without a formal organizational structure.

Introduction

In Chapter 2 you were introduced to the theory of pluralism, which asserts that power is widely dispersed throughout society to the extent that no single *interest group* holds absolute power. The pluralists were influential in drawing attention to the idea of government and wider state bodies arbitrating between competing interests as they develop policy. As a result, pluralists focused on interest groups in order to explain how policy is shaped, arguing that, although there are powerful elites, no elite dominates at all times. They contended that sources of power such as information, expertise and money are distributed non-cumulatively. While this may be true for routine matters of policy ('low politics'), pluralism has been criticized for not giving sufficient weight to the fact that major economic decisions which are generally part of 'high politics' tend to be taken by a small elite in order to preserve the existing economic and political regime. In these circumstances, pluralism is clearly 'bounded' and power unequally distributed in society. For example, interest groups wishing to replace a capitalist system of economic organization with a socialist one would not be invited to take part in the policy process.

Pluralists have also been criticized for focusing on Western liberal democracies and failing to recognize differences between countries, not all of which offer the opportunity for interest groups, particularly those from *civil society*, to put pressure on governments. In such countries, extra-governmental influences can be repressed or non-existent or derive from personal and family connections. Despite this, there has been a proliferation of NGOs, both national and international, in the health and development sectors in the last 40 years. They are difficult to enumerate, but Lawrence (2018) estimated that there were approximately 50 large international NGOs worldwide (defined as multi-mandate, multi-country NGOs) and 300,000 small international NGOs. Most of the latter are small organizations that focus on a single field (e.g. water) or a specific beneficiary group (e.g. blind people) and work in one or a handful of countries with an annual income in UK terms of £20 million or less. In part, this growth was due to waves of democratization leading to less authoritarian and elitist governments in a number of countries and, in part, to a concern to give greater opportunities to organizations outside government to make governments more accountable to their people. However, these developments are far from universal. Recent years have seen the return of more authoritarian regimes in countries such as Hungary, Turkey and Russia, severely limiting the scope for civil society activity.

Activity 4.1

Before reading any further, take a few minutes to think about your under-standing of what is meant by 'interest groups'. Write your own definition and a list of the groups that could come under the heading of 'interest groups' in relation to health policy.

Feedback

At its simplest, an 'interest group' promotes or represents a particular part of society (e.g. people suffering from blindness or manufacturers of pharmaceuticals) or stands for a particular cause (e.g. net zero carbon emissions or free trade). Different types of interest group are discussed later in the chapter.

Your list of 'interest groups' involved in health policy is likely to have contained organizations and groups such as those representing:

- staff, such as the medical, nursing and the allied health professions (e.g. physiotherapy, speech therapy);
- care providers, such as hospital associations;
- insurers such as sickness funds;
- payers such as employers' associations;
- different groups of patients;
- manufacturers/suppliers, such as pharmaceutical companies, medi-cal equipment manufacturers and food corporations;
- wider public health issues such as the climate crisis or widening socio-economic and health inequalities.

You may have wondered how different labels for organizations outside the formal system of government such as NGO, 'civil society group' and 'inter-est group' relate to one another. We will now try to clarify these different terms. Make notes of your own definitions as you go through this and modify them, if necessary.

Different types of interest groups

While there are varying definitions of 'interest groups', most would agree on the following features:

- They are voluntary – people or organizations choose to join them.
- They aim to achieve some desired goals.

- They are located outside the formal government and state machinery though they may work to influence government policy in support of their goals.
- They can be *private sector* (market-related, for profit) or civil society (not for profit) groups.

Unlike political parties that are also voluntary and goal-oriented, most interest groups do not generally plan to take formal political power (e.g. by putting forward candidates for election). Sometimes they evolve into political parties and become involved in policy making from within government – like the German Green Party, which began life as an environmental activist group. But interest groups exist outside government, even if some of them have very close relationships with government (as you will see in the discussion of 'insider' and 'outsider' groups, below).

Although there is some inconsistency in the way that interest groups are categorized in the policy literature and terminology has changed over time, currently, most policy analysts would distinguish *market-related interest groups* such as business, professional and employer associations from the wide range of non-profit *civil society groups* (e.g. campaigning groups on abortion, antenatal care, human rights, environment and conservation). This distinction is based on the understanding that market-related interest groups are intrinsically self-interested through the pursuit of profit (i.e. their orientation is *sectional* to protect and enhance the interests of their members), whereas civil society groups are far more likely to be *cause* groups pursuing altruistic goals without personal gain being foremost if the cause is successful.

Civil society groups

'Civil society' can be defined as 'a sphere located between the state and market' (Giddens 2001). According to this scheme, civil society lies in the social space not occupied by the family/household, the state or the market. Giddens (2001) goes on to make this supportive, rather optimistic claim about civil society, namely, that it represents 'a buffer zone strong enough to keep both state and market in check, thereby preventing each from becoming too powerful and dominating.' However, it is important not to assume that all civil society activity is necessarily benign and civil society groups can pursue goals that are controversial (e.g. those that support women's rights to abortion and those that wish to restrict these rights) (see below).

Non-governmental organizations (NGOs)

NGOs are the most familiar civil society organizations in the health and development sectors. The term NGO originally referred to any not-for-profit organization outside government but more recently has taken on the more specific meaning of a relatively large, highly structured organization with a headquarters and paid staff working in fields such as client advocacy or service delivery, in many cases providing a service that might have been provided directly by the state at an earlier stage. A good example is Médecins Sans Frontières (MSF).

Like many NGOs, MSF delivers services but it also takes a stance on policy. Its *Campaign for Essential Medicines* launched in 1999 challenged governments, international organizations, the pharmaceutical industry and other NGOs to improve the rate of development of, and access to, life-saving medicines, diagnostic tests and vaccines for patients in MSF programmes in LMICs. The Campaign contributed to the reduced price of anti-retroviral drugs for HIV and encouraged a greater focus on neglected tropical diseases such as sleeping sickness, leishmaniasis and Chagas disease.

Cause groups

Cause groups are civil society groups that aim to promote an issue that is not necessarily specific to the members of the group themselves, although it can be. For example, disabled people or people living with HIV or post-COVID-19 syndrome may form a pressure group to shape policy directly related to them. Nonetheless, people from all walks of life with a wide range of beliefs come together in organizations such as Greenpeace devoted to global conservation of species or Amnesty International, which highlights human rights abuses all over the world.

Since the mid- to late 1950s, in wealthier countries, membership of cause groups has risen and membership of political parties has tended to fall (Audickas et al. 2019). Some political scientists argue that this is a result of a growing disillusionment, particularly among younger people, with conventional Left–Right party politics and with the seeming remoteness of representatives in a democratic system. It is also a function of people's concern about large single issues such as environmental conservation and climate change (both with major health implications) that had not been given high or consistent priority by conventional political parties, often because of pressure from business interests backed up by threats to withdraw their funding from political parties.

Social movements

Interest groups may start simply as a group of people concerned about a particular issue with little or no formal organization. When a large number of people get involved with the same issue informally, sociologists talk of them as forming a '*social movement*'. For example, the popular protests against authoritarian rule in countries like Tunisia and Egypt that formed the so-called 'Arab Spring' of 2011 were among the first social movements to be largely orchestrated through the elaborate use of social media, particularly by young people. The governments in the region struggled to know how to react to such protests and particularly how to control social media such as Facebook, YouTube and Twitter. Such activities have become more commonplace, such as the farmers' blockade of Delhi orchestrated by a coalition of over 40 Indian farmers' unions known as Samyukta Kisana Morcha, formed in November 2020, to protest against three pieces of subsequently repealed farming legislation.

In Tunisia, video cameras in the mobile phones of demonstrators captured images of the first protests. These were widely transmitted through social media and contributed to spreading unrest elsewhere. The uploaded images also prompted Al Jazeera, the satellite television network, to begin focusing on the revolt, which toppled the Tunisian government and set the stage for the ensuing demonstrations in Egypt (Preston and Stelter 2011). In the past, the government could have simply closed newspapers, TV and radio stations, but highly distributed media were much more of a challenge, at least initially. However, governments since have become more adept at countering with their own social media, for example, flooding the public with counter-narratives and false information to damp down criticism and protests.

The private for-profit sector

Among interest groups, for-profit business (market-related) interests are generally the most powerful in most areas of public policy, followed by interest groups representing workers. This is because both capital and labour are vital to the economic production process. In capitalist societies, ownership of the means of production is concentrated in the hands of business *corporations* rather than the state. As a result, business has huge power vis-à-vis government, particularly in the current globally interconnected environment in which corporations can potentially shift their capital and production relatively easily between countries if their interests are threatened or being harmed by government policies (see Chapter 3).

There is a wide range of industrial and commercial interests involved in health policy. Even in health care systems where most services are provided in publicly owned and managed organizations, there will be extensive links with private sector actors who bring new ideas and practices into the public sector (e.g. improving safety procedures in operating theatres by learning from the aviation industry) as well as providing essential services (e.g. construction firms building hospitals and IT companies providing information systems).

The private for-profit (or commercial) sector is characterized by its market orientation. It encompasses organizations that seek to make profits for their owners. Profit, or a return on investment, is the central defining feature of the commercial sector. Many firms may pursue additional objectives related, for example, to social, environmental or employee concerns, but these are, of necessity, secondary and supportive of the primary profit interest. In the absence of profit, and a return to shareholders, firms cease to exist.

For-profit organizations vary considerably in scale. The sector consists of firms which may be large or small, domestic or *multinational*. In the health sector there are single doctor's surgeries and large group practices, pharmacies, generic drug manufacturers and major research and development pharmaceutical companies, medical equipment suppliers, logistics companies, management consultancies and private hospitals and nursing homes.

When thinking about the role of the commercial sector in health policy, it is often useful to broaden the scope of analysis to include some organizations that are registered as not-for-profit in their legal status but, in practice, represent for-profit interests. These may have charitable status but are established to support the interests of a firm or industry. These may include business associations or trade federations. For example, in the US, both PhRMA (Pharmaceutical Research and Manufacturers of America) and BIO (Biotechnology Innovation Organization) are advocacy organizations that act to promote the economic interests of their member firms while also emphasizing the health benefits flowing from their products. In Pakistan, there is a similar interest group for multinational pharmaceutical companies (Pharma Bureau) and a separate one for domestic firms.

A wide range of industry-funded think tanks, 'scientific institutes' and patient advocacy groups are engaged in the health policy arena. The public relations arms of large corporations and trade associations reason that their messages are more likely to be listened to by the public if they are articulated by apparently independent interest groups. Sometimes, organizations are set up at one remove from their underlying purpose. Thus the Global Warming Policy Foundation, a UK-based think tank set up by the former Conservative politician, Nigel Lawson, claims only to campaign against the costs and harms of policies advocated to halt global warming, not to question its existence and causes. After criticism from the charities regulator, the Foundation set up a campaigning subsidiary, which it rebranded in October 2021 as Net Zero Watch, to scrutinize and critique the UK government's plans to reach net zero emissions. Both organizations, regardless of their stated missions, have close links to individuals and organizations that actively seek to discredit the science of climate change.

Similarly, the tobacco industry supports libertarian organizations devoted to promoting the rights of smokers to smoke without hindrance from government *regulation*. For example, the tobacco company Philip Morris established the Institute of Regulatory Policy as a vehicle to lobby the US federal government and delay the publication of a report by the Environmental Protection Agency on environmental tobacco smoke

(Muggli et al. 2004). The food industry has funded seemingly independent research bodies such as the World Sugar Research Organization. Industry also organizes and supports patient groups to influence health policy decisions of governments. While such organizations usually present arguments that are pro-industry, these are not always influential. For example, Stuckler and colleagues (2016) show that the 2015 WHO sugars intake guideline was little changed following consultative submissions from bodies including the World Sugar Research Organization. However, there was more emphasis on the poor quality of evidence on the harms of sugar. The involvement of commercial interest groups in public health policy making is often unavoidable but poses challenges in managing potential conflicts of interest (see below).

✎ Activity 4.2

Find examples of the types of commercially linked or sponsored organizations listed below with a link to a health issue (either due to the goods or services they manufacture, promote, distribute, sell or regulate). For each example, identify the health issue in which they have an interest, what they manufacture, distribute, sell or promote, the relationship of these goods or services to health (either positive or negative) and the organization's activities designed to influence health policy.

The types of organization to consider are:

- small firm;
- multinational or transnational corporation;
- business association;
- professional association (e.g. medical association);
- think tank;
- patients' group;
- commercial scientific network;
- public relations firm;
- loose network.

Feedback

It should be evident that a wide range of organizations associated with the private sector are involved in trying to influence health policy. It may also be evident that these organizations vary tremendously in relation to their size (e.g. resources and staff), organizational form and interest in particular health policies.

The power of the private for-profit sector

While there is considerable debate over the meaning of 'power', it is generally regarded as describing both the ability to influence others and to achieve particular goals (see Chapter 2). Resources often confer power and, on that basis, the power of some industries and firms may be obvious to you given their huge resources. In 2017, 157 of the top 200 economic entities in the world by revenue were corporations, not countries, according to Global Justice Now and the percentage is rising as companies consolidate into ever larger, more powerful entities. The stock market value of the ten largest pharmaceutical companies is greater than the national income of over 50 LICs, but they also have global reach, large knowledge bases and paid lobbyists all over the world. Particularly striking in recent years has been the rise of the 'tech giants' (Apple, Amazon, Alphabet and Microsoft), with combined revenues of US$900 billion in 2019 – larger than the GDP of four of the 20 largest country economies in the world. If they had been countries, they would each have had larger economies than Saudi Arabia and the Netherlands. The 'tech giants' grew substantially absolutely and relatively during the pandemic. Their incomes dwarf the annual budget of the World Health Organization, which was approximately US$4.8 billion in 2020/21 (WHO 2019).

Firms provide governments with tax revenues, some are major employers in the economy, and wealthy country governments gain influence in international affairs on the back of their large corporations and are therefore interested in their success. In many sectors, firms have specialist knowledge (some of it generated originally by publicly funded research) which governments rely on when making policy. In many countries, large commercial entities have arisen in response to governments' goals to outsource activities that were previously undertaken by public bodies. Firms such as Serco, Capita and G4S have gained large government contracts especially in the fields of health, transport, justice, immigration, space and defence. For these reasons, small and large businesses are often important actors in policy debates.

Their activities can pose major regulatory problems for governments. The main social media platforms, in global order of popularity (October 2021) – Facebook, YouTube, WhatsApp, Instagram, Facebook Messenger and Tiktok – reach hundreds of millions of people daily. Yet, their parent companies such as Facebook, which owns four of the most popular platforms, initially resisted external regulation of misleading or harmful content arguing that they were not publishers. Belatedly, Facebook has recognized that it cannot self-regulate effectively, but governments have not so far managed to find a way to reconcile reasonable free speech with regulation of hate speech, deliberate falsehoods and incorrect information on social media platforms.

Public–private partnerships

In the last 25 years, the field of global health has been marked by the emergence of a wide range of public–private partnerships designed to align the interests of public, private and philanthropic sectors. The rationale is that the private sector brings business acumen and some finance, the development organizations bring technical knowledge and large philanthropies provide a varying share of the funds. The two most notable in policy terms are GAVI, the Global Vaccine Alliance, established in 2000 with core partners the World Health Organization, UNICEF, the World Bank and the Bill & Melinda Gates Foundation, and the Global Fund to Fight AIDS, Tuberculosis and Malaria set up in 2002. The Global Fund is primarily a financing mechanism with 95 per cent of its income coming from public sources and 5 per cent from the private sector. GAVI develops the market for vaccines and helps countries pay for vaccines in proportion to their wealth over the long term so that manufacturers have the confidence to increase production and countries to adopt vaccine programmes knowing that they will be able to be paid for. Public–private partnerships are complex to govern and manage. The main *governance* issues relate to the intrinsic differences in motivation and objectives of the partners, fair sharing of risks and responsibilities, ensuring transparency of processes and the different external expectations placed on the partners (e.g. public bodies accountable to tax payers and businesses accountable to shareholders). Critics of public–private partnerships argue that they effectively entrench *conflicts of interest* in the policy process and that they can never be designed fully to eliminate these conflicts, which can prejudice the behaviour of both the public and private sector participants. All health systems with mixed public and private interests are vulnerable to conflicts of interest and these can be difficult to identify and remove (Rahman-Shepherd et al. 2021).

Professional interest groups

In most sectors of policy, including health care delivery, professional interest groups tend to have the closest contacts with government and exercise the strongest influence since the provision of health services depends on them, while consumer groups tend to have less influence, principally because their co-operation is less central to the implementation of policies. A large part of the activities of influential, well-organized professional interest groups in the health sector such as medical or nursing associations is market-related since they act as trade unions to improve the pay and conditions of service of their members. The power of these professional groups lies in the fact that their members have a monopoly over service provision. For example, the Nigerian Association of Resident Doctors, representing trainees, was able to organize strikes over pay in 2020–2021 because

40 per cent of doctors across the country were members, including 90 per cent of those in teaching hospitals, and because pay bargaining was nationally determined.

In health care policy, the medical profession was traditionally regarded as occupying a dominant position not just in controlling the delivery of health care (particularly who is permitted to carry out which tasks), but also in shaping policy. In HICs, physicians controlled and regulated their own training and day-to-day clinical work for much of the twentieth century. This is still true in many LMICs where the state has struggled to standardize the training and validation of doctors. For example, in India and Pakistan, private medical schools are still able to determine their own standards (Aftab et al. 2021).

The scope of practice of other health workers such as nurses depended on the consent of doctors, and their role was seen primarily as supporting doctors rather than acting independently. In the eyes of the public, the medical profession was seen as the most authoritative source of advice on health-related matters whether at the individual, community or national levels. Health care systems tended to be organized in deference to the preferences of medical interest groups (e.g. systems of reimbursement in public systems that mirrored the fee-for-service arrangements in private practice). However, starting gradually in the 1950s and gathering pace in the 1980s, there was a significant, multi-pronged challenge to the medical profession's privileged status.

✎ Activity 4.3

What have been the major challenges to the dominant position of doctors in health care and policy over the last 40 years?

Feedback

Your answer probably included a number of different challenges coming from different sources. Here are some of the challenges you may have identified:

- Governments and insurers attempted to control doctors' use of resources by imposing budget caps, limiting the range of drugs that they could prescribe, or restricting patient referral to the least cost or most efficient providers.
- Governments and insurers brought in stronger management and encouraged competition (e.g. between public hospitals and between public and private providers) to try to make services more responsive and efficient.

- Governments developed systems for assessing the quality of clinical care and promoted evidence-based medicine rather than relying on individual clinical judgement
- The so-called 'medical model' of disease, which explains ill health in biological terms and the appropriate response in individual, curative terms, was challenged by the 'primary care approach', which emphasized intersectoral action beyond treatment of individuals and outside the health care system, and community involvement to make services more responsive to people's needs.
- There was a growing recognition that patients themselves have valuable expertise in relation to their own ill health, derived from their own experiences that required doctors to share decisions with patients.
- Nurses and other health care workers became better educated and organized, and governments moved to widen the range of clinical tasks they were permitted to undertake, sometimes at the expense of doctors.
- More publicity and media attention was given to cases of medical malpractice and criminality.

While it is undoubtedly true that medical interests have been challenged and have lost some influence in most countries, the knowledge and authority with which medical organizations speak is still a key resource enabling them to influence health policy (Johnson 1995). In poorer countries, professional associations have not played such an important role in health policy although this may be changing. In part, this is because most publicly paid-for health care and preventive activity is undertaken not by doctors but by nurses and community health workers in these settings. The medical profession largely serves the small urban elites through private practice. Doctors are influential in public health policy in such countries, but often as civil servants in the MoH or as health ministers rather than through the medical associations.

Resources and strategies of interest groups

 Activity 4.4

In what you have read so far in this chapter, you will have begun to appreciate the resources available to different interest groups. Think of a range of different interest groups that you are familiar with and list their attributes and resources.

Feedback

The resources that interest groups can mobilize vary widely. Some of the resources you may have listed include:

- *Their members* – the larger the number of members, all other things equal, the more influence an interest group is likely to have, though in the case of patient groups, their personal experience may give them even greater legitimacy. Interest groups composed of other organizations, particularly where they are representative of these other associations (known as 'peak' or 'apex' associations), are particularly likely to have more influence and often draw on a wide range of skills, knowledge and contacts from within their constituent organizations.
- *Their level of funding* – funding affects all aspects of an interest group's activities such as its ability to hire professional staff to organize campaigns and work with the media, prepare critiques of government policy and develop alternatives, contribute to political parties, organize rallies and demonstrations, and so on. This explains, in large part, why health producer interest groups tend to be better organized than consumer groups since their members are often prepared to pay large subscriptions to ensure that their key economic and professional interests are well represented and defended.
- *Their knowledge about their area of concern* – some of this information and understanding may be unavailable from any other source. For example, a government may be dependent on a commercial interest group for access to confidential information about the likely financial impact of a proposed policy on its members that may be essential to justify the policy.
- *Their persuasive skills* in building public support for particular positions or policies by stimulating activity by others, such as the mass media.
- *Their contacts and relationships* with policy makers, officials, ministers, opposition parties, the mass media, celebrities and social media influencers.
- *The sanctions, if any, at their disposal* – for advocacy groups, these could range from embarrassing the government in international fora or the mass media to organizing consumer boycotts thereby harming the domestic economy.
- *Their monopoly power* – this is especially relevant to the medical profession, which generally has the right to restrict others from entering their part of the health care market thus making governments dependent on the profession for the delivery of health care.

Some interest groups have political influence which far exceeds the support for their views among the general public. How do they achieve this? A notable example is the National Rifle Association (NRA) in the US. The majority of Americans support stricter gun control, and a large proportion support banning of weapons with high-capacity magazines. However, only about 1 per cent puts gun control as their number one policy priority. This allows an advocacy group with a highly concentrated agenda to exert huge influence over the public and legislators using a three-pronged strategy: publicly grading politicians on their voting records related to the constitutional second amendment guaranteeing the right to bear arms; generously resourcing candidates who favour NRA policies of laxer gun controls against candidates showing any signs of supporting tighter regulation of firearms; and funding lobbyists to pressurize legislators to vote down any bills that might increase regulation (Gift 2022).

Relations between interest groups, and the state and government

'Insider' and 'outsider' group strategies

Interest groups can also be analysed in terms of how far they are recognized or legitimized by the state and governments, which, in turn, relates to their aims and their strategies. Grant (1984) identified two basic categories in this respect – *insider* and *outsider* groups. Insider groups are groups which are not officially part of the machinery of government but are regarded as legitimate by government policy makers, are consulted regularly and are expected to play by the 'rules of the game'. For example, if they accept an invitation to sit on a government committee, they can be relied upon to respect the confidentiality of the discussions that take place there until ministers are ready to make a statement about the agreed direction of policy. Insider groups thus become closely involved in testing policy ideas at an early stage. Typically, in health policy, producer groups such as medical and nursing associations expect to be consulted at an early stage or directly involved from the outset in policy developments and frequently are, even if they do not always get their own way.

In the UK, the Association of the British Pharmaceutical Industry (ABPI) has traditionally had insider status on the grounds that the government is both concerned to promote the UK pharmaceutical industry and to ensure that safe and effective medicines are available at the earliest opportunity to patients. There are regular meetings between the industry, senior officials and ministers. Like so many sectional interest groups, the ABPI has also recruited retired civil servants to help it negotiate with government over drug regulation and prices, thereby improving its insider knowledge of the policy-making process.

Outsider groups, by contrast, are either organizations that reject a close involvement in government processes on ideological or strategic grounds, or have been unable to gain a reputation as legitimate participants in the policy process. Perhaps the highest profile outsider groups in the contemporary health field are anti-abortion and anti-vivisection organizations because of the vehemence of their views and their reputation for taking direct action against clinics, laboratories and sometimes those who work in them. Another is Extinction Rebellion, or XR, which campaigns and takes direct action to pressurize governments to take rapid action to avert climate catastrophe. Direct action such as protestors gluing themselves to busy roads or disrupting commuter trains or school boycotts has been controversial. Although it has been high profile, direct action has generated hostility towards the activists and the cause. By attempting to reach the attention of the general public through its actions, XR has been criticized for not directly targeting the activities of transnational corporations driving climate change.

Interest groups may shift their strategies over time. For example, in its early life, Greenpeace favoured direct action as a way of drawing attention to conservation issues. Most notably it disrupted the activities of whaling vessels. More recently, Greenpeace has adopted a less flamboyant and confrontational strategy through scientifically based advocacy though it does still use peaceful direct action from time to time. In the process, it has developed closer relations with governments, though is probably not regarded as a full insider group. Groups that shift their strategies or positions are known as *thresholder* groups.

The Treatment Action Campaign (TAC) in South Africa successfully used a wide range of insider and outsider strategies over time to advance a human rights approach to access to medicines for HIV, combining negotiation with government and outspoken criticism, constitutional litigation, alliance building with civil society organizations internationally, engagement with scientists and the media, and social mobilization including demonstrations, civil disobedience and campaigns (Robins 2004; Heywood 2011). Over time TAC's success in embarrassing and pressurizing the government led to close involvement in drafting the National Strategic Plan on HIV, AIDS and Sexually Transmitted Infections, 2007–2011, which committed the government to a large increase in spending on anti-retrovirals (see below).

✎ Activity 4.5

Obtain information on a number of health-related interest groups (perhaps in a field of health that you are interested in) and try to work out what sorts of strategies they are using, their range of activities and whether they could be regarded as insider, outsider or thresholder groups.

Feedback

The orientation of an organization will not always be apparent from its literature or website, but there are some clues you can look for. For example, the slogans of an organization give an indication of its attitude towards government. If the organization is 'fighting' for animal rights, it is more likely to be an 'outsider' group than one that claims to be 'working' for animal welfare. Similarly, an organization that lists its main activities as organizing demonstrations and mobilizing the media is likely to be pursuing an 'outsider' strategy, while an organization that describes its participation in government committees and consultations, or its links to elected representatives is more likely to be following an 'insider' track.

Policy networks, communities and sub-systems

Political scientists have observed that when it comes to policy formulation and implementation in health (as opposed to getting an issue onto the agenda in the first place – see Chapter 8) the participants (actors) are usually individuals and organizations with an enduring interest and knowledge of the field, even if, conceivably, a far wider range of actors could potentially be involved. Who is involved, for what reasons and how their relationships are structured have been the subjects of much research on what have been referred to at various times as 'policy networks', 'policy communities' and 'policy sub-systems'. The terminology and classifications can be confusing and even contradictory. The main point to grasp is that these are all forms of network linking governments with 'insider' interest groups. By definition, 'outsider' groups are excluded from these networks or very peripheral since they seek influence at a distance and through challenging the government.

A *network* in a policy area consists of organizations that have resources important to others in the policy area such as information, skills and influence, but which are dependent on others in the network for other resources (e.g. money, access to government decision makers). They thus have to exchange resources to achieve their goals (Rhodes 1997). The government within a country becomes part of these networks depending on the degree to which it depends on interest groups to develop, support and/or implement its policies. *Policy networks* can also be international or global (Shiffman 2018). Analyses of policy areas as networks of actors or interests are common (stakeholder analysis described in Chapter 11 is often used as part of a network analysis). However, network analysis is criticized for failing adequately to explain how policies change and how some interest groups gain or lose power (see Chapter 2 for more on power).

Marsh and Rhodes (1992) identify a *'policy community'* as a particularly highly integrated, tightly knit form of policy network involving a limited number of participants each controlling some valued resources, with some groups excluded, and marked by stable and frequent interactions, continuity of membership and consensus in terms of values and policy preferences. The characteristic feature of a policy community is that there is sustained interaction between the participants through a web of formal and informal relationships (Lewis 2005). By contrast, *'issue networks'* are loosely inter-dependent, unstable networks comprising a large number of members whose interaction fluctuates. There is a lack of consensus and there may be conflict within the issue network. Its members have very different levels of resources and power. This can hamper negotiations within the network and weaken its negotiating position vis-à-vis government. Such networks usually draw attention to issues and help with agenda setting, whereas the predominant form of interaction in the policy community is one of bargaining over policy developments and implementation.

In health care policy, organizations and individuals representing practitioners (health professionals), users, the public, researchers (from laboratory sciences to the social sciences), commentators (journalists and policy analysts), businesses (drug companies, medical equipment manufacturers), hospitals and clinics, insurers, politicians and international organizations are involved with government to differing degrees depending on their resources and the issue at stake. Some sets of relationships are closer to the integrated policy community end of the spectrum and others are closer to the fluid issue network end.

✎ Activity 4.6

Think of a tight 'policy community' or loose 'issue network' around a specific health policy issue in your own country. It could be focused on any public health issue such as whether or not condom use should be promoted to prevent HIV infection or that the marketing of breast milk substitutes needs greater government oversight. List those interest groups known to be or likely to be critical of the current policies in your country and those likely to be supportive.

Feedback

Obviously your answer will depend on the policy network and issue you considered. For example, if you chose the issue of condom use and HIV, your answer will reflect the precise arrangements for HIV prevention in your country and the groups involved in trying to influence policy in this field. The list might include the following:

- In support of policies to increase condom use: MoH, national HIV commission or programme, interest groups of people living with HIV and their supporters, men who have sex with men, sexual and reproductive health NGOs, family planning associations, employers (those aware of the economic costs).
- Against policies to increase condom use: some religious groups, some international donors (i.e. those promoting abstinence), sections of the media (others may be supportive), certain professional associations.

Another related way of understanding the formal and informal network relationships between government and non-government (interest group) actors is to identify the *policy sub-system* in which they interact. At its simplest, a policy sub-system is a recognizable sub-division of public policy making comprising the individuals and groups most often involved in decisions in that field (very similar to the concept of the 'policy community'). In health policy, for example, mental health policy formulation is distinctively different from policy on environmental health issues and involves different actors. Some sub-systems, known as *iron triangles*, are small, very stable and highly exclusive three-way sets of relationships usually between politicians, bureaucrats and a commercial interest. In the case of food and agriculture policy in the US, the triangle is constituted by the Department of Agriculture, politicians from farming regions and agribusiness (the food industry), and leads to the continuing subsidy of types of food production that are unhealthy for both people and planet. Other sub-systems are typically larger (i.e. involving more entities), more fluid and with less clear boundaries (e.g. children and young people's mental health).

The policy sub-system or Advocacy Coalition Framework (ACF)

The ACF is a general approach to understanding the policy process and policy change within policy sub-systems developed by Paul Sabatier with a series of colleagues (Sabatier and Jenkins-Smith 1993). Policy change is seen as a continuous process that takes place within policy sub-systems bounded by relatively stable limits (e.g. the attributes of the problem, fundamental socio-cultural values and structure of a society) and shaped by major external events (see Figure 4.1). Within the sub-system (e.g. mental health policy), the same actors interact over considerable periods of time. The actors include all those who play a part in the generation,

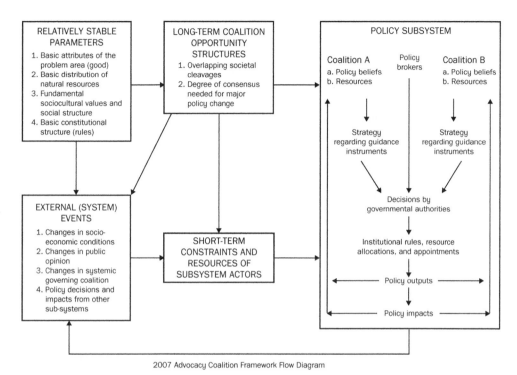

2007 Advocacy Coalition Framework Flow Diagram

Figure 4.1: The Advocacy Coalition Framework
Source: Weible et al. (2009)

dissemination and evaluation of policy ideas. Sabatier does not include the public in any policy sub-system on the grounds that ordinary people as individuals rather than as members of organizations do not generally have the time or inclination to be direct participants.

The large number of actors and relationships within each sub-system are organized into a smaller number of 'advocacy coalitions', in conflict with one another. Each competes for influence over government institutions by advocating its solutions to policy problems. An 'advocacy coalition' is a group distinguished by a distinct set of norms, beliefs and resources, and can include politicians, civil servants, members of civil society organizations, researchers, journalists and others. Advocacy coalitions are defined by their *ideas* rather than by the exercise of self-interested power (see Chapter 10 for more on their role in bringing ideas from research to bear on policy). Within advocacy coalitions there is a high level of agreement on fundamental policy positions and objectives, though there may be more debate about the precise means to achieve these objectives. Sabatier argues that the fundamental (or 'core') norms and beliefs of an advocacy coalition change relatively infrequently and in response to major changes in the external environment such as shifts in macro-economic conditions or the replacement of one political regime by another. Otherwise, less fundamental, 'normal' changes in policy beliefs occur as a result of policy-oriented learning in which a coalition tests and refines its beliefs either in order to achieve its goals or in response to challenges or changing environments. The changes take place through the interaction between advocacy coalitions within the policy sub-system.

The final element in Sabatier's model is to identify the existence of so-called *'policy brokers'*; that is, actors concerned with finding feasible compromises between the positions advocated by the multiplicity of coalitions (a role similar to that of 'policy entrepreneurs' in agenda setting – see Chapter 5). 'Brokers' may be civil servants experienced in a particular sub-system or bodies designed to produce agreement, such as committees of inquiry.

Subsequent empirical work has shown that the advocacy coalition framework works fairly well in explaining policy change over a decade in Western democratic settings, especially relatively open, decentralized, federal, pluralistic political systems such as the US, but works less well in political systems such as the UK's which are more hierarchical and closed, and where there is less interplay between advocacy coalitions. It is beginning to be used to explain policy change in LMICs and in places where policy making is or has been relatively authoritarian and elitist. The ACF is potentially applicable in any setting where the rule of law exists that will permit coalitions to act without repression either from the government of the day or their opponents. The basic elements in the theory tend to be confirmed in LMICs, such as the importance of policy core beliefs to advocacy coalitions as against support for specific policy interventions. Not surprisingly, compared to applications of the approach in Western democracies, international organizations play a larger role in coalitions or even act as policy brokers in LMICs. In authoritarian countries, state actors were the sole or dominant actors in bringing about policy change (Osei-Kojo et al. 2022).

Looking at its utility in specific policy sub-systems, the ACF appears to fit well with sub-systems such as AIDS policy and other aspects of public health where government typically has to try to reach agreement among conflicting advocacy coalitions. It is less applicable to the policy sub-systems of 'high politics' such as defence and foreign policy (e.g. decisions to go to war) where policy decisions are normally made within a small and tightly defined elite since the national interest as a whole may be perceived to be at stake.

An application of the ACF that conveys its ability to explain how policies change over time is the analysis of government policy towards the use of illicit drugs in Switzerland in the 1980s and 1990s by Kübler (1999). Over this period, policy shifted from a predominantly prohibitionist position in the early 1980s to a harm reduction position with some moves to decriminalizing the use of drugs. How and why did this change occur? Until the mid-1980s, drug policy was dominated by an 'abstinence coalition' of prosecutors, judges, police and public health specialists. As a result, access to needles and syringes for drug use was made as difficult as possible despite the risk of needle sharing and associated infection. The arrival of AIDS in the mid-1980s – a major change in the external environment – changed the debate; unlike hepatitis, there was no vaccination or cure for AIDS, and there was the risk of the spread of HIV to the general population through drug-related sex work. As a result, some health experts who had supported the abstinence coalition began to advocate a change in policy on the grounds that an abstinence-oriented policy was ineffective in preventing HIV. The idea that controlling HIV was more important than abstinence rapidly led to embrace of the concept of harm reduction and a coalition of public health and infectious disease specialists, plus social workers. This coalition was soon supported by leftist local politicians, and began to press for harm reduction facilities. In the late 1980s and early 1990s, needle exchanges and safe injection rooms were set up in the large cities with local funding, but the federal (national) government also began to be interested in testing harm reduction approaches scientifically thereby allowing it to contribute resources.

The harm reduction coalition's political strategy was two-pronged: on the one hand to lobby local and national governments for a change in their policies; and on the other to produce change without waiting for the active support of local government by mobilizing finance and expertise that allowed the establishment of harm reduction facilities by NGOs. The goal of the latter was to demonstrate that harm reduction was the correct policy and thereby attract additional support. By the early 1990s, the harm reduction coalition was driving drug policy decision making in most parts of Switzerland, but faced a further challenge as a result of the emergence of a third advocacy coalition concerned with quality of life in cities. Plans for new harm reduction facilities usually led to protests from local residents and businesses fearing that facilities would not only attract drug users but also disorder, crime and debris (e.g. used needles). Neighbourhood quality of life advocates frequently allied with the abstinence coalition so as to be able to claim that their opposition to harm reduction facilities was more than simple self-interest.

The harm reduction coalition was forced to confront the public order implications of its position, and some members began to advocate an approach that gave equal weight to public order and drug users' health so as to rescue the harm reduction approach. The idea of *Stadtverträglickeit* ('city compatibility'), or the search for an equilibrium between repression and harm reduction interventions, became a substantial secondary element in the harm reduction coalition's belief system. The re-balancing of the objectives of local drug facilities proved a practical success. As a result, neighbourhood quality of life advocates no longer supported the abstinence coalition and withdrew from drug policy, and the harm reduction coalition was able to consolidate its dominant position.

✎ **Activity 4.7**

Which external event fundamentally altered the debate and actors involved in the above case study of drug policy in Switzerland in the 1990s? Describe the advocacy coalitions involved and their policy core beliefs. Which part of Sabatier's Advocacy Coalition Framework did not appear to be present in the Swiss case study?

Feedback

The AIDS epidemic fundamentally altered the range of policy ideas at play in the drug field and mobilized a new set of actors – the harm reduction coalition. This coalition began to press local and national governments to change direction away from abstinence and prohibition towards a policy focused on the health of people who use drugs.

There were two major advocacy coalitions competing in the drug policy sub-system: the abstinence coalition, which believed in repression of drug use and making drug use as unattractive as possible; and the harm reduction coalition, which believed in improving the health and social situation of people who use drugs and reducing the harm associated with drug use as a way of motivating users to come off drugs. A third minor coalition (the urban quality of life coalition) entered the policy sub-system for a time. It believed in policies to improve the experience of living in cities and to enhance the economy of cities.

There were no obvious 'policy brokers' at work in the Swiss case study trying to produce a deal between the abstinence and harm reduction coalitions, perhaps because their belief systems were so incompatible. Only when the public order issue arose did some members of the harm reduction coalition try to identify a consensus between their own beliefs and those of the quality of life advocates, though only at the level of secondary aspects of the respective belief systems.

Political scientists argue that the increasing significance of policy networks in public policy represents an important change in the process of governing, or making decisions. Policy networks reduce the ability of governments to act alone and require politicians and bureaucrats to learn new skills of working with and through interest groups in a less hierarchical and more negotiated, less controlling way. This trend is sometimes summed up as representing the transition from a world of *government* to one of *governance*. Where once governments were perceived to be largely responsible, there has been a re-arrangement of responsibilities, so that organizations outside government are also involved in health-related decision making. A key skill of government in such a world is the ability to co-ordinate and hold to account a disparate set of actors, many of which are far from its direct control. In turn, external actors need to be able to hold governments to account for their performance. One set of forces driving this transition relates to globalization, which reduces, but by no means eliminates, the power of national governments as they become increasingly dependent on international agreements, agencies and business corporations (see Chapter 9).

The contribution of civil society to health policy making

It is increasingly apparent that interest groups are playing a more influential role in health policy including in poorer countries where they have traditionally been weak or absent. Of course, the extent of influence on policy from outside government varies from place to place and from issue to issue. This changing relationship between government and interest groups can be seen as part of the wider shift in the way that governments operate, discussed above, from a hierarchical, directive and controlling mode towards operating through networks of government, civil society and private sector organizations (the shift from *government* to *governance*).

The history of the role of civil society groups in global policy to combat AIDS and prevent HIV

The history of the global response to HIV is noteworthy for the very high level of involvement and influence of civil society organizations. 'Nothing about us; without us' was a common rallying cry leading to the institutionalization of the 'GIPA' principle (greater involvement of people living with AIDS). As a consequence, 'Never before have civil society organizations – here defined as any group of individuals that is separate from government and business – done so much to contribute to the fight against a global health crisis, or been so included in the decisions made by policy-makers' (Zuniga 2005). The HIV history is also notable for the diversity of interest group activities, the large number of national HIV organizations involved in policy making (over 3,000 in 150 countries in the mid-2000s), the shift of activism from the high- to low- and middle-income countries and the eventual globalizing of the movement for access to treatment (Table 4.1).

Table 4.1 The history of the role of civil society groups in global policy to combat AIDS and prevent HIV

Phase of activism	Main activities of advocacy groups	Main advocacy group demands	Impact
Early 1980s in US and Western countries: civil rights activism	Protest, lobbying and activism modelled on US black civil rights movement of 1960s.	Protection of human and civil rights; PLHIV are not to blame; inclusion of PLHIV in policy process – inclusion and partnership.	Traditional STI approach of isolation, surveillance, mandatory testing and strict contact notification replaced by rights-based model promoted by WHO from 1987.
Mid-/late-1980s in US and Western countries: aggressive, scientific activism	New more aggressive organizations such as ACTUP and TAG lobbying politicians; simultaneous street protests and scientific debates with government; AIDS pressure groups winning places on government committees.	Government funding for treatment and price reductions for early ART.	Access to effective treatment for PLHIV; showed that new drugs did confer benefits and that early trials did not warrant denying treatment to PLHIV; ensured that trials included women, minorities, etc.
1990s in US and Western countries: institutionalized and internalized activism	US/Western activist groups shrinking because of success; activists increasingly accepted and working within health policy system; established CSO role in provision.	Ensuring that HIV remains a policy and resource allocation priority in the West; attention should be given to HIV in poorer countries.	Increased awareness of distribution of HIV and AIDS globally.
Later 1990s in LMICs: growing activism	Overseas funding to raise awareness and educate people, and support CSOs; explosion of CSOs; North–South co-operation between CSOs.	Franker public discussion of HIV and AIDS; better leadership; concerted government responses; provision of AZT and treatment of co-infections.	Notable impact in pioneer countries such as Brazil and Uganda; latter showed that ART could be provided with good results and that comprehensive response could save health care costs.

Table 4.1 (Continued)

Phase of activism	Main activities of advocacy groups	Main advocacy group demands	Impact
Late 1990s/early 2000s: global movement for treatment access	Period of advocacy sparked by successful CSO protest and resistance to attempt by US/SA pharmaceutical companies to prevent SA government from offering low-cost, generic ART; growing international coalition of NGOs pushing for low-cost ART by promoting production of generic drugs and pressurizing pharmaceutical companies to reduce their prices in low-income settings.	Universal access to affordable treatment as a human right; HIV to be seen as a security and development issue with major negative economic consequences.	CSOs contributed to recognition that public health considerations had some weight alongside trade and intellectual property considerations in WTO; new funding initiatives (Global Fund to Fight AIDS, TB and Malaria, and US President's Plan for AIDS Relief – PEPFAR); gradual roll-out of ART helped by lower drug prices.
2000s: advocacy alongside service delivery	Advocacy continues but complemented by an increasing role in service delivery – particularly with funds from Global Fund and PEPFAR.	Demand for universal access to HIV prevention, treatment and care; PEPFAR and Global Fund should finance generic ARVs; recognition of men who have sex with men, sex workers and people who inject drugs as higher risk groups.	Mobilization of resources – from US$1.6 billion in 2001 to US$16.7 billion in 2010; unprecedented roll out of treatment coverage in LMICs from 300,000 in 2001 to 6.6 million in 2010; drop in new infections from 3.1 million in 1999 to 2.6 million in 2010; high-risk groups identified for first time in 2011 UN General Assembly Declaration Challenge to traditional pharma from producers of low-cost generic ARVs for LMICs.

(Continued)

Table 4.1 (Continued)

Phase of activism	Main activities of advocacy groups	Main advocacy group demands	Impact
2010s and 2020s: 'treatment as prevention'	Development of community and mHealth services; hospital services developed as part of sexually transmitted disease services; in response to advocacy, targets set in 2014 for 2020: 90 per cent of PLHIV on treatment, 90 per cent of whom in HIV care and on ARVs, and 90 per cent of all PLHIV in the country virally suppressed, 500,000 new adult infections, zero discrimination; targets for 2030, were 95 per cent of all PLHIV on treatment and virally suppressed; 200,000 new adult infections, zero discrimination.	Demand for further roll-out of ARV and recognition of the cost-effectiveness ART to prevent HIV transmission; increased demand for pre-exposure prophylaxis (PREP) as part of 'Treatment as Prevention'	Use of injectable, long-acting ARVs for treatment and prevention with rapid roll-out in HICs, slower in LMICs; PLHIV increased from 30.8 million in 2010 to 37.8 million in 2020 while PLHIV on ART increased from 7.8 million to 27.2 million; use of PREP increasing, especially in HICs; HIV resources increased from US$16.7 billion in 2010 to US$27.2 billion in 2020; HIV deaths decreased from 1.4 million in 2010 to 650,000 in 2020; number newly infected with HIV decreased from 2.2 million to 1.5 million; many LMICs unable to reach the 2020 targets; COVID-19 pandemic disrupted many services, especially in LMICs.

Key: ACTUP, AIDS Coalition to Unleash Power; ART, anti-retroviral treatment; ARVs, anti-retroviral drugs; AZT, Azidothymidine; COVID-19, disease caused by the SARS-CoV-2 virus; CSO, civil society organization; LMICs, low- and middle-income countries; mHealth, health services using mobile phones, patient monitoring devices, personal digital assistants and other wireless devices; PLHIV, people living with HIV; STI, sexually transmitted infection; TAG, Treatment Action Group; SA, South Africa; WTO, World Trade Organization.

Sources: Seckinelgin (2002); Zuniga (2005); UNAIDS (2011, 2022)

Activity 4.8

Why has the HIV policy arena attracted such a high level of civil society group involvement over the decades?

Feedback

A number of factors help to explain the high level of interest group activism, particularly in the early stages of the pandemic in HICs, which inspired later activism in LMICs:

1. The demographic profile of the early affected population and most subsequent infections – HIV tended to affect young adults and in countries like the UK, it initially affected relatively affluent gay men in cities.
2. HIV, and even AIDS before therapy was available, is not an immediate killer, allowing an opportunity for activism, unlike some other diseases.
3. Spill over from other social movements – in the US and Western Europe, the most affected population group was gay men who had recent experience of the gay rights movement of the 1970s. They used some of the same civil rights strategies and refused to play the role of 'patients'. In LMICs subsequently, HIV activism was inspired by and allied itself to wider social justice movements such as those for debt relief or took inspiration in South Africa from the anti-apartheid movement and its practices.
4. The slowness of the official response in HICs – it took between two and four years, and sometimes longer, between the first diagnosis and the development of official awareness campaigns. It also took time before drug manufacturers were willing to reduce costs for LMICs.

 Activity 4.9

Why do you think HIV activism was less prominent in poorer countries in the 1980s and early 1990s?

Feedback

There are a number of inter-related explanations. You may have written down some or all of the following:

1. Unresponsiveness of political leaderships, especially in undemocratic countries in Africa (which were more common in the 1980s).

2. Denial by governments of the prevalence of the disease in countries, popular views that HIV was a Western, alien problem only affecting gay men and concerns in some countries that it might affect tourism.
3. The fact that HIV in these countries did not affect a cohesive, well off group such as gay men in the US but poor people who could easily be silenced and ignored.
4. Other diseases and their interest groups competing for policy attention as traditionally funded with external assistance.
5. Lack of donor interest and funding to NGOs in HIV.

Does interest group participation always lead to 'good' policy making?

Up to now, the involvement of interest groups and the evolution of networks have been analysed largely without attempting to judge their positive or negative consequences for policy making. Generally, in liberal democratic societies, the involvement of organizations outside the government in policy processes is seen as a good thing. However, there are potential drawbacks from a normative perspective (see Chapter 3) as well as some practical challenges that could affect policy outcomes.

Activity 4.10

List the possible positive and negative consequences of having a wide range of interest groups involved in the shaping of health policy.

Feedback

Your lists will probably have included some of the possible advantages and drawbacks shown in Table 4.2.

Conflicts of interest are a particular concern when involving commercial interests in public health policy making.

There is a strand of more authoritarian policy thinking that regards 'open' policy making as unnecessary and inefficient. Lee Kuan Yew, prime minister of Singapore from 1959 to 1990, argued that his illiberal and paternalistic style of government was not only very successful but built on what he called 'Asian values' and thus was justified. In crude summary, these values were a deep respect for social hierarchy and the rights of the state based on the interdependence of human beings ahead of the Western

Table 4.2 Possible advantages and drawbacks of interest group involvement in shaping health policy

Potential advantages of 'open' policy processes	Potential negative consequences of 'open' policy processes
Wide range of views is brought to bear on a problem including a better appreciation of the possible differential impacts of policy on different groups.	Difficult to reconcile conflicting and competing claims for attention and resources of different interest groups.
Policy-making process includes information not accessible to governments.	Adds to complexity and time taken to reach decisions and to implement policies.
Consultation and/or involvement of a range of interests gives policy greater legitimacy and support so that policy decisions may be more likely to be implemented and more sustainable.	Groups may be neither representative of the wider public nor of their members or supporters and lack accountability.
New or emerging issues may be brought to governments' attention more rapidly than if process is relatively 'closed'.	Less well-resourced, less well-connected interests may still be disadvantaged in 'open' processes.
	Groups may not be capable of providing the information or taking the responsibility allocated to them.
	Conflicts of interest may not be made transparent (e.g. big business supports 'front' groups providing multiple covert channels of influence).
	Interest groups can be self-interested, badly informed, abusive and intimidatory – being in civil society does not confer automatic civility or virtue.

emphasis on the rights of the individual (Barr 2000). There is a strong element of self-justification in such arguments, but they draw attention to an old debate in policy about the extent to which the means are acceptable as long as the ends (goals) are met. Irrespective of how you judge Yew's views and decisions, this is also a reminder that policy norms vary between countries and over time (see Chapter 8).

Summary

There are many groups outside government that try to influence health policy during the policy process. In some countries, there are many of these groups and they are strong; in other countries there are few

non-governmental actors and their influence on policy makers is relatively limited. Until the 1990s, policy in many poorer countries was
dominated by elites closely affiliated with the government of the day
(including representatives of donor agencies). However, from the 1990s,
the number of different groups and alliances of groups trying to influence government policies generally grew, and governments increasingly
came to recognize that they needed to listen more widely. NGOs that
had previously confined themselves to delivering services became more
involved in policy advocacy – as did local and foreign researchers.
Alliances between interest groups in different countries have become
more prominent in their efforts to influence governments' policies in the
health field.

Interest groups differ in the way they are treated by governments. Some
are given high-legitimacy, 'insider' status and are regularly involved in
policy development. Market-related groups often fall into this category
because they are powerful and can employ economic sanctions if they do
not approve of a government's policy. In contrast, cause groups may be
consulted but have less recourse to sanctions. They may be perceived as
'outsider' groups or even deliberately pursue an 'outsider' strategy organizing demonstrations and ensuring a high level of media coverage in a bid
to embarrass or put pressure on governments.

The increasing significance of interest groups organized within policy
networks around particular areas of public policy represents a challenge to
the assumption that governments can act alone, and requires politicians
and bureaucrats to learn new skills of working in a less hierarchical and
more negotiated way. This trend has been referred to as a shift from 'government' to 'governance'. A key skill of governments in such a world is the
ability to co-ordinate and hold to account a diverse set of actors, many of
whom are far from its direct control.

Further reading

Harris, J. (2019) Advocacy coalitions and the transfer of nutrition policy to Zambia, *Health Policy*, 34(3):
    207–15. https://doi.org/10.1093/heapol/czz024
Hoffman, S.J. and Cole, C.B. (2018) Defining the global health system and systematically mapping
    its network of actors, *Globalization and Health*, 14: 38. https://doi.org/10.1186/s12992-018-
    0340-2
Kaufman, J. (2012) China's evolving AIDS policy: the influence of global norms and transnational
    non-governmental organizations, *Contemporary Politics* 18: 225–38. https://doi.org/10.1080/
    13569775.2012.674343
Knai, C., Petticrew, M., Capewell, S. et al. (2021) The case for developing a cohesive systems approach
    to research across unhealthy commodity industries, *BMJ Global Health* 6: e003543. https://doi.
    org/10.1136/bmjgh-2020-003543
Shearer, J.C., Abelson, J., Kouyaté, B. et al. (2016) Why do policies change? Institutions, interests,
    ideas and networks in three cases of policy reform, *Health Policy and Planning*, 31: 1200–11.
    https://doi.org/10.1093/heapol/czw052

References

Aftab, W., Khan, M., Rego, S. et al. (2021) Variations in regulations to control standards for training and licensing of physicians: a multi-country comparison, *Human Resources for Health*, 19: 91. https://doi.org/10.1186/s12960-021-00629-5

Audickas, L., Dempsey, N. and Loft, P. (2019) *Membership of UK Political Parties*, House of Commons Library Briefing Paper Number SN05125, 9 August. London: House of Commons. Available at: https://researchbriefings.files.parliament.uk/documents/SN05125/SN05125.pdf (accessed 24 April 2023).

Barr, M.D. (2000) Lee Kuan Yew and the 'Asian values' debate, *Asian Studies Review*, 24(3): 309–34. https://doi.org/10.1080/10357820008713278

Giddens, A. (2001) Foreword, in H. Anheier, M. Glasius and M. Kaldor (eds.) *Global Civil Society*. Oxford: Oxford University Press. Available at: www.academia.edu/4164817/Introducing_Global_Civil_Society (accessed 24 April 2023).

Gift, T. (2022) Guns in the US: why the NRA is so successful at preventing reform, *The Conversation*, 1 June. Available at: https://theconversation.com/guns-in-the-us-why-the-nra-is-so-successful-at-preventing-reform-184180 (accessed 24 April 2023).

Grant, W. (1984) The role of pressure groups, in R. Borthwick and J. Spence (eds.) *British Politics in Perspective*. Leicester: Leicester University Press.

Heywood, M. (2011) South Africa's Treatment Action Campaign: combining law and social mobilization to realize the right to health, *Journal of Human Rights Practice*, 1: 14–36.

Johnson, T. (1995) Governmentality and the institutionalisation of expertise, in T. Johnson, G. Larkin and M. Saks (eds.) *Health Professions and the State in Europe*. London: Routledge, pp. 7–24.

Kübler, D. (1999) Ideas as catalytic elements for policy change: advocacy coalitions and drug policy in Switzerland, in D. Braun and A. Busch (eds.) *Public Policy and Political Ideas*. Cheltenham: Edward Elgar, pp. 116–221.

Lawrence, P. (2018) *Whither Large International Non-Governmental Organisations? Plowden Fellowship Report*. Birmingham: Third Sector Research Centre, University of Birmingham. Available at: www.birmingham.ac.uk/Documents/college-social-sciences/social-policy/tsrc/working-papers/working-paper-142.pdf (accessed 19 October 2022).

Lewis, J. (2005) *Health Policy and Politics: Networks, Ideas and Power*. Melbourne: IP Communications.

Marsh, D. and Rhodes, R.A.W. (1992) Policy communities and issue networks: beyond typology, in D. Marsh and R.A.W. Rhodes (eds.) *Policy Networks in British Government*. Oxford: Oxford University Press.

Muggli, M.E., Hurt, R.D. and Repace, J. (2004) The tobacco industry's political efforts to derail the EPA report on ETS, *American Journal of Preventive Medicine*, 26(2): 167–77.

Osei-Kojo, A., Ingold, K. and Weible, C.M. (2022) The Advocacy Coalition Framework: lessons from applications in African countries, *Politsche Vierteljahresschrift*, 63: 181–201. https://doi.org/10.1007/s11615-022-00399-2

Preston, J. and Stelter, B. (2011) Cellphones become the world's eyes and ears on protests, *New York Times*, 18 February. Available at: www.nytimes.com/2011/02/19/world/middleeast/19video.html?_r=1&ref=tunisia (accessed 19 October 2022).

Rahman-Shepherd, A., Balasubramaniam, P., Gautham, M. et al. (2021) Conflicts of interest: an invisible force shaping health systems and policies, *Lancet Global Health*, 9: e1056.

Rhodes, R.A.W. (1997) *Understanding Governance*. Buckingham: Open University Press.

Robins, S. (2004) 'Long live Zackie, Long Live': AIDS activism, science and citizenship after Apartheid, *Journal of Southern African Studies*, 30: 651–72.

Sabatier, P.A. and Jenkins-Smith, H.C. (eds.) (1993) *Policy Change and Learning: An Advocacy Coalition Approach*. Boulder, CO: Westview Press.

Seckinelgin, H. (2002) Time to stop and think: HIV/AIDS, global civil society, and the people's politics, in H.K. Anheier, M. Glasius ands M. Kaldor (eds.) *Global Civil Society Year Book, 2002*. New York: Oxford University Press.

Shiffman, J. (2018) Agency, structure and the power of global health networks, *International Journal of Health Policy and Management*, 7: 879–84.

Stuckler, D., Reeves, A., Loopstra, R. and McKee, M. (2016) Textual analysis of sugar industry influence on the World Health Organization's 2015 sugars intake guideline, *Bulletin of the World Health Organization*, 94: 566–73.

UNAIDS (2011) *AIDS at 30: Nations at the Crossroads*. Geneva: UNAIDS.

UNAIDS (2022) *In Danger: UNAIDS Global AIDS Update 2022*. Geneva: UNAIDS.

Weible, C.M., Sabatier, P.A. and McQueen, K. (2009) Themes and variations: taking stock of the Advocacy Coalition Framework, *The Policy Studies Journal*, 37: 123.

World Health Organization (2019) *Programme Budget 2020–2021*. Geneva: WHO.

Zuniga, J. (2005) Civil society and the global battle against HIV/AIDS, in E. Beck, N. Mays, A. Whiteside and J. Zuniga (eds.) *Dealing with the HIV Pandemic in the 21st Century: Health Systems' Responses, Past, Present and Future*. Oxford: Oxford University Press, pp. 706–19.

Agenda setting

5

This chapter looks at how issues are identified as a matter of concern for policy making. Why do some issues gain attention to the extent that action is likely to be taken? According to the simple 'stages model' of the policy process introduced in Chapter 1, problem identification is the first step in the process of changing and implementing policy. However, it can be surprisingly difficult to explain how and why some issues become prominent in the eyes of policy makers and others recede from view. In terms of the health 'policy triangle', also set out in Chapter 1, the explanation most often relates to changes in the policy context which enable the policy actors concerned to change policy by persuading others that action should be taken. Objective conditions, such as changes in disease patterns, rarely straightforwardly determine the health policy agenda. The focus in this chapter is on how and why governments choose to act on some issues but not on others. It also discusses how the global public health agenda is set. The chapter further looks at the range of interest groups that contribute to agenda setting, paying particular attention to the role of the mass and social media since they often play an important part in shaping issues so that they are more or less likely to find their way onto the policy agenda.

Learning objectives

After working through this chapter, you will be better able to:

- define what is meant by the *policy agenda*
- understand three different theories explaining how issues get onto the policy agenda and how certain issues get priority for policy development over others
- compare the respective roles of a range of interest groups in setting the policy agenda.

Key terms

Agenda setting Process by which certain issues come onto the policy agenda from the much larger number of issues potentially worthy of attention by policy makers.

Feasibility   A characteristic of those issues or policy options or solutions considered practical in a particular political context.

Frames   Concepts and images by which policy issues are described and understood.

Framing   The process by which policy issues are constructed and given particular 'frames' that relate to the values and/or goals of different interests.

Infodemic   An excess of information about a health issue that is often invalid, rapidly disseminated and hampers an effective response.

Legitimacy   A characteristic of those issues which public policy makers see as appropriate for government to act on.

Policy agenda   List of issues to which an organization, usually the government, is giving serious attention at any one time with a view to taking some sort of action.

Policy stream   The set of possible policy solutions or alternatives developed by experts, politicians, bureaucrats and interest groups, together with the activities of those interested in these options (e.g. debates about the merits of different solutions).

Policy windows   Points in time when the opportunity arises for an issue to come onto the policy agenda and be taken seriously with a view to action.

Politics stream   Political events such as shifts in the national mood or public opinion, elections and changes in government, social uprisings, demonstrations and campaigns by interest groups that influence the likelihood that a problem and its potential response will be acted on by government.

Problem stream   Indicators of the scale and significance of an issue which give it visibility, together with the activities of those interested in the issue.

What is the policy agenda?

In public policy making, the term *agenda* refers to:

> *the list of subjects or problems to which government officials and people outside of government closely associated with those officials, are paying some serious attention at any given time ... Out of the set of all conceivable subjects or problems to which officials could be paying attention, they do in fact seriously attend to some rather than others.* (Kingdon 2013: 3)

Agenda setting is the political process in which issues compete to be brought to the attention of policy makers.

 Activity 5.1

List some of the health-related subjects or problems that you are aware of to which the government in your country has recently paid serious attention. If you cannot remember any, have a look at the news reports for the last few months to see which health issues and policies are mentioned. This may provide an indication of the issues on, or near the policy agenda.

Feedback

Out of the potentially wide range of health and related issues that the government could be attending to, there is usually a shorter list of 'hot' topics actively under discussion and thus on or near to the official agenda. For example, the government could be concerned about regulating or banning junk food advertising to children, combating non-communicable diseases (NCDs) such as diabetes, addressing trends in sexually transmitted disease, providing care for frail older people, improving the recruitment and retention of nurses in hospitals, boosting the immunization rate in remote rural areas, or deciding whether nurses should be able to prescribe essential drugs.

Obviously, the list of problems under active consideration varies from one section of the government to another. The president or prime minister will be considering major items such as the state of the economy or relations with other countries. The minister and ministry of health will have a more specialized agenda, which may include a few 'high politics' issues, such as whether a system of national health insurance should be established, as well as a larger number of 'low politics' issues such as whether a particular drug should be approved for use and, if so, whether it should be paid for as part of the publicly financed health care system.

How and why do issues get onto the policy agenda?

Sometimes it is obvious why policy makers take particular issues seriously and then act upon their understanding of them. For instance, once a pandemic is recognized, the government would normally rapidly recognize this as a problem requiring a concerted government response. This sort of identification and reaction to a crisis, however, is not typical of most policy making. Most policy making is, as Grindle and Thomas (1991) put it, related to 'politics-as-usual changes': a response to routine, day-to-day problems that need solutions, usually adaptations of existing policies. Given that there are always more such problems being publicly discussed than government has the capacity for, where does the impetus for change or response to a particular problem come from when there is no crisis?

The role of policy 'frames' in agenda setting

It is tempting to assume that public policy problems, in contrast with issues that individuals and families are expected to deal with themselves, are defined in purely objective terms based on indicator data, such as, the lethality of a pathogen. From this perspective, governments act in a rational manner, for example, when a phenomenon threatens the well-being of the population and the role of the government is judged to include protecting the population (see Chapter 2 for more on the rational model of policy making). According to this explanation, governments actively scan the horizon, identify issues using data and from this identify the most 'important' issues for serious policy attention (e.g. in health terms, all governments would focus on the diseases responsible for the greatest share of illness, death and disability, perhaps with the proviso of focusing particularly on those where there was some prospect of intervening effectively). A more sophisticated variant of this approach is to argue that the issues that eventually reach the policy agenda are more a function of long-term changes in socio-economic conditions which produce a set of issues to which governments have to respond eventually, even if there is no systematic assessment of their likely importance. From this perspective, countries with ageing populations will have to respond eventually to the implications of this trend for retirement pensions, health services, long-term care, transport and so on.

By contrast, political scientists and sociologists emphasize the importance of power (especially Lukes' second and third 'faces' of power), and of values and ideas (e.g. through appeals to national security and sovereignty) rather than a linear rational process of problem identification (see Chapters 2, 7 and 8 for more on power, values, and the role of ideas and evidence, respectively) (Smith 2013). Policy problems are seen as socially constructed through their representation, debate and advocacy rather than emerging fully formed on the basis of taken-for-granted, objective indicators. Ideas matter because recognizing something as a problem for government to respond to involves defining what is 'normal' in a society and thus what is an unacceptable deviation from normality that could potentially require policy attention (Berger and Luckmann 1975). This perspective draws attention to the ideologies and assumptions that determine how different governments operate and how these shape what is defined as an issue for government attention.

The manner and form in which problems are understood and described (or *'framed'*) are important influences on how they will eventually be tackled by policy makers (van Hulst and Yanow 2016). So, for example, if the problem of people with mental illness is largely 'framed' by the media in terms of the risk these people pose to themselves, this will have quite different consequences for the way in which mental health enters the policy agenda than if the problem is articulated as one of protecting the public from the threat posed by people with mental illness. In neither scenario is the prevalence and incidence of mental illness central to the question of whether the issue will be taken seriously, the priority it will receive and how it will be responded to.

Not everyone will necessarily agree on how a phenomenon should be framed (i.e. what sort of a problem it is and how it should be understood) and, indeed, whether it should even be a matter for government action at all. Important policy actors can clash and compete in attempting to persuade government not only to put an issue on, or take it off, the agenda but also in the way they wish to see it presented and dealt with. For example, rival *'frames'* are apparent in the way that HIV and AIDS have been conceived. Rushing (1995) identified three different conceptions, and noted how these 'frames' have affected the response over time:

- archaic – AIDS as a punishment for moral failings attracting stigma;
- metaphorical – AIDS as something to be fought against as in a 'war';
- medical scientific – covering a range of conceptions including a gradual shift from a fatal to a chronic disease, a virus or a sexually transmitted infection.

For example, the first two conceptions tend to be associated with discriminatory and exclusionary approaches to tackling HIV and AIDS.

At the level of global health priorities, Shiffman and Shawar (2022) identify three not dissimilar *framings* often determined by global health elites:

- 'securitization' – framing an issue as an existential threat;
- 'moralization' – framing an issue as an ethical imperative;
- 'technification' – framing an issue as a wise investment to meet a problem that science can solve.

Khan et al. (2019) show how global health organizations compared with LMIC governments promote rival explanations of, and potential responses, to the high-profile global issue of antimicrobial resistance (AMR). International policy documents frame AMR primarily as a threat to human health security and the global economy whereas countries themselves emphasize the human development and equity aspects (Khan et al. 2019).

Thus, different policy 'frames' enable or constrain different sorts of policy responses to a perceived issue (Townsend et al. 2020). Some framings are helpful and others can be misleading or even harmful to an effective policy response. For example, there is considerable doubt as to whether describing the policy response to cancer as a 'war' has been beneficial including to those suffering from cancer over the last 50 years. Similar militant language was used in the COVID-19 pandemic, characterizing the response as the 'fight' against the virus, thereby downplaying the fact that the impact of the virus depended on the social and economic conditions within the societies it entered as much as the intrinsic characteristics of the virus itself (Kohlt 2020).

Theories explaining how and why issues get onto the policy agenda

There are a number of theories of agenda setting that attempt to make sense of these processes. Three of the most prominent and widely used are described now.

Hall and colleagues: legitimacy, feasibility and support

This approach proposes that only when an issue and likely response score highly in terms of their *legitimacy*, *feasibility* and *support* do they get onto a government agenda. Hall and colleagues provided a relatively simple, quick to apply way of analysing which issues might be taken up by governments (Hall et al. 1975).

Legitimacy is a characteristic of those issues with which governments believe they should be concerned and in which they have a right or even obligation to intervene. At the high end of a spectrum of legitimacy, most citizens in most societies would expect the government to keep law and order and to defend the country from attack. There would be more debate about the role of government in other issues such as whether it was necessary for the government to own hospitals to ensure that care was provided equitably or enforce strict quarantine during a pandemic.

✎ Activity 5.2

Briefly list those health-related government policies and programmes that are generally regarded as highly legitimate.

Feedback

Probably the most widely accepted role for government in relation to health is to act to reduce the risk of infectious disease becoming established and spreading through the population. Another is regulating air and water pollution. Even in these areas, there is usually some debate about the precise nature and limits of government action as seen during the COVID-19 pandemic.

However, there are many other areas where legitimacy is much more contested. Legitimacy varies greatly from country to country and changes over time. Things that were not seen as the domain of government regulation in the past (e.g. control of smoking in work places) are now increasingly accepted as legitimate and vice versa (e.g. removal of laws prohibiting gay sex in many countries). Typically, in times of perceived external threats, the public and politicians are more willing to curb valued individual liberties because they may believe that such actions will protect the community from worse harm.

Feasibility refers to the potential for implementing the policy. It is defined by prevailing technical and theoretical knowledge, resources, availability of skilled staff, administrative capability and existence of the necessary infrastructure of government. There may be technological, financial or workforce limitations in a particular setting that suggest that a particular policy may be impossible to implement, regardless of how legitimate it is seen to be. If a potential policy cannot be shown to pass a test of feasibility, it is unlikely to find its way onto the policy agenda.

✎ Activity 5.3

What policies would you like to introduce into the health system in your country but which are likely to face major feasibility problems?

Feedback

You may have made all sorts of suggestions. One common one is to try to achieve geographical equity of provision and use of health services since this commonly encounters the reluctance of health care professionals to work in 'less desirable' areas such as remote, rural locations. Another common feasibility problem relates to health care financing in LICs. Their governments may wish to introduce more public finance into their health care systems but frequently lack robust tax systems to raise the revenue because so many people work in the informal sector of the economy.

Finally, *support* refers to the elusive but important issue of public support for the government of the day, at least in relation to the issue in question. Clearly, more authoritarian and non-elected regimes are less dependent on popular support than democratic governments, but even dictatorships have to ensure that there is some support among key groups, such as the armed forces, for their policies. If support is lacking, or discontent with the government as a whole is high, it may be very difficult for a government to put an issue on the agenda and do anything about it.

Thus, the logic of Hall and colleagues' model is that governments will estimate whether an issue falls at the high or low end of the three continua of legitimacy, feasibility and support. If an issue has high legitimacy (government is seen as having the right or even duty to intervene), high feasibility (there are sufficient resources, personnel, infrastructure) and high support (the most important interest groups are supportive – or at least not obstructive), then the odds of the issue reaching the policy agenda and faring well subsequently are greatly increased.

Of course, this does not rule out more tactical reasons for putting an issue onto the policy agenda. Sometimes, governments will publicly state their position on a particular issue to demonstrate that they care, or to appease donors who demand a response as a condition of aid, or to confound the political opposition, even when they do not expect to be able to translate their concern into a policy that could be implemented because it has low feasibility and/or support.

John Kingdon: policy windows and three streams within the policy process

John Kingdon's (2013) approach focuses on the role of policy 'entrepreneurs' inside and outside government who take advantage of agenda setting opportunities – known as *policy windows* – to move items onto the government's formal agenda. The theory suggests that the characteristics of issues combine with the features of political institutions and circumstances, together with the development of policy solutions, in a process that can lead to the opening and closing of 'windows of opportunity' necessary to shift an issue from a matter of some concern onto the official agenda. He conceives of policy emerging through the interplay of three separate, continuous 'streams' of activity or processes – the *problem stream,* the *policy stream* and the *politics stream*. Policies are only taken seriously by governments when the three streams converge (Figure 5.1). Kingdon's 'windows' are the metaphorical launch 'windows' at the start of a space mission. Blast-off can only occur when all three conditions are favourable.

The *problem stream* refers to activities that shape the perceptions of problems as public matters requiring government action and is influenced by previous efforts of government to respond to problems. Officials learn about issues such as trends in socio-economic conditions through indicators, research, feedback from existing programmes, pressure groups, or sudden,

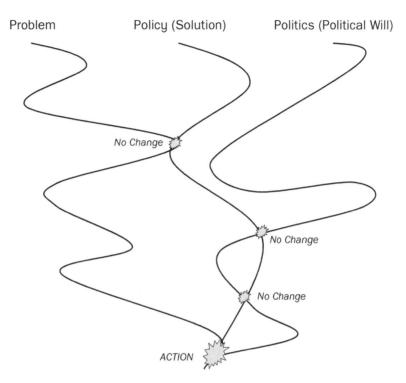

Figure 5.1: Kingdon's three stream model of agenda setting
Source: adapted from Kingdon (2013)

focusing events such as crises. Indicators may include routine health statistics – for example, showing an increase in childhood obesity or a return of TB to a population previously free of the disease. However, such facts rarely if ever 'speak for themselves' and lead directly to action (see Chapter 7 for more on the links between evidence and policy), though governments can use the definition, timing of release and interpretation (including framing) of official statistics (e.g. on unemployment) to attempt to shape the policy agenda.

The *policy stream* consists of the ongoing analyses of problems and their proposed solutions together with the debates surrounding these problems and possible responses. In this stream of ideas, a range of possibilities is explored and, at times, may be progressively narrowed down or promoted. For an idea or solution to get to the surface, it must be technically feasible, consistent with dominant social values, be capable of handling future feasibility constraints (such as on finance and personnel), be publicly acceptable and resonate with politicians.

The *politics stream* operates quite separately to the other two streams and is comprised of events such as swings of national mood, changes of government and campaigns by interest groups that influence the likelihood that a problem and its potential solution will be acted on.

Kingdon identifies visible and hidden participants affecting the coming together of the streams. The visible participants are organized interest groups which highlight a specific problem, put forward a particular point of view, advocate a solution and use the mass and social media to get attention. Visible participants may be inside or outside government. For example, a new president or prime minister may be a powerful agenda setter because they have only recently been elected and are given the benefit of the doubt by the electorate. Other highly visible participants include UN 'goodwill ambassadors' on particular issues such as James Chau, Chinese broadcaster and writer, who was appointed in 2016 as goodwill ambassador promoting the SDGs. The hidden participants are more likely to be the specialists in the field – the researchers and consultants who work predominantly in the policy stream – developing and proposing options for solving problems which may get onto the agenda. They also include business lobbyists. Hidden participants may play a part in getting issues onto the agenda, particularly if they work with the mass media. Increasingly, universities, which are competing with one another for research funds, encourage their staff to promote their research findings in the mass media. This may mean that some academics shift from hidden to more visible roles in the agenda setting process.

According to Kingdon's model, the three streams flow along different, largely independent channels until at particular times, which become *policy windows*, they flow together. This is when new issues get onto the agenda and policy is highly likely, but not guaranteed, to change. From this perspective, policies do not get onto the agenda according to logical stages. The three streams flow simultaneously, each with a life of its own, until they meet or align, at which point an issue is likely to be taken seriously by policy makers. The meeting of the streams cannot easily be engineered or predicted though 'policy entrepreneurs' work to take advantage of favourable conditions such as a change of government to bring this about.

✎ Activity 5.4

Suggest possible reasons why the three streams might meet, leading to a problem moving onto the policy agenda. Locate each possible reason in one of Kingdon's three 'streams'.

Feedback

The main reasons why the three streams might converge and open a policy window include:

- the activities of key players in the *political stream* who work to link particular policy 'solutions' to particular problems and at the same

time create the political opportunity for action. These people are known as *policy entrepreneurs* since this is the political version of the activity of bringing buyers, sellers and commodities together on which commerce thrives;
- media attention to a problem and to possible solutions (*problem* or *policy streams* influencing the *politics stream*);
- a crisis such as a serious failure in the quality or safety of a service or other unpredictable event such as a pandemic (*problem stream*);
- the dissemination of a major piece of research (*problem or policy stream*);
- a change of government after an election or other regular, formal landmarks in the political process (e.g. budgets) (*politics stream*).

Thus, in reality, participants in the policy process rarely proceed from identification of a problem to seeking solutions. Alternative courses of action are generated in the policy stream and may be promoted by experts or advocates over long periods before the opportunity arises (i.e. before the policy window opens) to get their problems and their solutions onto the agenda.

Shiffman and colleagues: explaining the health priorities of individual countries and at the global level

Despite an international, shared body of knowledge about public health issues and potential responses, the policy agendas and priorities within those agendas of different countries can differ substantially. Aware of this phenomenon, American political scientist, Jeremy Shiffman, carried out a series of studies in the 1990s and 2000s to try to explain why the priority given to the issue of reducing maternal mortality differed across countries. He explained these differences in terms of efforts by international agencies to establish a global norm about the unacceptability of maternal death; the agencies' provision of financial and technical resources within countries; the degree of cohesion among national safe motherhood policy promoters; the presence of national political champions to promote the cause; the availability and strategic use of credible evidence to show policy makers that a problem existed; the generation of clear policy options indicating that the problem was surmountable; and the organization of attention-generating events to raise the national visibility of the issue (Shiffman 2007).

Shiffman and his colleague Stephanie Smith then took their work to the international level to try to explain why the global Safe Motherhood Initiative to reduce maternal mortality, launched in 1987, had not received much attention and remained a relatively low international public health priority. Shiffman and Smith (2007) developed a framework based on four elements: the strength of the actors involved and their cohesion; the power of the ideas used to portray the issue; the way that the political context either inhibited or enhanced support for the issue; and the characteristics of the issue itself (see Table 5.1 and Figure 5.2).

Table 5.1 Shiffman and Smith's framework of determinants for understanding the political priority of different global health initiatives

	Description	Factors shaping political priority
Actor power	The strength of the individu- als and organizations concerned with the issue	1. Policy community cohesion: the degree of coalescence among the network of individuals and organizations that are centrally involved with the issue at the global level. 2. Leadership: the presence of individuals capable of uniting the policy community and acknowledged as particularly strong champions for the cause. 3. Guiding institutions: the effectiveness of organizations or co-ordinating mechanisms with a mandate to lead the initiative. 4. Civil society mobilization: the extent to which grassroots organizations have mobilized to press international and national political authorities to address the issue at the global level.
Ideas	The ways in which those involved with the issue understand and portray it	5. Internal frame: the degree to which the policy community agrees on the definition of, causes of, and solutions to the problem. 6. External frame: public portrayals of the issue in ways that resonate with external audiences, especially the political leaders who control resources.
Issue characteristics	Features of the problem	7. Credible indicators: clear measures that show the severity of the problem and that can be used to monitor progress. 8. Severity: the size of the burden relative to other problems, as indicated by objective measures such as mortality levels. 9. Effective interventions: the extent to which proposed means of addressing the problem are clearly explained, cost effective, backed by scientific evidence, simple to implement and inexpensive.
Political contexts	The environ- ments in which actors operate	10. Policy windows: political moments when global conditions align favourably for an issue, presenting opportunities for advocates to influence decision makers. 11. Global governance structure: the degree to which norms and institutions operating in a sector provide a platform for effective collective action.

Source: adapted from Shiffman and Smith (2007: 1371)

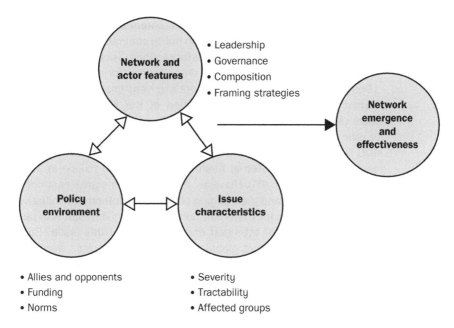

Figure 5.2: A framework on the emergence and effectiveness of global health networks
Source: Shiffman et al. (2016)

The Safe Motherhood Initiative was hampered in all four respects. In relation to the power of the interest groups most involved with maternal mortality, Shiffman and Smith found that, among other things, they were divided over the intervention strategy that should be adopted, reducing their credibility with international and national political leaders. There were no strong guiding organizations or leaders who could engineer consensus, and civil society organizations were weakly mobilized.

At the level of ideas, the contrasting approaches to 'framing' the issue of maternal mortality led to confusion. For example, some viewed it as a human rights issue, others in terms of its adverse economic consequences, yet others as harming children and families. In some countries the issue of child survival generally took precedence over that of mothers though not without controversy. There was also confusion over whether maternal mortality or maternal health should be the focus, what the appropriate interventions should be and how the issue related to other women's health concerns such as reproductive health.

In terms of issue characteristics, Shiffman and Smith argued that maternal mortality failed to become a priority because maternal death was not as common as other causes of death (e.g. from communicable diseases), was difficult to measure and there was no single, simple intervention that was readily available to avert maternal deaths. The evidence supporting interventions was also weaker than for other competing health programmes.

In relation to the global policy context, potential policy 'windows' opened periodically, but the safe motherhood policy community was not well placed to take advantage of them. For instance, there was no single or obvious 'home' within United Nations (UN) organizations for safe motherhood.

Despite these difficulties, a potentially very important 'policy window' opened in 2000 with the promulgation of the Millennium Development Goals (MDGs). MDG 5 was the reduction of the global maternal mortality ratio by 75 per cent over 1990 levels by the year 2015. Influenced by MDG 5, countries such as the UK increased their allocation of development resources to maternal health (e.g. from £0.9 million in 2001/02 to £16.2 million by 2005/06). However, it seems that the greater priority resulting from the MDGs and the merging of the Safe Motherhood Initiative into a broader partnership for maternal, newborn and child health was beginning to pay off in terms of attention and resources for this issue. By 2010, it was being suggested that global maternal mortality rates were beginning to decline although some countries had made little progress (Hogan et al. 2010). The greater priority was sustained by the Every Woman Every Child (EWEC) initiative launched in 2010 by the former UN Secretary-General H.E. Ban Ki-moon and the 2015 SDGs.

Activity 5.5

What is notable about Shiffman and Smith's approach to explaining the political priority given to maternal mortality both within countries and at the international level from the perspective of the 'rational' approach to policy making described in Chapter 2?

Feedback

Only part of the explanatory framework relates to the influence of objective data such as indicators of the scale of the problem of maternal death and the (cost-) effectiveness of potential interventions to reduce it which, according to the rational approach to policy should be central to deciding on priorities. Instead, the main factors contributing to the priority given to maternal death as a public health issue are social and political, relating to the inter-relationships between the main organizations operating in the field, the wider political context and the way that influential people and agencies view, and project the issue.

Walt and Gilson (2014) reviewed a wide range of other studies of agenda setting in order to assess the ability of Shiffman and Smith's theory to identify the factors shaping the policy agenda at national and international levels. They found that the approach was widely applicable but would benefit from some refinement. For example, 'issue characteristics' should include the degree of conflict related to the problem being considered and the concept of 'guiding institutions' should be split between guiding organizations, and the formal and informal legal and political norms and rules present in the specific policy context. Depending on the issue and the degree of contestation, the role of the private sector would need to be given more explicit consideration, as in the example of food policy (Baker et al. 2018).

✏ Activity 5.6

Read the following account, based on Colombini et al. (2016), which describes getting the issue of domestic violence onto the policy agenda in Nepal. Apply the theories of agenda setting described above to this case study to explain the events that took place.

Getting the issue of gender-based violence onto the policy agenda in Nepal

In the 1990s, the democratization process exposed Nepal to widening awareness of international commitments towards gender equality and facilitated the rise of influential women's organizations that started to campaign for gender equity and reduction of discrimination – including gender-based violence (GBV). The Ministries of Women and of Social Welfare advocated for legal changes to end GBV. Women's NGOs also contributed significantly to help place violence on the national policy agenda since these Ministries were not very influential acting alone. Women's groups developed gender equity and development frames to advocate for GBV reduction. Despite that, there was little political recognition of the negative health impact of violence on women's lives or the role of the health sector in preventing GBV. Instead, the government's focus at the time was on women's safety and security (due to the armed conflict ongoing since 1996), and on maternal mortality reduction and safe abortion (in the early 2000s) – particularly influenced by the related MDGs. The Nepalese Safe Motherhood movement, supported by NGOs and international donors, became a catalyst to ensure recognition of GBV as a health issue contributing to maternal mortality, though evidence on such a link was scarce. In the early 2000s, women's organizations and researchers collaborated to study the negative effects of GBV on maternal health to influence the new government's position on violence (which adopted a human rights frame). This contributed to the prohibition of GBV under the new constitution of 2006 and the development of service guidelines by the MoH to address GBV. However, these events were neither sufficient to legitimize GBV as a health priority nor the MoH's role in responding to it. One explanation could be the government's focus on rehabilitation and reconstruction after the end of the armed conflict in 2006. In the late 2000s, international donors and UN agencies supported the MoH to undertake further research that more clearly demonstrated the link between violence against women (VAW) and ill health. In response, in 2010, the prime minister declared GBV a critical concern that deserved policy attention, which subsequently led to the adoption of a Domestic Violence Act and a National Plan of Action against gender-based violence.

Feedback

Applying the Hall model

The policy on gender-based violence had *legitimacy* because the Office of the Prime Minister declared it as a priority. It was a new democratic government after decades of armed conflict and the democratization processes legitimized these new policies. There was strong support from international donors and UN agencies, which further legitimized the importance of addressing GBV.

It was *feasible* to introduce a National Plan on GBV because it had the official support of the prime minister and the MoH had already developed guidelines for service delivery which paved the way for the implementation of the plan at service delivery level.

Support was available from women's NGOs and academics, and initially from less influential ministries like Women and Health. As international donors and agencies got involved (with production of evidence) so support for the policy grew.

Applying the Kingdon model

The problem of gender-based violence had been floating in the *problem stream* for some time, but without any action being taken. However, numerous political events contributed to the increasing prioritization of GBV including the resolution of the decade-long armed conflict and the democratization process, which led to a new constitution in 2006 (change in the *politics stream*) and to proposed solutions by women's groups (legislation to criminalize GBV) and subsequently by the MoH (health services to address GBV) that appealed to the prime minister's office (*policy stream*). Women's NGOs and academics acted as initial catalysts for GBV recognition, but they needed the political support of Ministries to influence high-level decision making. The MoH missed some opportunities to integrate GBV earlier into its Safe Motherhood plan, but acted as policy entrepreneur when it involved international donors to gain the support of the prime minister, recognizing an opportunity to get GBV as a health issue on the government agenda.

Applying the Shiffman model

In relation to the *power of the interest groups* most involved with GBV, NGOs and the Women's Ministry were mobilized but less influential, while the MoH was interested in service delivery changes but did not have any policy champions. It was when they joined forces with international donors that they became more influential.

In relation to *ideas*, the framing of GBV by various actors evolved from gender equity and development (initially used by women's NGOs in line with the government's frame) to human rights (promoted by influential women's groups and accepted by the prime minister's office – which gave GBV a higher political profile) to public health (adopted by the MoH and international donors after it became possible to implement policy on GBV following adoption of the new legislation).

In terms of *issue characteristics*, GBV became a visible priority when evidence produced by women's NGOs, academics and UN agencies became available linking GBV to the already high-profile issue of maternal mortality.

In relation to the global *policy context*, potential policy 'windows' opened periodically, but it was only when the Domestic Violence Bill became law that the MoH was able to take a legitimate role in the national response to GBV. Despite initially limited political leadership and will to address GBV, the strong support from international donors and agencies eventually allowed for a health response to GBV.

The three approaches to understanding agenda setting that you have just read about (Hall et al., Kingdon, and Shiffman et al.) were developed to be applied retrospectively to understand particular instances of agenda setting, including how some issues fail to reach the policy agenda and why. However, they also provide insights that can be used prospectively, for example, by policy advocates. It is also possible to use more than one theory (i.e. 'multiple lenses') to explain different aspects of a process, thereby enriching the analysis (Cairney 2007). Parkhurst and Vulimiri (2013) used the three theories summarized in this chapter plus Geneau et al.'s (2010) modified 'political process model' for chronic diseases to try to explain why cervical cancer had received relatively little political attention at the global level. They show that each of the theories produce a number of overlapping insights relevant to cervical cancer, namely, the importance of a clearly visible problem and solution; a network of policy actors with the power to advocate effectively; resonant 'framing' of the issue; and identifying the favourable moments to push the issue onto the agenda.

The impact of *focusing* events on agenda setting

You have seen that a perceived crisis is one reason why policy windows open. Crises are a form of *focusing event*, meaning sudden, rare events such as disasters and scandals that can produce external shocks to a settled policy agenda. Policy making in times of crisis is different from ordinary, business-as-usual policy making since crises provide opportunities for groups that may have been struggling to advance an issue to come to prominence. Crises can force radically different policies onto established agendas, provided that there is both a clear notion of the problem and of potential solutions (Birkland 2020). For example, the COVID-19 pandemic led even some right-wing, free market governments hastily to give serious consideration to providing income support to millions of workers through so-called furlough schemes to avoid the collapse of many businesses. In health care, virtual consultations became the norm overnight in many settings.

A crisis exists when important policy makers perceive that one exists; in other words, when they believe that they face a real and threatening set of circumstances, and that failure to act could lead to even more disastrous consequences. Events that do not have all these perceived characteristics are not likely to be considered a crisis. However, where the gravity of the situation is confirmed by pressure from outside government, such as a dramatic increase in prices of basic foodstuffs or the rapid spread of a severe infectious disease, and the government has access to corroborating information from its own experts, then the chances are that the government will see the problem as a crisis, and pay it serious attention. However, governments will vary in the nature and extent of evidence that they regard as proving beyond doubt that there is a crisis to which they may need to respond. This recognition may or may not eventually lead to a change of policy.

Since crises are defined by the intersection of 'objective' conditions and perceptions of the gravity of those conditions, there is always scope for interest groups and governments to heighten the sense of crisis in order to pave the way for changes they particularly want to introduce. The reverse can also be the case with politicians and related interest groups arguing that talk of a crisis is an over-reaction and that 'business as usual' should prevail. In large parts of Europe, libertarian politicians joined forces with the hospitality industry to resist or reduce the scale of restrictions planned or implemented to halt the spread of COVID-19. At different times and places, they used a range of arguments including that the virus was less severe than the public health community's account, that livelihoods would be permanently put at risk by closures of venues, that the needs of the economy had to be fairly balanced against the protection of the public health and so on.

Non-decision making

While both crisis and politics-as-usual models are useful for helping explain how issues come onto the policy agenda and are acted upon, or why eventually they are not (because they may lack legitimacy, feasibility or support or because the three policy streams do not come together in favourable circumstances to provide a 'window of opportunity'), observable action provides an incomplete guide to the way all policies are decided. In other words, you need to think about the possibility of *non-policy making*, or *non-decision making* when thinking about what gets onto the public policy agenda (see Chapter 2 for a fuller discussion of this in relation to Lukes' dimensions of power). According to Bachrach and Baratz (1963), the power to keep things off the policy agenda is as important as the power to push certain issues onto the government's agenda. For instance, those with enough power (e.g. economic elites) are not only capable of stopping items reaching the agenda; they are also able to shape people's wishes so that only issues deemed acceptable and non-threatening to their interests are discussed, never mind acted on.

✎ Activity 5.7

Until the 1970s, stopping smoking was widely seen as almost entirely an individual matter (except for deterring children from smoking). As a result, there was not even discussion about the possibility of limiting where smoking could take place in the health interests both of smokers and non-smokers.

Do you think the lack of discussion of restrictions on smoking before the 1970s is an example of non-decision making through force, prevailing values or avoidance of conflict on the part of governments? Why do you think governments subsequently gradually began to act to curb tobacco consumption?

Feedback

The main reason for non-decision making related to the prevailing values of the time, which, in turn, were supported by the tobacco industry and its advocates (see Chapter 8 on values). In addition, governments

were reluctant to face conflict with the tobacco industry and invite public unpopularity. Governments were also concerned about the economic
consequences and the impact on tax revenues of reducing tobacco consumption. This anticipation of conflict with the industry and with voters
kept the issue off the agenda for many years.

Although the strong association between tobacco smoking and disease,
particularly lung cancer, had been known since the 1950s, the tobacco
industry had been highly effective in calling this knowledge into question
(e.g. by arguing that the links were not causal in the absence of randomized controlled trials) and limiting the flow of information reaching the
public (e.g. on the harmful effects of environmental tobacco smoke)
over decades. Eventually, the accumulation of evidence and concerted
advocacy compelled governments to act. This was further encouraged by
revelations of the extent to which the tobacco industry had concealed its
knowledge about the harmful effects of tobacco (see Chapter 7 for the
role of evidence in policy).

Currently, there is an unresolved struggle of ideas and material interests between the gambling industry, and public health researchers and
advocates about the harms of gambling and whether gambling should be
considered ('framed') as a public health issue rather than a matter of personal consumption (van Schalkwyk et al. 2021). Up to now, the gambling
industry has been largely successful in keeping mandatory regulation off
the policy agenda of most governments.

Who sets the agenda?

In the rest of this chapter you will explore how the main actors in the policy
process, particularly the government and the media, put issues or keep
issues on the policy agenda. Since government policy making is covered in
Chapter 3 and the business community, the medical profession and other
interest groups are covered in Chapter 4, more time will be spent here on
the role of the media than any of the other actors in agenda setting. Furthermore, in most circumstances, the media's primary role in policy making
is likely to be in helping to set the policy agenda by shaping and structur-
ing issues rather than in other aspects of the process. However, it must be
recognized that business interests can be very influential in keeping issues
off the policy agenda or delaying them reaching the agenda (see above)
and that business interests, media and politicians may pursue agendas
which may not be in the wider interests of the public. They frame public
health issues in ways that favour their interests, for example, portraying
them as matters of individual responsibility and choice rather than societal
and regulatory action.

✏ **Activity 5.8**

From what you know, how would you say alcohol and its use and misuse are framed by the drinks industry in contrast to how the same issues are presented by public health advocates in order to shape the policy agenda? How different is the presentation of gambling by the gambling industry?

Feedback

The alcohol industry and its lobbyists tend to frame alcohol consumption as a much valued, enjoyable part of everyday life and alcohol abuse as harmful use by a small group of susceptible or ignorant individuals. Public health practitioners would tend to frame alcohol as a powerful legal drug that causes extensive social harm and which should be tackled through population-wide measures rather than by targeting individuals. They would tend to favour government regulation (e.g. raising the price of drinks through taxation) while the industry would tend to favour voluntary codes encouraging responsible drinking (e.g. by putting sensible drinking advice on posters advertising alcoholic drinks). The gambling industry encourages a very similar framing of gambling as a normal, fun activity.

Donors and global philanthropy

Control of financial resources is generally the main way in which public or philanthropic external donors influence the policy agenda and priorities of poor countries (Khan et al. 2018). In the field of global health and development, private charitable donors have come to the fore as agenda setters, particularly in relation to poor countries and their governments due to the relatively large resources they control with limited or no external accountability. The Bill & Melinda Gates Foundation, for instance, is increasingly recognized as both influencing the process and, in some cases, setting the global health agenda through the size of its annual disbursements. The Foundation has advocated and invested in its own ambitious strategies to eradicate polio and malaria rather than supporting more conventional prevention and control programmes. Critics argue that the Foundation is inappropriately altering the international priority given to different diseases and responses.

Governments as agenda setters

Governments, particularly of large, wealthy countries, can be very influential in setting the international policy agenda. For example, PEPFAR, the United States President's Emergency Plan for AIDS Relief, US President

George W. Bush's initiative to combat the global epidemic of HIV, actively promoted its 'ABC' ('abstain, be faithful and use a condom') strategy for HIV prevention within the international public health community and high-prevalence countries, particularly in sub-Saharan Africa, in the face of criticism from many experts and activists. It was able to do so because of the large sums of money it was making available for HIV prevention and the conditions it applied to the use of these funds.

Within their own countries, governments are plainly crucial agenda set-ters since they control or at least shape the legislative process and often initiate policy change. The detailed institutional arrangements within dif-ferent countries affect the power of government (the executive) to set and control the agenda (see Chapter 3). For example, in the United States, the committees of Congress (the lower house of representatives) have the right to bring proposals to a vote by the legislature. The president as leader of the executive cannot do so in the same way. By contrast, in the British Parliament, the government (the executive) largely initiates and controls this process, giving it much greater influence over the policy agenda and eventual legislation.

Because there are always more issues competing for attention than governments can attend to at any one time, why would any government pursue an active programme of issue search – looking for items to go on the policy agenda? Hogwood and Gunn (1984) argue that governments *should* do so because they need to anticipate problems before they occur in order to minimize any adverse consequences or avert a potential crisis. Perhaps the most obvious reasons for engaging in issue search lie in the external environment such as demography, disease, climate change and technology. In almost all countries, the growing numbers and proportion of older people in the population have to be considered in setting health policy in areas such as paying for services, long-term care of frail people and the management of chronic diseases. New technical solutions become available to old problems such as linking patients' records kept by differ-ent providers. New problems begin to assume clear contours such as the potential effect of climate change on food supply and on public health. As well as serving the elected government of the day, one of the functions of a responsible civil service is to provide reports identifying and drawing long-term policy issues to the attention of ministers, such as the effects of global warming. However, there is no guarantee that the government of the day will wish to respond to what it may perceive to be an issue that its successors can deal with or a highly uncertain threat to health which may never come about.

There is also the cost of putting issues on the agenda and then acting on them, which may act as a deterrent. For example, provision of PPE for health care staff for use during a potential future pandemic was on the UK policy agenda to the extent that the stockpile was reviewed a few years before COVID-19, but it was decided not to update or increase the stockpile on the grounds that it would be too costly given the uncertainty surrounding its ever needing to be used and the overall financial situation. The UK was not alone in having insufficient PPE at the start of the pandemic. By contrast, in the wake of the severe acute respiratory syndrome epidemic in 2003 and the avian flu outbreak in 2008, a number of Asian countries had either maintained their stocks or had plans rapidly to increase local production of PPE (Feinmann 2021).

The media as agenda setters

How far and in which circumstances do the mass media guide attention to certain issues and influence what we think about and what ends up on the government's agenda? How much influence do they have on policy makers in their choice of issues of political concern and action? What role do social media play? How does their contribution differ from conventional mass media?

The conventional mass media serve a range of vital functions: they are sources of information; they function as propaganda mechanisms; they are agents of socialization (transmitting a society's culture and instructing people in the values and norms of society); and they serve as agents of legitimacy, generating mass belief in, and acceptance of, dominant political and economic institutions such as democracy and capitalism. They can also criticize the way societies and governments operate, bringing new perspectives to the public. In the past, the role of the media tended to be underestimated in policy making. However, the conventional mass media such as television, radio and newspapers have had a major influence over many years on governments' policy agendas through their ability to raise and shape, if not determine, issues and public opinion which, in turn, influences governments to respond.

The way the mass media function is shaped by the political system. In some countries, newspapers and television stations are entirely state-owned and censor themselves, fearing government reprisals for covering issues in a way that might be considered inappropriate, thereby prejudicing their impartiality. In others, media are notionally independent of the state, but editors and journalists are intimidated, gaoled, expelled or worse – a notable example being Jamal Khashoggi – a critical Saudi journalist who was murdered by the Saudi Arabian state in Turkey in 2018. The Internet and satellite broadcasting are less easy for individual regimes to influence or undermine than television and radio, which are easier to control, though the Chinese state actively censors the Internet. Even in liberal democracies, the mass media may be controlled in more or less subtle ways beyond simple ownership. Governments, increasingly concerned about their image in the media, can favour certain more co-operative broadcasters over others, giving them exclusive news stories and advance warning of policy announcements to boost their viewer numbers in return for generally favourable coverage – for example, former US President Donald Trump's close relationship with Fox News and dismissive attitude towards more critical media.

Most mass media organizations are part of large conglomerates with a wide range of media interests in many countries. Some of the best known are owned by business magnates, such as the late Silvio Berlusconi (who was also Italian prime minister) and Rupert Murdoch. Their personal political values (almost entirely on the political Right) and their commercial goals shape the orientation of the news reporting and political commentary provided by their television channels and newspapers without the proprietors necessarily having to direct their journalists on a day-to-day basis. Most commercial media are also dependent to some degree on advertising. Taken together, the pattern of ownership and the requirements of advertisers mean that in most countries the majority of newspapers and television stations adopt broadly right-of-centre, pro-capitalist, political positions. Advertisers and commercial interests can also, on occasions, influence the content of media directly – for example, through the sponsorship of newspapers and the placement of articles in the press apparently written by neutral journalists but intended to promote the industry's interests (e.g. enthusiastic reports of the latest pharmaceutical innovation). Politicians and powerful media actors often become unhealthily enmeshed in compromising personal relationships – for instance, former UK Prime Minister Tony Blair is the godfather to one of Rupert Murdoch's daughters.

Despite being largely controlled by the state and major commercial interests, the media can, sometimes, put an issue on the policy agenda which researchers or interest groups unconnected with the state or business are concerned about. For example, *The Guardian* newspaper in the UK is unusual in being able to pursue independent investigations (e.g. into the Edward Snowden files that revealed evidence of the US National Security Agency's mass electronic surveillance), often in the face of government or commercial resistance, because it is owned by Guardian Media Group, with one shareholder – the Scott Trust – which exists to secure its financial and editorial independence in perpetuity.

One of the most notable campaigns on an unjustly neglected issue in the UK was the *Sunday Times'* successful campaign in the 1970s to win higher compensation for children with birth defects after their mothers had taken the tranquillizer thalidomide to control their nausea in pregnancy. The newspaper's researchers succeeded in showing that the risk of congenital malformations had been foreseeable (Karpf 1988).

By contrast, in liberal democracies, the conventional mass media generally acts ideologically to contribute to reproducing and reinforcing the capitalist economic order (see Chapter 2). Under more authoritarian regimes, the role of the media in maintaining the status quo is more explicit. For example, state-controlled television remains the main source of information and news for the majority of Russians, especially older people, and voices little or no criticism of the regime.

The arrival of social media in the 2000s has both amplified and made more complicated the role of media, most obviously because of the huge volume of largely unregulated information and opinion propagated globally at low cost by a vast range of groups and individuals driven by every conceivable material and ideational interest. Unlike mass media, the amount of content on social media platforms, together with producers' ability to target particular demographic groups and consumers' ability to select their own content, has led to 'narrow casting'. As a result, different groups in society can exist in separate 'echo chambers' in which their prejudices are amplified and their assumptions never questioned. The rise of extreme political partisanship and increasingly divergent views within countries has been linked to these 'echo chambers'. Social media have enabled the mobilization and channelling of public opinion to governments and sometimes to big corporates in ways that they cannot easily predict or control, but which they may have to respond to in some way (e.g. the #MeToo international campaign against sexual harassment of, and violence against, women). Electronic media such as more conventional websites, blogs, social networking sites like Facebook and different forms of messaging from short message service (SMS) to Twitter are now also used by governments and interest groups to target different demographic groups, the former to justify their policies, the latter to promote their arguments. One consequence of the increase in media platforms is that different sub-groups in the population tend to choose different news and information sources that reinforce their beliefs. There are concerns that this is leading to greater political polarization. Authoritarian governments attempt to shut down social media if they provide a platform for political opponents, as in Putin's Russia.

In many respects, use of new media has lowered the cost of entry into policy debate enabling a wider range of groups to have a voice (e.g. via Twitter). A good example is Avaaz (meaning 'voice' in several languages), which has used the internet since 2007 to organize political campaigns on the issues its millions of members (70 million in 194 countries in 2022, according to its website, www.avaaz.org) judge to be important. Each year, Avaaz sets overall priorities through all-member polls and tests ideas for specific campaigns using weekly polls of 10,000 members drawn at random. Issues that find a strong response at 'tipping-point moments of crisis and opportunity' become large-scale campaigns. Avaaz claims that hundreds of thousands of its members can take part in signing petitions, funding media campaigns and direct actions, emailing, calling and lobbying governments, and organizing protests within days or even hours.

There have been calls for both mass and social media to become more responsible in their coverage of public health issues. Research in the UK on media coverage of health issues shows that the amount of news coverage of a topic is unrelated to the risk posed to the public health

(Harrabin et al. 2003) and, indeed, the diseases with the lowest risk to population health frequently received the highest level of coverage and vice versa. For example, coverage of vCJD, or mad cow disease in humans, bore no relationship to its extreme rarity. Yet, as the same research showed, politicians changed their priorities in response to media coverage rather than on the basis of the scientific evidence of what was in the best interest for public health. The same is true in other countries.

During the COVID-19 pandemic, public health experts criticized the social media companies for tolerating or failing to remove a huge amount of misinformation and 'fake news' about all aspects of the pandemic and its response, including conspiracy theories that the pandemic was a hoax designed to enable governments and global figures such as Bill Gates to increase surveillance and control of people, exaggeration of the probability of harms from COVID-19 vaccines, promotion of bogus cures and preventive measures against the virus, etc. While misinformation clearly affected the views and behaviour of millions of people, and some was propagated by governments themselves, overall, it had little impact on the policies of governments and global health organizations except to stimulate them into mounting campaigns to counter misinformation (the term '*infodemic*' was coined and often used by WHO leadership and staff). In addition, there is some evidence that public trust in mainstream mass media rose during the pandemic as people increasingly sought reliable, responsible sources of information to help them make sense of the cacophony emanating from social media.

Overall, the extent of direct media influence on government policy makers is open to question. Policy makers have many different sources of information and can use the media themselves to draw attention to a particular issue rather than the other way around. For example, often, the contents of government press releases will be reported verbatim by busy journalists. Concerted action by the press may make a difference, but in a competitive media environment, there is unlikely to be a unified view of an issue and the news media particularly are always looking for novelty.

It is difficult to separate different strands of influence shaping what gets onto the agenda. This is because the media are both part of the process itself and outside it, and they are not alone in shaping the agenda. Mostly, the conventional mass media highlight movements that have started elsewhere – that is, they help to delineate an issue, but they do not necessarily create it. For example, in the late 2000s, the mass media in most European countries helped raise concern about the need for government action to protect the population from the potential harm of an impending pandemic of swine flu. Yet, when it became apparent that the outbreak was less severe than predicted, the media in some countries switched their attention to highlighting government overreaction in the shape of unused vaccine stocks. They also accused the pharmaceutical industry of exaggerating the pandemic threat for profit. Interestingly, the swine flu pandemic led journalists and editors to question and criticize their own behaviour. They had been the targets of widely followed social media posts accusing mainstream media of exaggerating the risks of swine flu in the early stages of the pandemic. At each stage, mass and social media were following events while also shaping their interpretation and thus people's reactions to events, in a context of high epidemiological uncertainty about the course of the virus. As Nerlich and Koteyko (2012: 716) put it, 'media do not simply transmit and translate expert knowledge to lay publics but are an important and active (even self-critical and reflexive) player'.

Just as there are examples of the media inspiring policy shifts, so there are clear examples of politicians and their officials resisting media pressure to change policy. The controversy over the combined mumps, measles and rubella (MMR) vaccine is a good example of the latter (see Chapter 7). It showed how the mass media can provide a misleading picture of the relative weight of scientific evidence on a public health issue. While the vast majority of scientific evidence indicated that the MMR vaccine did not cause any significant harm, the sceptics' voices were heard relatively loudly in the mass media, perhaps because they injected drama and controversy into what could have been a relatively dull public health discussion (Boyce 2007).

So, there are no simple answers to questions such as: how much do the mass and social media influence public opinion and/or policy makers? The content of the policy issue, the political context and the process by which the debate unfolds and the policy issue is decided, all have a bearing on how influential the various forms of media will be. It is clear, however, that media framing makes an issue comprehensible in a particular way to a large number of people. It can shape the boundaries of public policy debate and identify who is or is not a legitimate commentator or participant in the debate. It opens up some policy solutions while effectively ruling out others (Hawkins and Holden 2013)

Summary

You have learned about the wide range of actors involved in agenda setting but that governments are usually central to the process. The policy agenda may change at times of crisis or through 'politics-as-usual'. A crisis will have to be perceived as such by policy elites and officials close to them, and they will have to believe that failure to act will make the situation worse. In 'politics-as-usual', many different problems and reforms compete continuously for policy makers' attention. Which ones reach the policy agenda will depend on a number of factors, including who is likely to gain and who lose in the change. Each of the three theoretical approaches to explaining the agenda setting process described in this chapter starts from the observation that objective indicators of the nature of a problem and evidence about possible solutions play a part, but far from fully determine why some issues get onto the policy agenda and attract high priority. The prominence of an issue is a product of how well actors in the relevant policy community work together, construct a persuasive account of the issue and its solution, and take advantage of opportunities to draw attention to the issue. Thus, timing is important. The media can be important for drawing attention to issues and encouraging governments to act but this is more likely in relation to 'low politics' issues. On major, or 'high politics' topics (such as economic policy or threats to national security), the media tend to shape and structure issues rather than bringing them to attention in the first place.

Further reading

Koon, A.D., Hawkins, B. and Mayhew, S.H. (2016) Framing and the health policy process: a scoping review, *Health Policy and Planning*, 31: 801–16. https://doi.org/10.1093/heapol/czv128

Rossa-Roccor, V., Giang, A. and Kershaw, P. (2021) Framing climate change as a human health issue: enough to tip the scale in climate policy?, *Lancet Planetary Health*, 5: e553–9. https://doi.org/10.1016/S2542-5196(21)00113-3

Shiffman, J. (2007) Generating political priority for maternal mortality reduction in 5 developing countries, *American Journal of Public Health*, 97: 796–803. https://doi.org/10.2105/AJPH.2006.095455

Shiffman, J. and Smith, S. (2007) Generation of political priority for global health initiatives: a framework and case study of maternal mortality, *Lancet*, 370: 1370–9. https://doi.org/10.1016/S0140-6736(07)61579-7

Stone, D. (2002) *Policy Paradox: The Art of Political Decision Making*, revised edn. New York: W.W. Norton, Part III (Chapters 6–10).

References

Bachrach, P. and Baratz, M.S. (1963) Decisions and nondecisions: an analytical framework, *American Political Science Review*, 57: 641–51.

Baker, P., Hawkes, C., Wingrove, K. et al. (2018) What drives political commitment for nutrition? A review and framework synthesis to inform the United Nations Decade of Action on Nutrition, *BMJ Global Health*, 3: e000485. http://dx.doi.org/10.1136/bmjgh-2017-000485

Berger, P.L. and Luckmann, T. (1975) *The Social Construction of Reality: A Treatise on the Sociology of Knowledge.* Harmondsworth: Penguin.

Boyce, T. (2007) *Health, Risk and News: The MMR Vaccine and the Media*. New York: Peter Lang.

Birkland, T.A. (2020) *An Introduction to the Policy Process: Theories, Concepts and Models of the Public Policy Process*, 5th edn. Routledge: New York and Abingdon, Chapter 6, pp. 205–46.

Cairney, P. (2007) A 'multiple lenses' approach to policy change: the case of tobacco policy in the UK, *British Politics*, 2: 45–68. https://doi.org/10.1057/palgrave.bp.4200039

Colombini, M., Mayhew, S.H., Hawkins, B. et al. (2016) Agenda setting and framing of gender-based violence in Nepal: how it became a health issue, *Health Policy and Planning*, 31(4): 493–503. https://doi.org/10.1093/heapol/czv091

Feinmann, J. (2021) What happened to our national emergency stockpiles?, *British Medical Journal*, 375: n2849. http://dx.doi.org/10.1136/bmj.n2849

Geneau, R., Stuckler, D., Stachenko, S. et al. (2010) Raising the priority of preventing chronic diseases: a political process, *Lancet*, 376: 1689–98. https://doi.org/10.1016/S0140-6736(10)61414-6

Grindle, M.S. and Thomas, J.W. (1991) *Public Choices and Policy Change: The Political Economy of Reform in Developing Countries*. Baltimore, OH: Johns Hopkins University Press.

Hall, P., Land, H., Parker, R. and Webb, A. (1975) *Change, Choice and Conflict in Social Policy*. London: Heinemann.

Harrabin, R., Coote, A. and Allen, J. (2003) *Health in the News: Risk, Reporting and Media Attention.* London: Kings Fund.

Hawkins, B. and Holden, C. (2013) Framing the alcohol policy debate: industry actors and the regulation of the UK beverage alcohol market, *Critical Policy Studies*, 7: 53–71. http://dx.doi.org/10.1080/19460171.2013.766023

Hogan, M., Foreman, K.J., Naghavi, M. et al. (2010) Maternal mortality for 181 countries, 1980–2008: a systematic analysis of progress towards Millennium Development Goal 5, *Lancet*, 375: 1609–23.

Hogwood, B. and Gunn, L. (1984) *Policy Analysis for the Real World*. Oxford: Oxford University Press.

Karpf, A. (1988) *Doctoring the Media*. London: Routledge.

Khan, M.S., Durrance-Bagale, A., Legido-Quigley, H. et al. (2019) 'LMICs as reservoirs of AMR': a comparative analysis of policy discourse on antimicrobial resistance with reference to Pakistan, *Health Policy and Planning*, 34: 178–87.

Khan, M.S., Meghani, A., Liverani, M. et al. (2018) How do external donors influence national health policy processes? Experiences of domestic policy actors in Cambodia and Pakistan, *Health Policy and Planning*, 33: 215–23.

Kingdon, J. (2013) *Agendas, Alternatives and Public Policies.* Updated edition with an epilogue on health care. Pearson New International Edition, 2nd edn. London: Pearson, Longman Classics.

Kohlt, F.E. (2020) 'Over by Christmas': the impact of war-metaphors and other science-religion narratives on science communication environments during the Covid-19 crisis. SocArXiv. Preprint, 10 November. https://doi.org/10.31235/osf.io/z5s6a

Nerlich, B. and Koteyko, N. (2012) Crying wolf? Biosecurity and metacommunication in the context of the 2009 swine flu pandemic, *Health & Place*, 18(4): 710–17. https://doi.org/10.1016/j.healthplace.2011.02.008

Parkhurst, J.O. and Vulimiri, M. (2013) Cervical cancer and the global health agenda: insights from multiple policy-analysis frameworks, *Global Public Health*, 8: 1093–1108. https://doi.org/10.1080/17441692.2013.850524

Rushing, W. (1995) *The AIDS Epidemic: Social Dimensions of an Infectious Disease.* Boulder, CO: Westview Press.

Shiffman, J. (2007) Generating political priority for maternal mortality reduction in five developing countries, *American Journal of Public Health*, 97: 796–803.

Shiffman, J., Quissell, K., Schmitz, H.P. et al. (2016) A framework on the emergence and effectiveness of global health networks, *Health Policy and Planning*, 31: i3–16. https://doi.org/10.1093/heapol/czu046

Shiffman, J. and Shawar, Y.R. (2022) Framing and the formation of global health priorities, *Lancet* 399: 1977–90.

Shiffman, J. and Smith, S. (2007) Generation of political priority for global health initiatives: a framework and case study of maternal mortality, *Lancet*, 370: 1370–9.

Smith, K.A. (2013) *Beyond Evidence Based Policy in Public Health: The Interplay of Ideas.* Basingstoke: Palgrave Macmillan.

Townsend, B., Schram, A., Baum, F. et al. (2020) How does policy framing enable or constrain inclusion of social determinants of health?, *Critical Public Health*, 30: 115–26. https://doi.org/10.1080/09581596.2018.1509059

van Hulst, M. and Yanow, D. (2016) From policy 'frames' to 'framing': theorizing a more dynamic, political approach, *The American Review of Public Administration*, 46(1): 92–112. https://doi.org/10.1177/0275074014533142

van Schalkwyk, M.C.I., Petticrew, M., Cassidy, R. et al. (2021) A public health approach to gambling regulation: countering powerful influences, *Lancet Public Health*, 6: e614–19. https://doi.org/10.1016/ S2468-2667(21)00098-0

Walt, G. and Gilson, L. (2014) Can frameworks inform knowledge about health policy processes? Reviewing health policy papers on agenda setting and testing them against a specific priority-setting framework, *Health Policy and Planning*, 29: iii6–22. https://doi.org/10.1093/heapol/czu081

Policy implementation

6

It will now be apparent that the policy process is complex and interactive: many groups and organizations at local, national and global levels try to influence what gets onto the policy agenda and how policies are formulated. Yet policy making does not come to an end once a course of action has been determined. It cannot be assumed that a policy will be implemented as intended since decision makers typically depend on other actors as well as resources and other contextual factors to see their policies turned into action. This chapter describes and analyses processes of implementation and the ways these have been studied by policy scholars including a focus on 'implementation science' over recent years.

Learning objectives

After working through this chapter, you will be better able to:

- contrast 'top-down' and 'bottom-up' theories of policy implementation
- understand other approaches to analysing policy implementation including those that attempt to synthesize insights from both 'top-down' and 'bottom-up' perspectives
- identify some of the tensions affecting implementation between international bodies and national governments, and between central and local authorities within countries (Chapter 10 also discusses these issues)
- understand the principal–agent problem in policy implementation and the development of New Public Management (NPM) designed to sharpen policy implementation
- describe some of the factors that facilitate or impede the implementation of policies and how policy goals can be shifted by 'street level bureaucrats'.

Key terms

Bottom-up approach to understanding policy implementation Approach to explaining policy implementation that focuses on how local actors and contextual factors influence policy implementation.

Implementation   Process of turning a policy into practice or action.

Implementation gap   Difference between what the policy architect intended and the end-result of a policy.

Implementation science   The study of methods and approaches designed to embed evidence-informed policies, programmes and practices in regular use.

Policy instrument   One of the range of options at the disposal of the policy maker in order to give effect to a policy goal (e.g. privatization, regulation, subsidy, etc.).

Principal–agent theory   Theory of organizational and government behaviour that focuses on the relationship between principals (e.g. purchasers) and their agents (e.g. providers), together with the contracts or agreements that enable the principal to specify what is to be done (e.g. service provision) and check that this has been accomplished.

Street-level bureaucrats   Frontline staff involved in delivering public services to members of the public who have some discretion and agency in how they apply the objectives of policies handed down to them.

Top-down approach to understanding policy implementation   Sees policy implementation as a linear, rational process in which policy initiated at higher levels of the policy system (e.g. national government) is subsequently executed at subordinate levels.

Upstream interventions   Policies involving collective action that focus on structural change in society, with the potential to affect large groups of people, for example, government regulation.

Introduction

Implementation has been defined as 'what happens between policy expectations and (perceived) policy results' (DeLeon 1999 ; Ferman, Barbara 1990). Until the 1970s, policy scientists had tended to focus their attentions on the agenda setting, policy formulation and decision-making 'stages' of the policy process (see Chapter 1 for an overview of these 'stages' and Chapters 3, 4 and 5 for analyses of agenda setting and policy formulation shaped by interests within and outside government). As you will recall, while the notion of there being formal 'stages' is far from the messy reality of most policy processes, it remains a useful device for drawing attention to different activities and actors, and for organizing the collection of data about policy.

For many years, the changes that followed policy decisions had been relatively neglected. However, it became increasingly apparent that many public policies had not worked in practice as well as their proponents had hoped. A series of studies in the late 1960s of anti-poverty programmes, initially in the US, led to an increasing focus by practitioners and analysts on showing the effects of policies and explaining why their consequences were often not as planned (Pressman and Wildavsky 1984). Throughout the 1980s, 1990s and into the new century, many governments and policy scholars focused more closely on the challenges of making policy 'work' in tandem with the increasingly influential evidence-based policy (EBP) and NPM movements of the period (Nilsen et al. 2013).

It has become commonplace to observe an *'implementation gap'* between what was planned and what occurred. For instance, consider the policy of routine vaccination programmes such as MMR for children or seasonal influenza for adults. In England, routine vaccinations are delivered by primary care general practitioners (GPs). A study by Crocker-Buque et al. (2018) explored why some GP practices are more successful in implementing routine vaccinations than other GP practices. The study found that whilst the clinical elements of vaccine delivery were very similar across GP practices, the administrative elements were very different. Some GP practices were much more effective in systematically sending reminders to patients to encourage them to attend appointments. Another factor in increasing implementation of routine vaccination programmes related to staff management and task allocation practices – essentially, ensuring that the right staff are able to use their skills in the most effective ways at the most valuable times.

As demonstrated in the example above, and as you will see later in this chapter, implementation is often linked to issues of administration and management in health policy. However, implementation is also linked to wider political and cultural issues. Staying with the example of vaccination, extensive international media coverage of one small study from 1998 published in the *Lancet* of the potential risk of autism associated with receiving the MMR vaccination led to many parents refusing to have their children vaccinated. A subsequent systematic review of the evidence proved that the link between autism and MMR was almost certainly non-existent and the article itself was eventually retracted by the *Lancet*. Despite the retraction and abundant evidence about the safety of MMR vaccination, more than two decades on, a third of Americans falsely believe that childhood vaccines can lead to children developing autism (Motta and Stekula 2021). This further exacerbates the implementation gap in relation to routine vaccinations as some parents remain wary about the possible side effects of the vaccine so may refuse to have their children vaccinated.

If routine policies such as vaccination remain difficult to implement, you can imagine that more ambitious, larger-scale ones such as the United

Nations Millennium Development Goals of 2000 and the subsequent SDGs of 2015, which set out a global vision for health and societal improvement, are likely to suffer from implementation challenges. They also relate to the links between global, regional and national policy, as discussed further in Chapter 10.

Across many countries, the past 30 years have witnessed the development of systems that increase the likelihood that government policies will be implemented in the way that ministers intended and that provide information on the impact of policies. 'Delivery units' for instance, are small teams that support policy implementation working for national or local policy makers through close data monitoring and troubleshooting. These have proliferated globally with some impressive results – for instance, improving childhood immunization rates in the Punjab region of Pakistan and helping reduce infant mortality in Maryland, US (Gold 2017).

 Activity 6.1

Think about some of the challenges and opportunities in relation to delivering SDG3 (*Ensure healthy lives and promote well-being for all at all ages*). What kinds of obstacles might ministries of health face in implementing policies to attain such a goal?

Feedback

There are a range of reasons that may include:

- limited government capacities – including lack of resources for staffing and staff training;
- shifting government goals and priorities that may reduce the importance of SDG3 for policy makers at some times;
- scale of the ambition leading to difficulties knowing how and where to start;
- unforeseen confounding issues such as COVID-19, or the impacts of global instability such as war;
- achievement of this target depending on wide-ranging action in sectors other than health such as employment, commerce, etc.;
- difficulty of measuring progress when not all countries have data to populate indicators of progress;
- misalignment between external donor interests and those of local actors – for example, national experts may not agree with the global priorities their leaders signed up to.

Early approaches to explaining policy implementation

'Top-down' approaches

'*Top-down*' approaches to understanding and thereby, it is hoped, improving policy implementation are closely allied with the rational model of the policy process, which sees policy making as a linear sequence of activities in which there is a clear division between policy formulation and policy execution (implementation). The former is seen as explicitly political and the latter as a largely technical, administrative or managerial activity. Policies set at a national or international level are communicated to subordinate levels (e.g. health authorities, hospitals, clinics, the community), which are then charged with putting them into practice. The 'top-down' approach was developed by policy analysts in the 1960s and 1970s focusing on the 'implementation deficit' or 'gap' to provide policy makers with a better understanding of what systems they needed to put in place to minimize the 'gap' between aspiration and reality (i.e. to make the process approximate more closely to the rational ideal from a policy maker's perspective). These studies were empirical attempts to understand and explain implementation but also included more normative recommendations for change. Thus, according to Pressman and Wildavsky (1984), the key to effective implementation lay in the ability to devise a system in which the causal links between setting goals and the successive actions designed to achieve them were clear and robust. Goals had to be clearly defined and widely understood, the necessary political, administrative, technical and financial resources had to be available, a chain of command had to be established from the centre to the periphery, and a communication and control system had to be in place to keep the whole system on course. Failure was caused by adopting the wrong strategy and using the wrong machinery. Much of this early work focused on implementation *failure* – sometimes being labelled 'misery research' (Nilsen et al. 2013). It is worth noting that much of the initial policy implementation research was conducted in the pluralist democratic political context of the US in the second half of the twentieth century. It for the most part did not lead to similar studies testing the applicability of these insights to LMICs or non-democratic or more autocratic political systems.

In a similar vein to Pressman and Wildavsky (1984), Sabatier and Mazmanian (1979) devised a list of six necessary and sufficient conditions for effective policy implementation, indicating that if these conditions were realized policy should be implemented largely as intended:

1. Clear and logically consistent objectives.
2. Adequate causal theory (i.e. a valid theory as to how particular actions would lead to the desired outcomes).

152

Making Health Policy

3. An implementation process structured to enhance compliance by implementers (e.g. appropriate incentives and sanctions to influence subordinates in the required way).
4. Committed, skilful implementing officials.
5. Support from interest groups and the legislature.
6. No changes in socio-economic conditions that undermine political support or the causal theory underlying the policy.

Proponents of this approach argued that it could distinguish empirically between failed and successful implementation processes, and thereby could provide useful guidance to policy makers in the future. Its most obvious weakness was that the first condition was rarely fulfilled in that most public policies have fuzzy, potentially inconsistent objectives. In addition, it is also very hard to fulfil all the criteria. A further criticism of the top-down approach in general is that it fails to adequately account for different contexts. For example, to return to the routine vaccinations example from earlier in this chapter, Crocker-Buque et al. (2018) demonstrated that it is hard in practice for policy makers to ensure that the third and fourth conditions can be met in practice as different GP practices, to use another example from health care policy, face different challenges depending upon local administrative systems, staffing mix, resource allocation and other work objectives notwithstanding patient attitudes and motivation. In essence – local contextual factors may mean that despite the best efforts of 'committed, skilful implementing officials' implementation may still not be achieved.

Activity 6.2

Given what you know already about policy in the health field, what criticisms would you level at the 'top-down' perspective to understanding implementation? How good an explanation of policy implementation does it offer, in your opinion?

Feedback

The main criticisms of the 'top-down' approach to the analysis of implementation were that:

- it gives too much weight to the perspective of central decision makers (those at the top of any hierarchy or directly involved in initial policy formulation) and not enough to the role and perspectives of other actors (e.g. NGOs, professional bodies, the private sector, communities) and factors shaping the behaviour of people at other levels in the implementation process (e.g. regional health authorities, front-line staff, patients) when designing implementation plans;

- as an analytical approach, it risks over-estimating the impact of government action on a problem compared with other social and economic factors;
- it is difficult to apply in situations where there is no single, dominant policy or lead agency involved – in many fields, there are multiple policies in play and a complex array of agencies implementing them;
- its distinction between policy decisions and subsequent implementation is analytically misleading since it ignored the possibility that policies might be changed as they were being implemented – and indeed in some cases, local adaptation is advantageous.

In essence, critics have argued that the reality of policy implementation was messier and more complex than even the most sophisticated 'top-down' approach could cope with and that the practical advice it generates on reducing the 'gap' between expectation and reality is, therefore, incomplete.

'Bottom-up' approaches

A number of 'bottom-up' approaches emerged throughout the 1980s and 1990s with a very different way of studying policy implementation and reaching different conclusions. The 'bottom-up' approach is rooted in an awareness that implementers often play an important function in implementation, not just as passive intermediaries to deliver policy handed down to them from above, but as active participants in a complex process that informs those higher up the system, and that policy should be made with this insight in mind. Even in highly centralized systems, studies show that subordinate agencies and their staff possess some power. The subordinate implementers often change the way a policy is implemented and, in the process, may even end up redefining the objectives of the policy.

One of the most influential studies in the development of the 'bottom-up' analytical perspective on implementation was by Lipsky (1980), who looked at the behaviour of what he termed 'street-level bureaucrats' in relation to their clients. These included frontline staff administering social welfare benefits, social workers, teachers, local government officials, doctors and nurses. His research suggested that even those working in the most rule-bound environments have some discretion in how they deal with their clients and that staff such as doctors, social workers and teachers have high levels of discretion, which enables them to get around the dictates of central policy and reshape policy for their own ends.

Lipsky's work helped re-conceptualize the policy implementation process, particularly in the delivery of health and social services, which is dependent on the actions of large numbers of professional staff, as a much more interactive, political process characterized by largely inescapable conflict and negotiation between interests and levels within policy systems. As a result, researchers began to focus their attention on the intermediate-level and local actors in the implementation process, their ideas, their goals, their strategies, their activities and their links to one another. Interestingly, 'bottom-up' studies showed that even in the rare situations where the conditions specified as necessary for the success of the 'top-down', rational model were in place (e.g. a strong chain of command, well-defined objectives, ample resources, and a communication and monitoring system), policies could be implemented in ways that policy makers had not intended. Indeed, well-meaning policies could make things worse, for example, by increasing staff workload so that they had to develop undesirable coping strategies (Wetherley and Lipsky 1977).

Studies of 'street-level bureaucrats' have provided useful insights about the realities of implementation across a wide range of settings. For example, Walker and Gilson (2004) studied how nurses in a busy urban primary health care clinic in South Africa experienced and responded to the implementation of the 1996 national policy of free care (removal of user fees). They showed that while the nurses approved of the policy of improving access in principle, they were negative towards it in practice because of the way it exacerbated existing problems in their working environment and increased their workload, without increasing staffing levels or the availability of drugs. The nurses were also dissatisfied because they felt that they had not been sufficiently included in the process of policy formulation. These findings were reinforced by further research showing that poor relationships and a lack of trust between mid-level managers and health workers can generate resistance to policies even when health workers stand to gain from a policy (Scott et al. 2011). The nurses in Walker and Gilson's (2004) study also believed that many patients abused the free system, and that some patients did not deserve free care because they were personally responsible for their own health problems. Such views were presumably at odds with the principles underlying the policy of free care and made nurses slow to grant free access to services to certain groups of patients. More recently, detailed international comparative research explored how street-level bureaucrats responded to the requirement to implement COVID-19 policy, highlighting the enduring utility of this as an analytical approach (Gofen and Lotta 2021). A recent study (see case study below) exploring agricultural policy and nutrition in Malawi has suggested an extension of the 'bottom-up' approach to understanding policy implementation from a focus not just on the role of *implementers* in shaping the policy process, but also the role of *those targeted by the policy* (Walls et al. unpublished manuscript).[1] Finally, bottom-up perspectives on policy implementation

---

1   Walls, H., Johnston, D., Matita, M. et al. The politics of agricultural policy and nutrition: a case study of Malawi's Farm Input Subsidy Programme (FISP). Unpublished manuscript, 2023.

are useful for highlighting the ways in which the relationships between central, regional and local agencies – and perhaps also those targeted by the policy – influence policy.

Agricultural policy and malnutrition in Malawi: exemplifying the role of *those targeted by the policy* in shaping policy implementation

Many LMICs, especially in sub-Saharan Africa, have invested in a potentially important *upstream* policy driver of food security and nutrition – agricultural input subsidy programmes (AISPs). AISPs are grants or loans given to farmers to reduce the cost of acquiring specific inputs used in agricultural production, such as inorganic fertilizer or hybrid seeds. These programmes have the aim of increasing agricultural productivity, household food security and the incomes of poor households. However, their impact is debated, and especially so in regard to their nutritional impacts.

Malawi's Farm Input Subsidy Programme (FISP), implemented between 2005 and 2020, was one of the most prominent AISPs globally. The FISP took up a large proportion (at times up to 75 per cent) of the Malawian government's agricultural budget. A mixed-methods study found little (if any) nutritional impact (Walls et al. 2023). To understand why, the researchers explored the political economy of the FISP and the policy processes shaping its potential nutritional impact. They did so by examining the perspectives of a range of actors, including those from central government health and agriculture departments as well as respondents from the rural farming communities targeted by the programme – and they draw on the kaleidoscope model (introduced in Chapter 1) for understanding policy change in LMIC contexts to examine the gap between FISP policy expectations and on-the-ground implementation.

The analysis (Walls et al. forthcoming) pointed to the way that on-the-ground decision making amongst the people targeted by a policy can critically influence its impact. In this case, the grassroots shaping of the policy outcomes was through the redistribution of coupons at community level. Policy makers had intended the coupons to be distributed to and used by randomly selected households. However, the study found, corroborating other studies of the FISP, a common practice of sharing and selling-on of coupons within communities. These practices potentially diluted the programme's effect.

In these poor rural communities, the coupons were often sold to wealthy farmers (potentially displacing the private purchase of fertilizer and seed). The coupons were sold to satisfy immediate financial needs – a priority to those targeted by the policy above longer-term use of the coupons as an input to agricultural production. The coupons were also often shared in the communities, sometimes between several households. Some participants spoke about the importance of this from an altruistic viewpoint.

Whilst targeting criteria had been developed and implemented by the central government to support identification of programme beneficiaries, the sharing of coupons suggests that such criteria are ignored where the maintenance of social cohesion is prioritized – in a context of severe poverty and food and nutrition security, with little in the way of mitigating social safety nets.

Some of these on-the-ground factors are driven by policy design, such as the limited number of coupons. However, the findings also reflect tensions between top-down and bottom-up policy implementation. Bottom-up understandings usually emphasize that policy implementers change a policy while implementing it – for example, see the identification in the kaleidoscope model of 'implementation veto players' who shape policy implementation. However, in this case, rather than it being the policy implementers who change the policy in its implementation, it was the intended beneficiaries themselves. Communities were using the programme in the way that best fitted their own needs, which included satisfying immediate financial concerns, as well as solidarity, provision of economic support and social cohesion. These needs are important for the community but not necessarily for the programme designers – central government. This consideration of the way that a policy is shaped by those it targets is an important extension to current models of policy implementation including the kaleidoscope model. It is also an important consideration for policy makers in sub-Saharan Africa and other regions considering AISP and other policy impact at the community level – and relates to the discussion in this chapter of the importance of local context and the co-production of knowledge and policy.

Activity 6.3

Write down in two columns the main differences between the 'top-down' and 'bottom-up' analytical approaches to understanding policy implementation. You might contrast the following aspects of the two approaches: where the analysis starts; how the main actors are identified; how the policy process is viewed; how the implementation process is evaluated; and the overall focus of the analysis.

Feedback

Your answer should have included some of the differences shown in Table 6.1.

Table 6.1 'Top-down' and 'bottom-up' approaches to analysing policy implementation

	Top-down approaches	Bottom-up approaches
Analytical starting point	Central government decision	Local implementation actors and networks of relationships.
Process for identification of major actors	From top-down and starting with government	From bottom-up, including both government and non-government actors, and potentially too those targeted by the policy.
View of the policy process	Largely rational, hierarchical process, proceeding from problem identification to policy formulation at higher levels to implementation at lower levels.	Interactive process involving policy makers and implementers from various parts and levels of govern- ment and outside, in which policy may change during implementation. Implementers are active participants in making policy, not just transmit- ters of policies made elsewhere.
Evaluative criteria	Extent of attainment of formal objectives rather than recogni- tion of unintended conse- quences.	Extent to which implementation processes are designed to consider local participants' views and influences on how policy unfolds.
Overall analytical focus	Designing the system to achieve what central/top policy makers intend – tends to focus on 'structure' and management (i.e. how systems and organizations can drive the implementation process using regulations, sanctions and incentives).	Recognition of strategic interaction among multiple actors in a policy network – focus on the culture and relationships between actors and their ability to shape their environ- ment and thus how policy unfolds.

Source: adapted and expanded from Sabatier (1986)

While the practical insights derived from the 'bottom-up' approach are likely to appeal to health care workers and middle-ranking officials because they bring their views and the constraints on their actions into view, the approach raises as many questions as the 'top-down' perspective both as an explanation of how policies are implemented and as a guide to action. One obvious question that both analytical approaches and their findings raise is whether the approach chosen by government to its policy making and particularly to implementation should be shaped predominantly by insights from the top-down or bottom-up perspective or some judicious mix of the two. Another question is how the divergence of views and goals between actors at different levels identified by 'bottom-up' analysis can or should be reconciled in practice. Specifically, in a democracy how much influence should unelected health professionals or managers, for example, have in shaping the eventual consequences of policies determined by elected governments? Should plans for policy implementation be equally informed by the perspectives and needs of, say, national policy makers and local implementers? And what of the role of those targeted by the policy themselves?

 Activity 6.4

Write down any other analytical drawbacks of the 'bottom-up' approach that you can think of.

Feedback

In addition to the value (normative) questions mentioned in the paragraph above, you could have listed:

- If policy is made largely through the process of its implementation as the bottom-up perspective indicates, then it becomes difficult to separate the influence of different levels of government and of elected politicians versus their subordinate staff on policy decisions and consequences. This is important for democratic and bureaucratic accountability.
- The approach risks under-emphasizing the indirect influence of higher levels of government in shaping the systems, structures and institutions within which lower-level actors operate and in giving them discretion over policy implementation.
- The approach may lead to divergent policy trends in different regions or locations with implications for equity across the population.

The list of drawbacks in the feedback above is a reminder that it pays to be cautious when judging one theory superior to another in such a complex field as policy. Most theory in policy science inevitably simplifies the complexity of any particular set of circumstances in order to bring greater understanding.

Other ways of understanding policy implementation influenced by economics and business management

The approaches discussed thus far have largely been developed by political scientists and sociologists. However, economists, management scholars, organizational psychologists and, in recent years, 'implementation scientists' have also been drawn to trying to explain why there are frequently gaps between policy intention and eventual outcomes, and how to reduce their scale and likelihood.

Principal–agent theory

Principal–agent theory focuses on the formal and informal contracts that constitute a system of policy implementation. From the principal–agent perspective, sub-optimal policy implementation is an inevitable result of the structure of modern government in which decision makers ('principals') at each level in the system have to delegate responsibility for the implementation of policies to 'agents' at the next level down who act on their behalf. Thus, ministers delegate responsibility to their officials (e.g. civil servants in the MoH) who, in turn, delegate to other 'agents' (e.g. managers, doctors and nurses in the health sector or private contractors) whom they only indirectly and incompletely control, and who are often difficult to monitor. These 'agents' have discretion in how they operate on behalf of their 'principals' and may not even see themselves as primarily engaged in making a reality of the wishes of their 'principals'. For example, publicly employed doctors may see themselves as members of the medical profession first and foremost rather than as public servants. Discretion opens up the potential for ineffective or inefficient translation of government intent into reality since 'agents' have their own views, ambitions, loyalties and resources which can hinder or alter policy implementation. The inherent problem for ministers is to get the compliance of their officials and others who are contracted to deliver services at all levels. The more levels of hierarchy there are, the more principal–agent relations there are, with each level dependent on the next level below, and the more complex the task of controlling the process of implementation.

The amount of discretion and the complexity of the principal–agent relationships are, in turn, affected by the following:

1. *The nature of the policy problem* – this can be, for example, macro versus sectoral or micro (affecting the scale of change required and size of the affected group), simple versus complex, ill-defined versus clear, with many causes versus a single cause, highly politically sensitive versus neutral politically, requiring a short or long period before impacts will become apparent, costly versus inexpensive and so on. In general, long-term, ill-defined, interdependent (goals affected by other policies and policy sectors), high-profile problems affecting large numbers of people

are far more difficult to deal with than short-term, specific issues with a single cause which are seen as largely technical rather than values driven. Most public policy debate focuses on the former, which are known, understandably, as 'wicked problems' or problems to which there is never likely to be an easy solution. A typical example would be how to balance the public desire to punish and deter criminals by giving them prison sentences with the evidence that prison does not help rehabilitate criminals and may even increase the odds of them reoffending.

2. *The context or circumstances surrounding the problem* – for example, the political situation, whether the economy is growing or not, the availability of resources and pace of technological change.

3. *The organization of the machinery required to implement the policy* – this includes the number of agencies and formal and informal relationships involved in making the desired change, and the skills and resources that have to be brought to bear.

✎ Activity 6.5

From the perspective of principal–agent theory, the three sets of factors listed above help explain why some policies are easier to implement than others. Take a health policy with which you are familiar and describe the nature of the problem, the context and the machinery required to implement the policy. Under each of the three headings, try to assess whether the factors you have listed are likely to make implementation of the policy easier or more difficult.

Feedback

Your answer will depend on the policy you chose to analyse. For example, if your chosen policy had simple technical features (e.g. introduction of a new drug), involved a marginal behavioural change (e.g. a minor change in dosage), could be implemented by one or a few actors (e.g. pharmacists acting alone), had clear, non-conflicting objectives (e.g. better symptom control with no cost implications) and could be executed in a short period of time (e.g. drugs were easy to source and distribute), you would be able to conclude that implementation *should* be relatively straightforward. Unfortunately, the majority of health policy issues and policies are more complex. Policy analysts are fond of contrasting the challenge of goals such as putting an astronaut on the moon with the stock-in-trade of public policy such as reducing poverty. The former was carried out in a tightly organized, influential, well-resourced organization focused on a single goal with a clear end point. The latter is driven by a large number of underlying causes, involves a wide range of agencies and actors and has inherently contestable objectives and means of achieving them (Howlett et al. 2009).

New Public Management: markets and performance payments

The insights of principal–agent theory led to a greater appreciation of the importance of the design of institutions and the choice of *policy instruments* for implementation, so that the 'top' had the information to monitor activities and hold to account the staff at 'street level' at reasonable cost. One aspect of this was a growing focus on the actual and implied *contracts* defining the relationships between principals and their agents in order to ensure that the principals' objectives were understood and followed by agents. From the 1980s, in a number of high-, middle- and low-income countries, the civil service and the wider public sector was reformed to make more explicit what officials were expected to deliver to elected officials and those they represent in return for their salaries and promotions. Multi-purpose ministries were restructured internally and new agencies outside these ministries, each with a smaller number of policy objectives, were set up with clear performance targets incorporated in contracts with the parent ministry. Performance indicators were used to assess whether their performance in meeting government objectives was improving or not. New payment systems were put in place such as paying hospitals for the number of treatments delivered, rather than giving them a fixed budget, with a view to improving implementation.

These developments were partly ideological and linked with the 'New Right' thinking of politicians such as President Reagan in the US and Prime Minister Thatcher in the UK. They were also linked to technological developments and the application of information technology to support data monitoring, audit and accountability. Better information flows encouraged a trend towards decentralization of parts of the decision-making function, from central to local levels, while reducing the number of tiers in the management hierarchy. In many jurisdictions, subordinate agents were given greater control over their own affairs on a day-to-day basis but, in return, were held more tightly accountable for the attainment of policy goals through the use of performance indicators. The theory was that this would free agents to pursue the objectives of their principals unfettered by unnecessary interference and allow principals to judge the performance of their agents objectively and remove from agents the excuse that their poor performance was the result of inappropriate interventions by principals.

As part of this process, the role of government as direct provider of services was critically reviewed in many countries with a view to improving the efficiency and responsiveness of services both to the objectives of ministers and the needs of citizens as consumers. The catchphrase of the reformers was that governments should be 'steering, rather than rowing' the ship of state (Osborne and Gaebler 1992). As a result, some services that had been directly provided in the public sector (e.g. by publicly owned hospitals) were contracted out to private for-profit or not-for-profit providers on the grounds that they would be better able to focus on delivering government policy objectives. The extent of such reform efforts varied internationally. Chile, New Zealand, the UK and US were at the forefront of many of these changes. Other countries – notably in continental Europe and Scandinavia, were less influenced by this intellectual fashion – maintaining higher levels of public service provision during this period (Pollitt and Bouckaert 2017). Internationally, the direct influence of NPM reforms was mixed, though influential global institutions such as the IMF, the World Bank and the WTO pursued what has been termed a 'neoliberal' reform agenda in many LMICs, which has similarities with elements of the NPM, exacerbating social inequality in many countries (Navarro 2007).

NPM thinking thus widened the range of policy instruments potentially available to governments to ensure the efficient delivery of goods and services, each entailing a differing scope of government involvement and of compulsion, as follows:

- *Information and persuasion* – this encourages changes in behaviour by providing non-mandatory guidance and feedback such as via performance indicators, clinical guidelines, training and programme evaluation.
- *Regulation* – this requires changes in behaviour by providing sanctions for those who do not comply with the regulations. Legislation is the most obvious form of regulation. Typical forms of regulation include licensing (e.g. of clinics and health professionals) and minimum standards (e.g. of nurse staffing levels), but others include redistribution such as through taxation, subsidy and reallocation of resources such as moving the clinical workforce from over-provided to under-provided geographic areas. Targets can be seen as a form of regulation if mandatory.
- *Public provision* – the government provides key public services itself or through publicly owned and directly managed agencies. This is particularly likely when the service has the features of a 'public good' (i.e. the benefits of the service accrue to everyone, and they depend on high population participation to be effective, such as defence and immunization).
- *Markets and market-like incentives* – these encourage behaviour change through using the incentives associated with markets such as introducing competition between different suppliers of public services where previously there was a public monopoly and allowing users greater choice of provider.

The NPM, as it became known, reflected the preference in mainstream economics for markets over other approaches to producing goods and services and the then fashionable public choice theory that the self-interested behaviour of voters, politicians and bureaucrats tends to lead to an increase in taxation, public spending and government activity, often unnecessarily and inefficiently, compared with the private sector (see Chapter 2). It was driven by economic critiques of policy implementation and the importation into the public sector of policy instruments and management techniques used in large private enterprises. Alongside the championing of *markets*, the NPM also called for greater *measurement* and more *managers* within public services including health services (Ferlie et al. 1996). As noted already, the reach and depth of NPM reforms internationally has been contested, though it is fair to say that these *three Ms* have increased in salience across most health systems over the past 30 years. In particular, market or market-like instruments (e.g. the separation of purchaser and providers within a publicly owned and financed health system or paying hospitals for the treatments they delivered) became more prominent in many countries leading to a more mixed set of policy instruments in sectors such as health. These included ways of giving patients more information and more choice over where and from whom they received their care. The supposition of reformers was that such arrangements would improve the implementation of policy designed to improve the efficiency and effectiveness of public services.

Another related, important policy instrument for service improvement allied to NPM thinking is performance-based funding, also known as payment for performance, or payment by results (PbR). In this approach a percentage of the revenue of a service provider is dependent on the achievement of pre-specified standards, targets, outputs or outcomes. The thinking behind this is that it will lead to improved services for users and the implementation of more effective practice since service providers will have to respond to the financial incentives or lose income.

PbR is well embedded into many health systems around the world. For instance, a proportion of the income received by general practices in the English NHS is linked to their performance in relation to a wide range of indicators, such as the proportion of their patients with normal blood pressure. Performance-based funding is also extensively used by a number of large development organizations, both public and philanthropic.

Given the challenge that principal–agent thinking and NPM posed for conventional ways of delivering public services, they have been extensively critiqued. The main criticisms in the health sector are that these reforms have increased administrative costs (e.g. associated with an increase in the number of specialized agencies, negotiating contracts, monitoring and managing performance, etc.); have focused disproportionately on efficiency of service delivery and aspects that can easily be measured and turned into targets (e.g. length of hospital stay) at the expense of other values such as humanity of care; and have led to fragmentation of services. D'Oliveira et al. (2020) argue that such reforms reduce the visibility of health issues where NPM has little to offer such as gender-based violence.

PbR has attracted significant critical attention, including in the health sector, since it embodies many of the limitations of principal–agent theory. It is very hard to design a perfect, or complete, contract between the principal and the agent that fully aligns the interests of each party. Poorly designed contracts may generate 'perverse incentives' and lead to 'creaming' (prioritizing those who are easiest to serve) and 'parking' (enrolling the neediest who attract the highest remuneration while offering them the least possible assistance). At the same time, there is good evidence that frontline workers delivering health and other social services, who tend to be motivated by professionalism and altruism, may resist following what they regard as perverse contractual incentives (Heinrich and Marsche 2010).

Public management thinking and practice have changed in response to some of these limitations, leading scholars to argue that the NPM era is over. Dunleavy et al. (2006) identified a new approach which they call Digital Era Governance. It responds to problems caused by NPM reforms such as disaggregation of public services by encouraging more collaboration rather than competition between services providers, alongside harnessing digital tools to increase the power of service users and their ability to communicate effectively with providers. Other scholars emphasize the endurance of NPM logics.

 Activity 6.6

Extract the main elements of the 'New Public Management' from what you have just read about principal–agent theory and related ideas.

Feedback

NPM is a hybrid of different intellectual influences and practical experience, and emphasizes different things in different countries, but the following elements are commonly seen as distinctive in NPM:

1. Clarification of roles and responsibilities for effective policy implementation by separating strategic (i.e. advising ministers on policy direction) from operational (i.e. service delivery) functions within the government machinery. For example, this has led to governments to set up agencies to run public services at arm's length from central government (e.g. courts, prisons and health services) with greater operational freedom and to limit central government ministries to providing policy advice.
2. Separation of the 'purchaser' from the 'provider' roles within public services in order to allow the contracting out of services to the private or voluntary sector if this is regarded as superior to in-house, public provision; the establishment of more independent public providers (e.g. turning English NHS hospitals into 'foundation trusts' at arm's length from direct government control); and greater competition between providers driven by giving users more choice.

3. Focus on performance assessment and incentives to improve 'value for money' and to ensure that services deliver what policy makers intended (e.g. including payment for performance, sometimes known as payment by results, or PbR).
4. Setting standards of service which consumers can expect to be delivered.

Implementation science

The past two decades have witnessed the emergence of a new field of implementation research – labelled 'implementation science' and distinct from the wider field of policy implementation research covered in this chapter. Nilsen et al. (2013) compared the two, finding some areas of convergence – but many of divergence. Implementation science seeks to apply scientific principles to the study of the uptake of research findings in health care organizations, and to a lesser extent in wider policy arenas. The roots of implementation science can be traced back to the 1990s and the emergence of the evidence-based medicine (EBM) movement (see Chapter 7 for more on this). Compared to policy implementation research, implementation science is less concerned with politics, and how policies are formed and implemented, and more concerned with how policies can be better implemented within organizations. Implementation science uses social science methods but typically adopts quite a narrow, positivist approach to questions of implementation compared to policy implementation research, which is often more interpretive. It tends to involve quantitative studies such as randomized experiments and has been criticized for viewing the research–practice relationship in rather unidirectional, or linear, ways (Nilsen et al. 2013). However, there are some useful sociologically informed models such as Normalization Process Theory (NPT) (May et al. 2009) which have emerged from implementation science and can inform health care professionals about effective ways to improve their practice. NPT centres on four theoretical constructs to help illuminate how processes may become routinized in health care settings. The first focuses on individual and collective 'sensemaking' that may promote or inhibit the coherence or understanding of an intervention to be implemented. The second focuses on the 'cognitive participation' and commitment of actors to the implementation of an intervention. The third recognizes the importance of shared 'collective action' amongst health care workers to implement an intervention. The final element highlights the importance of 'reflexive monitoring' for both individuals and teams as they evaluate their work and the extent to which an intervention has been implemented and subsequently routinized.

Implementing change through behavioural interventions

A further development over the past 20 years that is relevant to policy implementation is behaviourally influenced policy design. Known more colloquially as 'nudging' (Thaler and Sustein 2008), behavioural interventions focus specifically on individuals, and ways to subtly encourage them to act in ways that are consistent with policy goals. The approach exploits common human cognitive biases so as to increase the likelihood that individuals choose to engage in certain actions rather than others. The attraction of 'nudges' to policy makers is that they avoid the need for direct government action such as banning certain behaviours and are thus more likely to be acceptable to libertarians who are against state regulation on principle (see Chapter 8 for more on this).

Influenced by insights from behavioural psychology, these nudges can be beneficial – for instance by encouraging doctors to prescribe certain drugs rather than others through the use of digital reminders at the point of prescribing – thus improving the implementation of more clinically appropriate or more cost-effective prescribing practices. However, 'nudging' can be problematic. Petticrew et al. (2020) highlight that corporate actors – notably Big Alcohol – are adept at using 'dark nudges' which also exploit cognitive biases but in ways that encourage *unhealthy* behaviour. Chater and Loewenstein (in press), who were originally strong champions of the potential of behaviourally influenced policy design to improve public health, have highlighted both that the evidence of the effectiveness of these policies is weak and that the emphasis on individual behaviour change is ultimately damaging in that it downplays the need for, and the effectiveness of, systemic change – for instance, through government regulation of Big Alcohol.

Towards a synthesis of 'top-down' and 'bottom-up' perspectives

You have seen by now that both 'top-down' and 'bottom-up' approaches have strengths and weaknesses in explaining health policy implementation. A number of scholars have attempted to combine top-down and bottom-up approaches to generate a more comprehensive model of policy implementation that can be used both to understand policy implementation and to provide some guidance on how to improve the implementation process. An example of this approach is Matland's conflict–ambiguity matrix (Matland 1995).

Matland's matrix highlights two key factors that influence policy implementation. First, *conflict* – the extent to which policy actors may disagree about, or clash over the need for, or implications of, a policy. Second, *ambiguity* – the extent to which the motivation and (likely) outcomes of a policy are clear or not. Matland suggests that different degrees of conflict and ambiguity related to distinct policies may determine the type of policy implementation most likely to succeed and the key elements needed to foster successful implementation (or not). In Matland's view, the way these factors interact is crucial to understanding policy implementation diversity. Figure 6.1 shows in stylized fashion four ways in which conflict and ambiguity may interact and the type of implementation process that this may provoke.

Matland suggests that where there is low policy ambiguity and low policy conflict, *administrative implementation* is likely to be present and sufficient. Administrative implementation is achieved through good administrative processes and does not for example require excessive political force. This is the least complicated form of implementation, and the desired outcome is very likely to be achieved so long as sufficient resources are funnelled

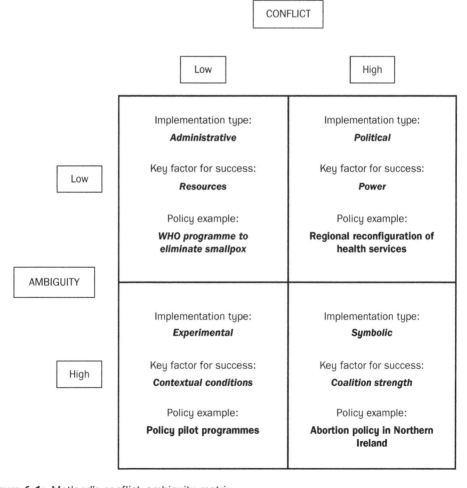

Figure 6.1: Matland's conflict–ambiguity matrix

Source: adapted from Matland (1995)

into the programme to deliver the policy. Matland uses the example of the WHO programme to eliminate smallpox. The means and goals of the policy were clear, the policy had a very high degree of support from key actors, standard processes were developed and replicated, and the programme was well resourced.

In situations of low ambiguity and high conflict, Matland argues that *political implementation* is likely to be present and necessary. In these situations, actors have clearly defined goals, but these goals may be incompatible, or there can be disagreement over the means by which a goal is to be achieved. The key driver in such scenarios is that implementation outcomes are decided by power – either one group of actors have sufficient power to impose their goals on others, or some kind of bargaining will take place that will lead to an agreement (see Chapter 2). An example of this might be a regional reconfiguration of health services. As discussed in Chapter 7, Fraser et al. (2017) show that whilst there was near universal support from clinicians, patient groups, managers and policy makers to reduce the number of London hospitals delivering acute stroke care to patients into fewer, more specialized centres, there was deep disagreement about which hospitals should host the new stroke units and which would not. This required the senior leaders of the health service in London to use their power to impose a decision about how many units were required and where they would be located – in a top-down way (which Matland describes as *political implementation*).

In situations with high policy ambiguity and low policy conflict, Matland suggests that *experimental implementation* will take place and be needed. In this situation, contextual conditions dominate the process of implementation. An example here might be when policy makers develop and fund policy pilot programmes in order to learn more about how policies develop in real-world settings (Ettelt et al. 2015), or when a policy is rushed out by a government before a coherent implementation plan can be devised so that the policy is no more than a set of goals. In these circumstances, for academic researchers a bottom-up approach to implementation analysis is superior to a top-down one as an emphasis on the agency of local actors to shape policy locally is most apparent.

Finally, when there is a situation of high policy ambiguity and high policy conflict, it is likely that *symbolic implementation* takes place. In these cases, local actors and local coalition strength are central to the shape that implementation takes – but their actions are highly dependent upon larger political factors. An example here might be abortion policy in Northern Ireland. This has remained a highly contested issue in Northern Irish life with decades of conflict between those who wish to expand or restrict access to safe and legal abortion services. There is also a high level of ambiguity in relation to the policy given that although abortion has been legalized, the government of Northern Ireland has not commissioned any abortion services. Women from Northern Ireland can, and can continue to access, safe, legal abortion services in the UK and the Republic of Ireland.

There are questions about why no services are yet in place, whose interests this situation serves, and its impact on women's health. Due to the
particular Northern Irish socio-religious and historical context, abortion
remains a sensitive and symbolic issue for many actors remaining more
politicized than in other parts of the Republic of Ireland or Great Britain.

Matland's approach is not without criticism – for instance, some have
highlighted (somewhat ironically) that there are ambiguities in his description of what 'successful' implementation should look like (Coleman et al.
2021). For instance, at what point in the implementation process should
success be judged, and in situations of conflict, success for one set of
actors may be interpreted differently by other actors, so how should these
issues be reconciled? His desire to move beyond the top-down and
bottom-up dichotomy is valuable, however – and has parallels with Sabatier and Jenkins-Smith's (1993) ACF, a general theory of policy change which
is discussed in more detail in Chapter 4. The ACF is useful for explaining the twists and turns of policy implementation over time. The concept
of 'advocacy coalitions' has the virtue of highlighting the possibility that
many of the most important conflicts in policy cut across the simple divide
between policy makers and those formally charged with putting policy into
practice.

What help to policy makers are the different approaches to understanding policy implementation?

Most of the research discussed in this chapter was not directly intended
to provide practical advice for policy makers, though some fairly simple
messages emerge. For example, there is little doubt that policies which
are designed to be incremental (with small behavioural change), are more
likely to be able to be delivered through a simple structure involving few
actors and those that have the support of frontline staff are more likely
to succeed than those that do not. However, this is no great help to those
charged with bringing about more fundamental policy change in complex
systems where conflicts of fact and values abound (see Chapter 8 for more
on values).

This chapter has highlighted the importance of considering resourcing,
the skills of implementers and the importance of local contexts alongside
the significance of coalitions of actors to champion certain policies and
their implementation. The chapter has described a range of frameworks for
analysing policy implementation, each of which has something valuable
to offer to those responsible for planning the implementation of policies.
Elmore (1985) argues that thoughtful policy makers should use a variety
of approaches to analysing the implementation process, inspired by both
'bottom-up' and 'top-down' understandings of how implementation is brought
about. A key skill is the ability to map the participants, their situations,
their perspectives, their values, their strategies, their desired outcomes

and their ability to delay, obstruct, overturn or help policy implementation (see Chapter 11 for more on this). Hudson et al. (2019) emphasize the importance of rigorous and clear policy design and preparation, regular monitoring and support of implementation processes, and ongoing reflection and review as key foci for policy makers who wish to secure effective implementation of their policies.

As a broad generalization, most governments are ambitious (i.e. they want to make a significant impact) in the main fields of health policy, but each of these fields is complex and governments have relatively modest levels of direct control over many of the key actors – for example, they are highly dependent on a range of influential professional groups whose views are more likely to be taken seriously than those of elected officials. This suggests that persuasion and bargaining will often be important parts of any strategy of implementation. Drawing these threads of advice together, Walt (1998) set out a strategy for planning and managing the implementation of change in the health sector, summarized in Table 6.2.

Table 6.2 Strategy for planning and managing the implementation of change

Activity related to implementation of policy change	Type of analysis and planning required
Macro-analysis of the ease with which policy change can be implemented	Analyse conditions for facilitating change and, where possible, adjust simplify, i.e. one agency, clear goals, single objective, simple technical features, marginal change, short duration, visible benefits, clear costs.
Making the values underlying the policy explicit	Identify values underlying policy decisions. If values of key interests conflict with policy, wide coalition of support will have to be built and costs to key interests minimized.
Stakeholder analysis	Review interest groups (and individuals) likely to resist or promote change in policy at national and institutional levels; plan how to mobilize support by consensus building or rallying coalitions of support.
Analysis of financial, technical and managerial resources available and required	Consider the distribution of costs and benefits; assess likely self-interested behaviour within the system; review incentives and sanctions to change behaviour; review need for training, new information systems or other supports to policy change.
Building strategic implementation process	Involve planners and managers in analysis of how to execute policy; identify networks of supporters of policy change including 'champions'; manage uncertainty; promote public awareness; institute mechanisms for consultation, monitoring and 'fine tuning' of policy.

Source: adapted from Walt (1998)

Summary

Implementation cannot be seen as a separate part of a sequential policy process in which political debate and decisions take place among politicians and civil servants, and then managers, administrators and health care professionals at a lower level implement these decisions. It is best viewed as a mostly complex, interactive process in which a wide range of actors influence both the direction of travel as well as the way that given policies are executed, within the constraints of existing institutions, prevailing ideas and competing interests. Implementation is a political process shaped by government capacity and system complexity. Experience suggests that the basic insight from the social sciences of the interplay of actors (agency) and institutions (structure) is still imperfectly built into plans for putting policy into practice. To avoid the gap between policy expectation and reality, policy makers should develop strategies for implementation that explicitly take account of financial, managerial and technical aspects of the policy (capacity) alongside an active interest in how actors who will deliver the policy can collectively influence the policy in positive ways.

Further reading

Alonge, O., Rodriguez, D.C., Brandes, N. et al. (2019) How is implementation research applied to advance health in low-income and middle-income countries?, *BMJ Global Health,* 4: e001257.

Nilsen, P., Ståhl, C., Roback, K. et al. (2013) Never the twain shall meet? A comparison of implementation science and policy implementation research, *Implementation Science,* 8(1): 1–12.

Ridde, V. (2009) Policy implementation in an African state: an extension of Kingdon's multiple-streams approach, *Public Administration,* 87(4): 938–54. https://doi.org/10.1111/j.1467–9299.2009.01792.x

Walker, L. and Gilson, L. (2004) 'We are bitter but we are satisfied': nurses as street-level bureaucrats in South Africa, *Social Science & Medicine,* 59: 1251–61.

Websites

Consolidated Framework for Implementation Research website: https://cfirguide.org

Normalization Process Theory website: https://normalization-process-theory.northumbria.ac.uk

References

Chater, N. and Loewenstein, G.F. (in press) The i-frame and the s-frame: how focusing on individual-level solutions has led behavioral public policy astray, *Behavioural and Brain Sciences.* https://doi.org/10.1017&am

Coleman, A., Billings, J., Allen, P. et al. (2021) Ambiguity and conflict in policy implementation: the case of the new care models (vanguard) programme in England, *Journal of Social Policy,* 50(2): 285–304.

Crocker-Buque, T., Edelstein, M. and Mounier-Jack, S. (2018) A process evaluation of how the routine vaccination programme is implemented at GP practices in England, *Implementation Science*, 13(1): 1–19.

DeLeon, P. (1999) The missing link revisited: contemporary implementation research, *Policy Studies Review*, 16: 311–38.

d'Oliveira, A., Pereira, S., Bacchus, L. et al. (2020) Are we asking too much of the health sector? Exploring the readiness of Brazilian primary healthcare to respond to domestic violence against women, *International Journal of Health Policy and Management*, 11(7): 961–72.

Dunleavy, P., Margetts, H., Bastow, S. et al. (2006) New public management is dead – long live digital-era governance, *Journal of Public Administration Research and Theory*, 16(3): 467–94.

Elmore, R. (1985) Forward and backward mapping, in K. Hanf and T. Toonen (eds.) *Policy Implementation in Federal and Unitary Systems*. Drodrecht, Netherlands: Martinus Nijhoff.

Ettelt, S., Mays, N. and Allen, P. (2015) The multiple purposes of policy piloting and their consequences: three examples from national health and social care policy in England, *Journal of Social Policy*, 44(2): 319–37.

Ferlie, E., Fitzgerald, L. and Pettigrew, A. (1996) *The New Public Management in Action*. Oxford: Oxford University Press.

Ferman, B. (1990) When Failure is Success: Implementation and Madisonian Government, in DJ. Palumboand and DJ. Calista (eds.) *Implementation and the Policy Process: Opening Up the Black Box*. West port, CT: Greenwood Press. Chap. 3.

Fraser, A., Baeza, J.I. and Boaz, A. (2017) 'Holding the line': a qualitative study of the role of evidence in early phase decision-making in the reconfiguration of stroke services in London, *Health Research Policy and Systems*, 15(1): 1–9.

Gofen, A. and Lotta, G. (2021) Street-level bureaucrats at the forefront of pandemic response: a comparative perspective, *Journal of Comparative Policy Analysis: Research and Practice*, 23(1): 3–15.

Gold, J. (2017) *Tracking Delivery: Global Trends and Warning Signs in Delivery Units*. London: Institute for Government. Available at: www.instituteforgovernment.org.uk/sites/default/files/publications/Global%20Delivery%20report.pdf (accessed 25 April 2023).

Heinrich, C. J. and Marschke, G. (2010) Incentives and their dynamics in public sector performance management systems, *Journal of Policy Analysis and Management*, 29(1): 183–208.

Howlett, M., Ramesh, M. and Perl, A. (2009) *Studying Public Policy: Policy Cycles and Policy Subsystems*, Vol. 3. Oxford: Oxford University Press.

Hudson, R., Hunter, D. and Peckham, S. (2019) Policy failure and the policy-implementation gap: can policy support programs help?, *Policy Design and Practice*, 2(1): 1–14.

Lipsky, M. (1980) *Street Level Bureaucracy: Dilemmas of the Individual in Public Services*. New York: Russell Sage Foundation.

Matland, R. E. (1995) Synthesizing the implementation literature: the ambiguity-conflict model of policy implementation, *Journal of Public Administration Research and Theory*, 5(2): 145–74.

May, C. R., Mair, F., Finch, T. et al. (2009) Development of a theory of implementation and integration: Normalization Process Theory, *Implementation Science*, 4(1): 1–9.

Motta, M. and Stecula, D. (2021) Quantifying the effect of Wakefield et al. (1998) on skepticism about MMR vaccine safety in the US, *PloS One*, 16(8): e0256395.

Navarro, V. (2007) Neoliberalism as a class ideology; or, the political causes of the growth of inequalities, *International Journal of Health Services*, 37(1): 47–62.

Nilsen, P., Ståhl, C., Roback, K. et al. (2013) Never the twain shall meet? A comparison of implementation science and policy implementation research, *Implementation Science*, 8(1): 1–12.

Osborne, D.E. and Gaebler, T.A. (1992) *Reinventing Government: How the Entrepreneurial Spirit is Transforming the Public Sector*. Reading, MA: Addison-Wesley.

Petticrew, M., Maani, N., Pettigrew, L. et al. (2020) Dark nudges and sludge in big alcohol: behavioral economics, cognitive biases, and alcohol industry corporate social responsibility, *The Milbank Quarterly*, 98(4): 1290–328.

Pollitt, C. and Bouckaert, G. (2017) *Public Management Reform: A Comparative Analysis-Into the Age of Austerity*. Oxford: Oxford University Press.

Pressman, J.L. and Wildavsky, A. (1984) *Implementation*, 3rd edn. Berkeley, CA: University of California Press.

Sabatier, P.A. (1986) Top-down and bottom-up approaches to implementation research: a critical analysis and suggested synthesis, *Journal of Public Policy*, 6: 21–48.

Sabatier, P.A. and Jenkins-Smith, H.C. (eds.) (1993) *Policy Change and Learning: An Advocacy Coalition Approach*. Boulder, CO: Westview Press.

Sabatier, P.A. and Mazmanian, D. A. (1979) The conditions of effective implementations: a guide to accomplishing policy objectives, *Policy Analysis*, 5(4): 481–504.

Scott, V., Mathews, V. and Gilson, L. (2011) Constraints on implementing an equity-promoting staff allocation policy: understanding mid-level managers' and nurses' perspectives affecting implementation in South Africa, *Health Policy and Planning*, 27(2): 138–46.

Thaler, R.H. and Sustein, C.R. (2008) *Nudge: Improving Decisions about Health, Wealth, and Happiness*. New Haven, CT: Yale University Press.

Walker, L. and Gilson, L. (2004) 'We are bitter but we are satisfied': nurses as street-level bureaucrats in South Africa, *Social Science & Medicine*, 59: 1251–61.

Walls, H., Johnston, D., Matita, M. et al. (2023) How effectively might agricultural input subsidies improve nutrition? A case study of Malawi's Farm Input Subsidy Programme (FISP), *Food Security*, 15: 21–39.

Walt, G. (1998) Implementing health care reform: a framework for discussion, in R.B. Saltman, J. Figueras and C. Sakellarides (eds.) *Critical Challenges for Health Care Reform in Europe*. Buckingham: Open University Press, pp. 365–84.

Wetherley, R. and Lipsky, M. (1977) Street-level bureaucrats and institutional innovation: implementing special education reform, *Harvard Educational Review*, 47: 171–97.

<table>
<tr><td>**7**</td><td># Evidence, evaluation and policy</td></tr>
</table>

Evidence, evaluation and policy

This chapter looks at the nature of evidence and the role it plays in the policy process. Different forms of evidence are central to political decisions about policy content and direction. Evidence derived from research embodies claims to truth and thus may have power to shape policy. At the same time, evidence is often contested and, as discussed in Chapter 8, people can have strongly held values that shape the evidence that they accept and their willingness to accept evidence that contradicts their world view. This chapter explores how research and evidence do or do not inform policy and practice, and highlights how and why the colonial origins of some evidence and research in global health have generated dissent and debate in recent years.

The chapter also explores policy evaluation. Evaluation draws on a set of research processes to help policy makers and practitioners to understand the effects of policy. Policy evaluation is often portrayed as occurring in the final stage of the policy cycle, but evidence, research and evaluation can influence policy throughout the policy process (e.g. helping define the nature and severity of problems and thereby helping get issues on the policy agenda or providing the basis to choose among policy alternatives in the formulation stage). It is useful to consider different models of the nature of the relationship between researchers and decision makers, and some of the steps that both are encouraged to take to improve the 'fit' between research and policy decisions. Evidence and evaluation both influence and are influenced by existing political contexts. The chapter explores some of the main barriers and facilitators to evidence use in health policy in different contexts and highlights theories that can help to understand these and strategies to encourage policy that is better informed by evidence.

Learning objectives

After working through this chapter, you will be better able to:

- define 'evidence', 'research' and 'evaluation', and the different ways 'evidence' of different types may be used in the policy process
- contrast different models of the relationship between research and policy, and their links to general perspectives on the policy process

- identify some of the barriers and facilitators to research uptake by policy makers and reasons why the relationship between research findings and policy decisions is rarely, if ever, direct and linear
- identify the impacts of epistemic hierarchies on the types of evidence used in health policy including how these may be influenced by neocolonial thinking
- critique the 'two communities' conceptualization of the relationships between researchers and policy makers and recognize the value of using other approaches such as the Advocacy Coalition Framework
- set out some of the strategies that researchers and policy makers are increasingly using in an attempt to close the 'gap' between research findings and policy decisions and assess their likelihood of success in closing the 'gap'.

Key terms

Audit   Examination of the extent to which an activity corresponds with pre-determined standards or criteria.

Colonization   The action or process of settling among and establishing control over the indigenous people of an area.

Dissemination   Process by which research findings are made known to audiences, including policy makers.

Downstream interventions   Policies or programmes focused on behaviour change at the individual level, not addressing the structural influences on individual behaviour.

Epistemicide   The destruction of certain forms of knowledge or ways of knowing – most often linked to colonialism in which knowledge practices from the Global North displaced indigenous ones.

Epistemology   The theory of knowledge which covers, in particular, the methods used to establish knowledge and the validity of that knowledge; i.e. how to distinguish between knowledge that is justified and mere opinion.

Evaluation   Research designed specifically to assess the operation and/or impact of a programme or policy in order to determine whether the programme or policy is worth pursuing, stopping or amending.

Evidence Any form of data, information or knowledge, including, but not confined to, research, that may be used to inform decisions.

Evidence-based medicine Movement within medicine and related professions to base clinical practice on the most rigorous and comprehensive scientific evidence available, ideally from randomized controlled trials of the effectiveness of interventions.

Evidence-based (or evidence-informed) policy Movement within public policy to give evidence greater weight in shaping policy decisions. It is better described as 'evidence-informed' policy than 'evidence-based', since evidence can only ever be one, albeit important, input to decision making.

Formative evaluation Evaluation in the early or pilot stage of a policy or programme designed to assess how well it is being implemented with a view to refining it to improve its longer term or full-scale implementation.

Knowledge transfer Strategy usually incorporating a variety of 'linkage' and 'exchange' activities designed to tighten the links between researchers and policy makers.

Monitoring Routine collection of performance data on an activity usually against a plan or contract.

Positivism A philosophical system that argues that knowledge can only come from observation and experience and rejects metaphysical speculation.

Power The ability to control resources and influence people, leading them to do things that they might otherwise not have done.

Research Systematic activity designed to generate rigorous new knowledge and relate it to existing knowledge in order to improve understanding of the physical or social world.

Summative evaluation Evaluation designed to produce an overall verdict on a policy or programme in terms of the balance of costs and benefits.

Technocracy A form of government led by an elite of technical experts.

Upstream determinants of health Structural features of society (e.g. socio-economic inequalities, urban design, taxation) that shape individuals' choices and health-related behaviour.

Upstream interventions Policies involving collective action that focus on structural change in society, with the potential to affect large groups of people, for example, government regulation.

Introduction

Evidence may be defined as information that enables actors to judge whether a proposition is true or not. This makes evidence a critically important currency for policy makers. However, there are different kinds of evidence, which are produced in different ways and have differential significance for different audiences in different contexts. For example, for some people, evidence is defined as only objective quantitative facts, for others it includes more subjective qualitative narratives. This means that the idea that evidence should guide policy – whilst seemingly straightforward – is an idea which is contested and complicated in practice (Boaz et al. 2019).

Evidence can be used to affect policy through introducing new ways of seeing the world, new techniques for improving health, or reasons for changing existing policies. *Research* is a sub-set of the wider category of evidence and is a systematic process for generating new knowledge and relating it to existing knowledge in order to improve understanding about the natural and social world. Research uses a wide variety of methods, theories and assumptions about what counts as valid knowledge. 'Applied' research takes new knowledge from 'basic' research and tries to apply it to solving practical problems. For some people, *evaluation* is distinct from research, but since evaluation uses research methods, it can also make sense to view it as a type of research, defined as:

Any scientifically based activity undertaken to assess the operation and impact of [public] policies and the action programmes introduced to implement those policies. (Rossi and Wright 1979)

With evaluation, it is common to make a distinction between *formative* and *summative* evaluations. The former is best thought of as evaluation designed to contribute directly to assisting those responsible for a programme to shape the programme while it is being developed or implemented. Formative evaluations generally take place during the early stages of a programme and focus on activities and processes with a view to providing advice directly to the policy makers that can be used to develop and modify the programme. By contrast, summative evaluations are designed to try to provide a verdict on a policy or programme in terms of its outcomes or ultimate impact. In other words, they focus on measuring the impact or outcome and costs, as well as the extent to which a programme has met its objectives. They tend to use quantitative methods but increasingly use a mix of quantitative and qualitative methods. Formative evaluations tend to use qualitative methods such as observation (e.g. of meetings or care delivery) and semi-structured interviews.

Evaluations are particularly policy-relevant forms of research since they are normally commissioned by decision makers or funders to assess whether or not policy implementation is going well and to what effect. Within the conventional device of the 'policy cycle', evaluation is portrayed as a fourth and final stage to assess whether a policy has been effective. However, since policy is a continuous process, evaluation can contribute at any stage. For example, an evaluation could show that a policy intervention was not working as intended and was generating unanticipated problems, thereby contributing to the first stage of problem identification in another policy cycle.

Policy makers have access to, and use, forms of evidence other than scientific research. For example, research is usually distinguished from *audit*, which examines the extent to which a process or activity corresponds with pre-determined standards or criteria of performance (e.g. checking that the facilities and staffing at a clinic are adequate to deliver babies safely). Research is also distinguished from *monitoring*, which constitutes the continuous, routine collection of data on an activity (such as health care treatments delivered) to ensure that everything is going according to plan. Policy agencies also commission and use the results of surveys, focus groups, stakeholder analysis and consultations with key interest groups, including service users (see Chapter 11).

There have been subtle but significant changes in the language used to describe the relationship between evidence and policy in recent years. Rather than using the term evidence-*based* policy, many proponents now talk of evidence-*informed* policy instead (Boaz et al. 2019). This discursive shift recognizes the limits of evidence, the enduring importance of other factors to guide policy – including values (as discussed in Chapter 8) and the benefits of a less *technocratic*, more open and deliberative approach to policy making. As discussed in Chapter 9 and as you will see later in this chapter, evidence transfer across international boundaries is more complicated than evidence use within a single setting, especially when it also involves prioritizing some forms of evidence, or ways of knowing, over others. Essentially, evidence may be useful to inform policy – but the process is often messy, contested and problematic.

How does evidence influence policy?

The relationship between evidence and policy has been much explored. Best and Holmes (2010) identify three generations of thinking about how research evidence can impact upon policy, each still valuable today:

- First-generation thinking is derived from the rational, linear approach to policy, which argues that policy choices should be made in the light of what works best. In this model, either a problem is identified by policy makers and 'solved' by researchers or new knowledge (e.g. of a previously unidentified health risk) is produced by researchers and policy makers act on this evidence by disseminating it to practitioners who change their behaviour. This is sometimes termed an 'engineering' or 'pipeline' model, which sees evidence as a 'product' passed through recognized stages leading to policy and practice improvements.

- Second-generation thinking draws on some rational linear principles but identifies that such an approach is often unrealistic and focuses instead upon relational approaches to improving research, policy and practitioner links. This emphasizes the importance of human interactions and networks of researchers and research users to share and disseminate evidence.
- Third-generation thinking emphasizes the importance of the wider systems and networks within which evidence and policy making interact. It highlights the complexity of these systems and encourages analysis of how organizational structures – for instance, hierarchies, bureaucracies, or networks-influence the ability of actors to use their own agency, or power, to fruitfully apply evidence to try to solve complicated issues. This approach encourages long-term thinking about how interactive evidence sharing organizations may be established. Examples of this approach in practice include the work of the *African Centre for Evidence* based at the University of Johannesburg as part of the Africa Evidence Network, and the network of *What Works Centres* established in the UK over the past two decades.

✎ Activity 7.1

Compare and contrast the three generations of thinking of evidence use by policy makers identified by Best and Holmes (2010). Think of some of the limitations of each approach as a guide to how to seek to improve research uptake by policy makers.

Feedback

Your answer is likely to have included the points outlined in Table 7.1.

Other studies of the complex way in which policy is made emphasize that research (and other forms of evidence) can be 'used' indirectly and in a variety of different ways by policy makers. For example, a study of evidence use in Cambodia by Walls et al. (2018) highlighted that evidence is not a uniform commodity for which more is better, but rather different pieces of evidence become relevant in relation to the features of specific health policy decisions. In relation to tobacco, large and expensive national prevalence surveys were considered necessary evidence for intervention, even given considerable evidence from smaller studies of a high prevalence of smoking in the country, and the irrefutable global evidence linking tobacco to numerous diseases and mortality. With HIV/AIDS, the dominance of global donors in supporting this health issue, and the apparent

Table 7.1 Differences between the generations of thinking about evidence to policy

	First-generation thinking	Second-generation thinking	Third-generation thinking
Relationship between research, evidence and policy making	Sees the relationship between research and policy as rational and sequential (sometimes referred to as the 'engineering' approach).	Sees the relationship between research and policy as indirect and not necessarily logical, predictable or neat – it emphasizes the importance of relationships between those producing and those using research.	Also sees the relationship between research and policy as indirect and not necessarily logical, predictable or neat. Sees strengths and limitations in both first- and second-generation thinking. Focuses on how the systems through which policy and research interact may constrain or improve evidence use.
Problem identification and location	A problem exists because basic research has identified it. Applied research is undertaken to help solve the problem. Research is then applied to helping solve the policy problem. Research produces a preferred policy solution.	Problems can be identified by different actors (researchers, policy makers, practitioners, patients). Knowledge about the problem can likewise come from different sources not just the researcher. Policy solutions are collectively negotiated iteratively and implemented, often locally.	Problems are located within complex health care or other health-related and less clearly health-related systems. Attempts to tackle problems within such systems requires a co-ordinated approach across multiple levels. Responding to certain problems may have impacts for other parts of the system.
Strengths of the approach	Strengths of this approach lie in its simplicity – for relatively simple changes with widespread support it can be feasible to act in this way.	Strengths of this approach lie in its focus on relationships and bringing different communities together to increase understanding.	Strengths of this approach lie in its comprehensiveness and focus, which goes beyond problem identification, research and relationships.
Weaknesses of the approach	Weaknesses of this approach lie in its simplicity when faced with the complexity of real-life policy formulation and implementation.	Weaknesses of this approach lie in its inattention to how wider systems impact upon problem understanding and research use.	Weaknesses of this approach lie in its overall complexity, which can become daunting in relation to specific problems and solutions.

limited contestation at a local level, led to the explicit embrace of epide-miological evidence that is widely held to be appropriate for HIV planning within the global health community. In the final case of performance-based financing, it was the government that drove both the initiation and imple-mentation of the policy response. This state-controlled process appeared to reflect a belief that national action must be taken to address an existing priority (in the form of an MDG). This, in turn, naturally led to a logic which saw relatively small studies focused on implementation to be the most relevant to policy. Although it is worth noting that, in the case of the Gov-ernment Midwifery Incentive Scheme, some believed that evidence was not perceived as important at all due to the policy being driven by higher level political authorities (Walls et al. 2018).

Researchers have also observed that new knowledge and insights appear to percolate through the political environment like water falling on limestone: the water is absorbed, disappears into multiple channels and then emerges unexpectedly sometime later elsewhere. Weiss (1979) suggested that it was more accurate to term this process one of *enlight-enment*. Concepts and ideas derived from research filter into the policy networks that shape the policy process in a particular field and have a cumulative, indirect effect rather than an immediate, direct effect on policy. Thus, the primary impact of research and researchers is at the level of ideas and ways of thinking about problems which are then taken up by others, rather than in providing specific answers to specific policy puzzles (Smith 2013).

Evidence, including evidence from research, can be used in entirely political ways by governments and powerful groups as an instrument to advance their interests. This *strategic* model views research as ammuni-tion to support predetermined positions or to delay or obstruct politically uncomfortable decisions (Weiss 1979). There is much empirical support for this view of the nature of politics and the use of research. A classic recurring example of the strategic use of research is for a government to argue that no decision can be made on a contentious issue without further research and analysis, and then to appoint a commission of enquiry taking several years to do the necessary work. The effect of this action is to take the issue off the policy agenda. With any luck, a different government will be in office when the awkward report arrives from the commission.

The presentation and use of evidence by senior policy makers reforming NHS stroke services in London in the early 2010s is a good example of the 'strategic' use of evidence. Whilst these reforms have proven to be benefi-cial for patients (Morris et al. 2014), the change process and the strength of the evidence used to justify how many hospitals would deliver hyper-acute stroke services and where they would be located was contested by many actors. Senior policy makers chose to prioritize evidence that justified their preferred model of care over evidence which might not, whilst emphasizing the evidence-based nature of their proposed changes to minimize actor discontent (Fraser et al. 2017).

The strategic use of evidence to decide the location of services between hospitals points to a wider issue in relation to evidence use and policy. Some forms of evidence are seen as more worthy, valuable or convincing to policy makers than others (Parkhurst and Abeysinghe 2016). Notably, experimental evidence created through randomized controlled trials (RCTs) is often seen by biomedical scientists and clinicians as the best evidence, irrespective of the type of research question. RCTs are very powerful tools for answering relative effectiveness questions on fairly narrow issues, especially comparing drugs and clinical interventions. However, there are power implications in such hierarchical thinking since effectiveness is not the only policy question, and not all policy issues lend themselves to the conduct of RCTs. There are some areas of health care and policy for which it is inappropriate or very difficult to conduct RCTs – often in relation to questions of equity. This has led to debates which have sometimes been termed as 'paradigm wars' between researchers who prioritize *positivist*, quantitative and experimental forms of knowledge and view systematic reviews of RCTs as the most valuable form of knowledge and other research-ers who espouse the value of interpretive, qualitative and non-experimental forms of knowledge. Whilst methodological and disciplinary differences sit at the heart of these debates about knowledge hierarchies, they also have significant power and privilege implications in respect of which questions can be asked, and who is authorized to answer them.

Epistemic injustice in global health research and implications for policy

You will see that different types of evidence are needed to answer dif-ferent research questions for policy and different types of evidence are considered relevant by different policy actors and in different policy con-texts. Hawkes et al. (2016) highlight how demand for evidence is created amongst policy makers and encourage greater understanding from their perspectives about what evidence counts. They outline three levels of capacity strengthening for evidence uptake – individual, organization and institutional. Epistemic debates, or arguments over how to accommodate different views about the validity and significance of systems of knowl-edge are particularly acute in global health because of the damaging legacies of European *colonization*. Colonial powers actively destroyed indigenous cultures and ways of knowing through practices of *epistemi-cide* (de Sousa Santos 2015) replacing these with a European, positivist *epistemology* in many countries. As described in Chapter 2, Lukes' third dimension of *power* is a useful lens to view how over time this colo-nial practice became normalized and European values in relation to what constitutes truth, knowledge and legitimacy have become internalized by those based in both the Global North and the Global South. Researchers from the Global South are increasingly challenging issues of epistemic injustice which have significant and enduring implications for research, evidence and policy (Bhakuni and Abimbola 2021; Naidu 2021; Koum Besson 2022).

Global health research is affected by unequal power dynamics rooted in global coloniality that manifest in the prioritization of outsiders' perspectives over local perspectives. These issues are visible in funding and publishing of research. Koum Besson (2022), drawing on Ndlovu-Gatsheni (2014) highlights that this injustice is linked to the following:

1. *Coloniality of power* – control over resources, research agendas and knowledge prioritization held by Global North governments and organizations. For example, the issues that are most often researched are those that funders in the Global North think are most important.
2. *Coloniality of knowledge* – epistemological colonialization of European and North American ways of thinking become dominant. This is also known as 'interpretive injustice', for example, where the experiences of those from the Global South are marginalized as they do not fit with concepts from the Global North.
3. *Coloniality of being* – legitimized inferiorization of non-European, non-North American ways of knowing. This is also known as 'testimonial injustice'. An example is the prioritization of research team members from the Global North over those from the Global South in terms of research tasks – whereby Global South researchers are tasked with data collection and Global North researchers are tasked with data interpretation. Also credit for research – such as author order in subsequent publications – where Global North authors frequently take the most prestigious positions.

Research funders from the Global North have been criticized for historically prioritizing research that is transferable and generalizable when commissioning research rather than promoting contextually focused research. Such research aims have been seen to favour research teams from the Global North (i.e. making them more likely to win competitive research funds) by encouraging multi-site international studies to the detriment of local research teams based in the Global South. This may compound existing biases and inequalities. It also means that local or national, contextually rich research that would be of value for local and national policy makers and populations remains harder to fund, and the research which is funded may be ignored by policy makers in the Global South as lacking relevance. Such research may be published in prestigious academic journals in the Global North but serves little use to the research subjects in the Global South who cannot often access papers published behind paywalls. A further issue has been labelled 'Northern ventriloquism', whereby LMIC scholars express HIC ideas in order to access competitive global funds or publish in high-impact journals based in HICs (Bhakuni and Abimbola 2021;

Naidu 2021; Koum Besson 2022). Whilst some research funders in recent years have tried to tackle some of these injustices by encouraging greater LMIC policy maker and community input into research design, the historical impacts of these injustices persist.

 Activity 7.2

How can some of these research funding and publishing problems be rectified? Consider at least two solutions that might be developed to challenge each of these problems.

Feedback

Your answers might include the following.

Funders:

- all funders being more thoughtful and explicit about the audience for the research and recognizing that what works in one context may not work in another one;
- funders inviting local researchers to provide additional information on their lived experience, knowledge practices and interpretive tools;
- funders promote equity and epistemic justice by creating space for marginalized interpretive perspectives to flourish and value local knowledge that meets local needs;
- reviewers of funding bids (often from the Global North) being required to be better aware of their own biases and positionality and be asked to consider the relevance of the research to local needs;
- increase the proportion of reviewers from the Global South.

Publishers:

- members of editorial boards of journals declaring their gender, racial, colonial and ancestral privileges and experiences in LMICs;
- allowing authors the space to write with emotion about personal and local identity perspectives in global health;
- publishing abstracts in LMIC authors' first languages and the indigenous languages of locations where research is done;
- supporting journal editors based outside the Global North with the support necessary for their work, while trusting, protecting and advancing the value of their previously neglected racial, gender, historical and personal perspectives in editorial decision making.

Source: Naidu (2021); Koum Besson (2022)

Barriers to the use of evidence in policy

Political and ideological factors

You should by now be familiar with the notion that 'policy' is a process that takes place in a particular context influenced by the values and interests of the participants. As a result, politics and ideology inevitably affect the way that evidence is used. For example, who initiates, undertakes, participates in and oversees an evaluation, and why it is wanted, are likely to influence how far it is used by policy makers. Different domestic governments will focus on policy issues that they deem more important than others, and this will impact upon the types of research they fund, the routine data they choose to collect, or evidence they choose to prioritize. These decisions, though seemingly mundane, are ideologically driven and often highly political.

Linked to, but beyond the purely political dimension, is how evidence often speaks to unisectoral policy solutions, e.g. policies from the health sector. It is more challenging to generate the evidence for multi-sectoral policy action, which is often the policy most relevant for addressing the more structural drivers of ill health such as housing, diet and transport. This is due to several factors. The interventions focusing on treatment or more '*downstream*' individual approaches, likely to be undertaken within a single sector, are easier to conceptualize, measure and evaluate. The assessment of potentially causal associations is more difficult for more '*upstream*' factors than for more downstream factors closer to the individual. This is because for upstream factors there is a greater 'distance' to a particular health outcome of interest and a larger number of intermediary and confounding factors, for instance between policies from a sector such as agriculture and impact on nutritional outcomes. Furthermore, the evidence in regard to the health outcome of interest, such as the prevalence or severity of particular nutritional concerns, may be generated from the health sector, and thus may not 'speak' to the values, beliefs and worldviews in the sectors such as finance or agriculture which may greatly impact it.

An example of multisectoral policy change is tobacco control policy in the UK. Despite the evidence highlighting the links between smoking and increased mortality and morbidity emerging as early as the 1940s, it took more than half a century before smoking was banned in indoor public places. Smith (2013) highlights how effective tobacco control policies were deemed politically infeasible for many decades. Factors included the power and influence of the tobacco lobby and the economic benefits of tobacco taxation and the wider tobacco industry for the UK Treasury throughout the twentieth century. In the early 2000s the New Labour government led by Prime Minister Blair, supported by anti-tobacco civil society and medical campaigners, was able to successfully challenge the consensus of the past decades and managed to change the context in relation to tobacco control. Ideas linked to the pernicious nature of passive smoking, and a refutation of the narrative that tobacco use generated an overall positive economic outcome for the UK, coalesced with government ideological goals to reduce heart disease, cancer and stroke. In this example, whilst the *evidence* did not change much over the course of 50 years or so, the *ideas* linked to, and politics of, tobacco usage did change, leading to radical legislation furthered in subsequent years by plain packaging and greater restrictions on tobacco availability. Notwithstanding these positive developments in tobacco control this century in the UK, other harmful products and pastimes such as alcohol, junk foods and gambling which also contribute to health inequalities remain less regulated despite evidence of their harms.

As you explored in Activity 7.2, global health research funding is bedevilled by colonial assumptions and priorities. In general, health research applied to the needs of people in LMICs is still under-resourced given the potential for such research to help reduce the large burden of preventable death and ill health in those countries. Yegros-Yegros et al. (2020) found that 80 per cent of health research is concentrated on HICs and focuses on diseases such as cancer, heart disease and depression historically particularly prevalent in those countries. Diseases linked to maternal health, HIV, malaria and diarrhoeal diseases – mostly affecting LMICs – are not funded to the same level. This should come as no surprise given the political nature of priority setting outlined in Chapter 9. They also found that research conducted by pharmaceutical companies focused on diseases prevalent in HICs. This should come as no surprise give the over-riding goal of the for-profit sector discussed in Chapter 4. Overall, diseases that affect HICs receive ten times more research attention than those affecting low-income ones – perpetuating Tudor Hart's inverse care law (Hart 1971) at a global level. Similar dynamics occur within countries driven by social norms and power imbalances, for example, affecting women and those whose sexual orientation is stigmatized.

Policy makers may have conflicts of interest which impinge upon their supposed neutrality in relation to evidence. Conflicts of interest can be subtle, hidden and hard to research. Conflicts of interest occur across all settings. Rahman-Shepherd et al. (2021) highlight how conflicts of interest impede the development of evidence-informed health policies to better structure and govern state and non-state health care providers. These may be linked to undeclared social or family interests of policy makers, undeclared financial flows between formal and informal providers and a desire on the part of policy makers to avoid regulating private providers for fear of popular resistance and exposure of public sector failings.

Of course, it is not just politicians whose approach to, and use of, research can be shaped by ideology and personal interests. Research requires resources and researchers have to apply to public and private sources of funds to support their projects. In turn, public and private funding bodies influence which sorts of research will be undertaken and which researchers will be selected to do the research. Notwithstanding the COVID-19 pandemic, globally, over the past 30 years the share of total health research funding from governments has been falling even though total spending has been rising in real terms. Similarly, large pharmaceutical firms are doing more research 'in-house' and funding less work in universities. The increasing proportion of pharma funding for research is especially problematic as pharma will generally not have an inherent interest in undertaking research on prevention or the social, economic and environmental determinants of ill health.

Scientific uncertainty and evidence uptake

All research findings carry a degree of uncertainty, but sometimes, there is a particularly high level of uncertainty affecting the way in which a piece of research can be used for policy. Mathematical modelling of the future trajectory and severity of an epidemic is important and highly valued by policy makers for planning an appropriate government response, but is intrinsically uncertain since it is dependent on current knowledge and assumptions about the future. This was apparent within and across many countries during the COVID-19 outbreak. Policy makers were forced to take high-stakes decisions about how to respond to a novel virus based on partial understanding and models that inevitably varied in their results. Leaders were supplied with models from different research teams generating different predictions and had to make decisions about which results to take on board and which to reject.

In relation to COVID-19 and more generally, a significant point of contention surrounding the interpretation and use of research relates to its generalizability and relevance to a particular policy context. Faced with research from another setting or country that does not support their policy line, policy makers tend to play down the relevance of the research. By contrast, scientists may tend to emphasize the generalizability of their findings to a wider range of settings, sometimes inappropriately.

It can be helpful to distinguish between genuine uncertainty and artificial, or manufactured uncertainty. An example of the former relates to debates amongst researchers during the early stages of the COVID-19 pandemic in relation to the effectiveness of facemasks to limit the spread of the virus. Despite a limited evidence base – and a lack of RCTs – some researchers argued passionately for policy makers to follow the 'precautionary principle' and mandate mask wearing in public spaces (Greenhalgh 2020). Other researchers, just as passionately put forward the counterargument that without robust evidence it could be counterproductive to argue for mass mask use (Martin et al. 2020). This was a genuine debate about how to best proceed when faced with limited evidence for an intervention – but in many countries mask wearing became a highly politicized issue with significant implications for the ability of governments to introduce or sustain mask mandates.

In contrast to genuine uncertainty, uncertainty may be manufactured by policy actors in order to further political or economic interests. This practice sits at the heart of strategies of corporations that produce fossil fuels. Companies such as ExxonMobil deliberately hid their in-house research that linked global temperature rises with fossil fuel use as early as the 1970s whilst paying for opinion pieces and taking out large adverts in newspapers to actively mislead the public into overestimating the level of uncertainty about the existence of global warming and its link to fossil fuel use across subsequent decades (Supran and Oreskes 2017). Similarly, populist politicians such as President Bolsonaro of Brazil and President Trump of the USA both advocated for the use of hydroxychloroquine during the COVID-19 pandemic in their respective countries despite the fact that there was no evidence for its effectiveness in combating the virus. Both these leaders clashed with health experts and government advisors in relation to hydroxychloroquine and other ineffective (and potentially dangerous) drugs increasing uncertainty rather than reducing it. Such an approach seeks to politically delegitimize expert knowledge as a means of distraction or part of a wider strategy of public misinformation.

In the case of policy or programme evaluations, interpreting and using the findings can be difficult for two reasons: the goals of the original programme are often deliberately broad and open to interpretation; and the effects are likely to be small in relation to all the other influences on the outcome(s) of interest. Indeed, it is now generally accepted that the better designed the evaluation, the smaller the effect it is likely to demonstrate. It can be difficult for policy makers to know whether the fact that an evaluation fails to show a programme achieving the results intended is due to the intrinsic methodological difficulty of disentangling the specific contribution of the programme from other factors, or whether the programme has genuinely failed to meet its objectives. This is particularly likely in relation to policies designed to tackle longstanding, complex, multi-causal problems such as child poverty or poor health in early life and their subsequent effects. These tend to be the most important programmes attracting a high degree of public interest and debate and highlight the practical complexities involved in using programme evaluation to inform policy making in a definitive sense.

Perceived utility of research

Researchers have been increasingly incentivized over recent years to make their work available and useful for policy makers. In many university systems, researchers are judged on the 'impact' that their work has on specific sectors and society more widely – for instance, this is an explicit element of the Research Excellence Framework within UK universities, which in turn affects the amount of government research funding each university receives. The ability of researchers to achieve impact partly depends on the kinds of information generated by their research. Weiss (1991) identified three basic forms of output from research, generated to differing degrees by different research styles:

- data and findings;
- ideas and criticism – these spring from the findings and typify the enlightenment model of how research influences policy;
- arguments for action – these derive from the findings and the ideas generated by the research but extend the role of the researcher into advocacy.

Each style of research is likely to be perceived as useful in different circumstances. Weiss argues that apparently objective data and findings are likely to be most useful when a clear problem has been recognized by all actors and there is already a consensus about the range of feasible policy responses. The role of research is then to help decide which option to choose. Ideas and criticism appear to be most useful in an open, pluralistic policy system distinguished by a number of different policy groupings in stable communication with one another when there is uncertainty about the nature of the policy problem (or, indeed, whether one exists worthy of attention) and where there is a wide range of possible responses.

Research as argument may be used when there is a high degree of conflict over an issue. In this case, the research group might decide to take an active role in the relevant policy community, which requires them to promote their findings in an explicitly political way if they are to have an impact. Its use depends on the lobbying skills of the researchers (or their allies) and whether the key policy audiences agree with the values and goals inherent in the research. If they do not, the research will be ignored. Thus, this is a high-risk strategy for researchers since, unlike simply letting the research percolate into policy and practice (following the 'enlightenment' model), it requires researchers to abandon their customary status as disinterested experts and enter the rough-and-tumble of political argument, which could be career-threatening.

When researchers disagree among themselves about research findings and offer conflicting advice to policy makers, this may reduce the likelihood that findings will be acted on by policy makers. The Kenyan 'worm-wars' (Stewart 2019), which saw a significant disciplinary disagreement between epidemiologists and economists about the value of deworming primary school children, provides an example. The epidemiologists cited systematic review evidence which showed there was a lack of high-quality evidence that community-based deworming programmes improve educational outcomes. They advised policy makers not to continue the programme. In contrast, economists were much more favourably disposed to the merits of deworming based on a single study (Miguel and Kremer 2004) in a high-impact economics journal that found deworming in schools had a significant impact on children's cognitive learning. This debate highlights the disciplinary differences between epidemiologists and economists and how far each group is willing to trust single study results compared to systematic findings.

Timing

Another factor affecting whether research is used in policy making is timing. As Chapter 5 shows, the insight that new issues get onto the government's policy agenda when 'windows of opportunity' open shows that researchers can do all they like to establish the nature of a problem and develop suitable responses, but their recommendations are unlikely to be taken up unless the political context is conducive. Frequently, a change of government with a secure political mandate provides this moment. In the UK, the New Labour years of 1997–2010 saw significant increases in funding for the NHS and dedicated strategies to tackle heart disease, cancer and stroke alongside public health measures to reduce smoking rates and childhood poverty. These years saw open policy windows to improve the health of the UK population and a commitment to use evidence in the policy-making process. In contrast, the years since 2010 have seen comparatively smaller gains in funding for health services and falls in life expectancy as Conservative-led governments pursued policies of economic 'austerity' before having to face the COVID-19 pandemic, which created an unusual context for policy maker–researcher relationships.

Decision makers often criticize researchers for taking too long to produce evidence or provide unequivocal advice when they are facing pressure to act. Sometimes, researchers have an influence because their findings happen to appear at just the right time in a policy development process, but it is difficult to predict this and build it into the plan of a research project. There may be a trade-off between the timeliness and the quality of research which is particularly apparent to the researchers as discussed earlier in relation to facemasks and COVID-19 transmission. However, high quality is no guarantee that policy makers will take notice of even the timeliest research when it suits them.

Communication and reputation

Alongside issues related to timing, the ways in which research is communicated and the perceived reputations of researchers also influence whether and how research may influence policy makers and other actors. An issue of wide public interest over recent years relates to data that show a fall in life expectancy in particular social groups in wealthy countries such as the US and the UK. This trend links with narratives about 'deaths of despair' in such countries (King et al. 2022). Such narratives are embarrassing to the government in power and, at the same time, politically useful to opposition politicians as they shape public views about the merits or otherwise of government policies such as 'austerity' in the UK from 2010. Research that engages with such issues often generates hostility from the government of the day – potentially with implications for the reputations of researchers.

Activity 7.3

List the main obstacles or barriers to evidence including research being accepted and used by policy makers discussed in this section.

Feedback

The main obstacles identified (Hyder et al. 2011; Andermann et al. 2016) are noted in Table 7.2.

Table 7.2 Obstacles to evidence use by policy makers

Political and ideological factors	• Vested interests and perceptions of conflicts of interest. • Political context, including the extent of civil and political freedom, political conflict and autonomy of policy officials. • Low priority in policy agencies to the use of research versus experience, political imperatives, etc. • Politically and ideologically controversial policy issues. • Findings that would require a major change in policy, organizations or professional practice.
Policy and scientific uncertainty	• Knowledge gaps and uncertainty. • Controversial, irrelevant and conflicting evidence. • High level of uncertainty associated with the research findings, and/or difficulties and differences in the interpretation of findings.
Different conceptions of risk	• Media storms and public concerns over specific issues.
Perceived utility of research	• Research which is not perceived as relevant in a given context (e.g. undertaken in a different country or offering solutions that are not practical in the given context).
Timing	• Missing windows of opportunity. • Decisions that need to be taken before research can be completed so that research lacks timeliness.
Communication and reputation	• Technical research reports written for other researchers, that are difficult to understand, and lack effective summaries and analysis of policy implications. • Limited access to research findings in policy agencies (e.g. lack of information services). • Lack of funds to pay for or synthesize or adapt relevant research. • Lack of communication channels between researchers and policy makers. • Low credibility of the researchers or the research (e.g. from outside the country or from institutes without a strong reputation or risk of bias from source of funding, or seen as politically motivated). • Poor quality research.

Activity 7.4

For each of the potential obstacles to evidence including research being accepted and used by policy makers, identify one or two possible ways of overcoming them.

Feedback

Many of the enabling or facilitating factors are the converse of the obstacles. Table 7.3 lists those that are widely regarded as helpful for getting evidence used in policy (Boaz et al. 2019; Innvaer et al. 2002).

Table 7.3 Facilitators for evidence use by policy makers

Political and ideological factors	• Increased lay participation and co-creation of evidence to increase wider evidence literacy and demand for policy-relevant research and evidence-informed policy making.
Policy and scientific uncertainty	• Development of formal and informal channels of communication and fora for interaction between researchers and policy makers to share knowledge and build trust to better integrate the generation and use of research (e.g. policy dialogues in which senior government officials, opposition parties, NGO representatives, academics and others are briefed and meet to discuss policy options).
Different conceptions of risk	• Policy staff and intermediaries such as specialist journalists who understand the principles and methods of research, and are open to discussing the implications of research for policy change.
Perceived utility of research	• Involve policy makers in the research process. • Getting research into the hands of influential third parties such as policy advocates, respected experts, NGOs, UN, etc.
Timing	• Timely, context-specific evidence that includes aspects relevant to decision making such as cost (not just effectiveness), acceptability to users and feasibility of implementation. • Approaches to doing research such as rapid appraisal, designed to match the pace of policy decision making.
Communication and reputation	• Offer of more diverse forms of knowledge and perspectives. • Systems for assuring the quality and integrity of research, including international support to local researchers. • Non-technical summaries of research that are widely accessible at low or no cost and written differently for different policy audiences. • Attention to ensuring that policy agencies have systems and staff incentives that encourage learning from a wide range of external sources including research and researchers.

Improving the relationship between evidence and policy

Since the mid-1990s in the health field, there has been an increased interest in using the insights from the different ways of understanding the evidence-policy relationship discussed above. An enduring idea is that there exist 'two communities' – researchers and policy makers – and that it is important to try to reduce the barriers between these two key actor groups in order to enhance the use of research in policy making in line with the goal of evidence-informed policy and practice. In the early stages of the evidence-informed policy movement (the first generation discussed above), the emphasis was on improving the flow of information to policy makers through better *dissemination* of research findings (e.g. researchers were encouraged to produce user-friendly summaries of their research findings and to try to draw out the policy and practical implications of their work). This emphasis was consistent with improving the functioning of the engineering model of research and policy. The focus then shifted to more active strategies of *'knowledge transfer'* (Denis and Lomas 2003), which began to focus attention on how the relationships between researchers and policy makers affect the extent to which the contribution of research is considered in the policy process and how these relationships can be improved (the second generation discussed above). Subsequent (third generation) work focuses on systems thinking to mobilize evidence research uptake through interlinked networks and specialist evidence intermediary organizations, closely attuned to how different contexts impact upon the relationships between policy actors and the complex ways in which evidence use can lead to unexpected outcomes whilst noting the value of the engineering and relational approaches (Best and Holmes 2010).

Nonetheless, the two communities model remains relevant and useful, even if it is a simplification, when considering the relationship between researchers and policy makers.

Activity 7.5

As a demonstration of the 'two communities' hypothesis, tabulate the main differences you can think of between university researchers and government officials in terms of the type of activities they engage in, their attitudes to research, who they are accountable to, their priorities, how they build their careers and obtain their rewards, their training and knowledge base, the organizational constraints they face and so on.

Feedback

Your analysis might look something like Table 7.4.

Table 7.4 The 'two communities' model of researchers and policy makers

	University researchers	Government policy makers
Work	Discrete, planned research projects using explicit, scientific methods designed to produce unambiguous, generalizable results (knowledge focused); usually highly specialized in research areas and knowledge; report findings using technical language.	Continuous, unplanned flow of tasks involving negotiation and compromise between interests and goals; assessment of practical feasibility of policies and advice on specific decisions (decision focused). Often required to work on a range of different issues simultaneously.
Attitudes to research	Justified by its contribution to valid knowledge; research findings lead to need for further investigations since there is always some uncertainty in findings.	Only one of many inputs to their work; justified by its relevance and practical utility (e.g. in decision making); some scepticism about the value of research findings versus their own experience; value research which supports their policy decisions and reinforces their world view.
Accountability	To scientific peers primarily, but also to funders.	To politicians primarily, but also the public, indirectly.
Priorities	Expansion of research opportunities and influence of experts in the world.	Maintaining a system of 'good governance' and satisfying politicians; may wish to protect or expand the role of their agency.
Careers/ rewards	Built largely on publication in peer reviewed scientific journals and peer recognition rather than practical impact though this varies by discipline and impact has recently become more important.	Built on successful management of complex political processes (as well as relationships) and involvement with 'successful' policy initiatives rather than use of research findings for policy.
Training and knowledge base	High level of training, usually specialized within a single discipline; little knowledge about policy-making processes.	Often, though not always, generalists expected to be flexible; often little or no scientific training.
Organizational constraints	Relatively few (except resources); high level of discretion, e.g. in choice of research focus.	Embedded in large, inter-dependent bureaucracies and working within political limits, often to short timescales; such organizations likely to be highly risk-averse.
Values/ orientation	Place high value on independence of thought and action, recognized by peers; belief in unbiased search for generalizable knowledge.	Oriented to providing high-quality advice, but attuned to a particular political and economic context and to informing specific decisions.

Practical steps inspired by the 'two communities' perspective to reduce the 'gap' between research and policy

Table 7.5 summarizes the practical steps which researchers and, importantly, policy makers, have been encouraged to take to improve incorporation of research into policy. In some cases, researchers and policy makers have a similar responsibility, such as in improving the quality of media reporting of research. In other cases, the onus lies on one group or the other.

Table 7.5 Practical steps advocated to reduce the 'gap' between research and policy

Steps to be taken by researchers	*Steps to be taken by policy makers who have capacity or interest seeking to evidential support for policy*
Provide a range of different types of research outputs including newsletters, executive summaries, short policy briefs, etc. all written in an accessible, jargon-free style and easily available.	Set up formal communication channels and advisory mechanisms involving researchers and policy makers working jointly to identify researchable questions, develop research designs, and plan dissemination and use of findings.
Stage conferences, seminars, briefings and practical workshops to disseminate research findings and educate policy makers about research.	Ensure that officials are able critically to appraise evidence, are familiar with the evidence in their area and are encouraged to use evidence in developing their policy advice. More strongly, require that major policy proposals demonstrate a basis in evidence.
Produce interim reports to ensure that findings are timely.	Be willing to fund researchers not just to produce research but also to take part in 'knowledge mobilization' activities.
Include specific policy implications in research outputs.	Ensure that all major policies and programmes have evaluations built into their budgets and implementation plans.
Identify opinion leaders and innovators, and ensure that they understand the implications of research findings for the issues they care about.	Identify opinion leaders and innovators, and ensure that they understand the implications of research findings.
Undertake systematic reviews of research findings on policy-relevant questions to enable policy makers to access information more easily.	Publish the findings of all public programme evaluations and view evaluation as an opportunity for policy learning rather than a threat.
Identify and keep in contact with policy actors including policy officials throughout the research process.	Commission research and evaluation and consider having additional in-house research capacity.

(Continued)

Table 7.5 (Continued)

Steps to be taken by researchers	Steps to be taken by policy makers who have capacity or interest seeking to evidential support for policy
Design studies to maximize their policy relevance and utility (e.g. ensure that evaluations include the experiences of those whom policies are intended to benefit and are of interventions feasible in a wide range of settings).	Establish 'clearing houses' and 'What Works Centres' to help summarize, package and disseminate evidence or agencies designed to increase the demand for, and use of, evidence.
Use a range of research methods, including 'action-research' (i.e. participative, practically oriented, non-exploitative research which directly involves the subjects of research at all stages with a view to producing new knowledge that empowers people to improve their situation) and other innovative methods.	Provide more opportunities for the public and civil society organizations to learn about research and to engage meaningfully in research and policy processes.
Research topics that are important and relevant for future policy development and give career recognition to researchers whose work is focused on practical application.	Encourage the mass media to improve the quality of reporting and interpretation of research findings and their policy implications through devoting more time and effort to media briefing.

Efforts to break down barriers between the 'two communities'

The steps outlined in Table 7.5 emphasize better communication and translation of research findings but offer little by way of a response to the political and ideological barriers to evidence uptake discussed earlier. Traditionally, many of the approaches to improving the use of evidence in and for policy see the problem of knowledge transfer and evidence-informed policy making as relating to the *separation* between the two worlds of research and policy making, hence the interest in techniques of brokerage and knowledge transfer as ways of making links (Gibson 2003). This fails adequately to consider the degree of conflict *among* both researchers and policy makers, and the *alliances* between sub-groups of both researchers and policy makers that can arise on specific issues in particular political contexts (see below and Chapter 4 on the Advocacy Coalition Framework). Rather than seeing researchers pitted against bureaucrats or politicians, advocacy coalitions are seen as comprising a diverse range of actors including politicians, civil servants, pressure groups, advocates and champions, journalists, researchers and others united by their beliefs and ideas for change. Each advocacy coalition thus interprets and uses research to advance its policy goals in different ways. For example, most academic disciplines are notable for controversies and disputes between rival groups of researchers. This is even more so in fields of enquiry occupied by different disciplines each of which brings different perspectives, assumptions and values to bear on each substantive topic (see the Kenyan 'worm-wars' example above). Gibson (2003) advocates the policy process analyses that abandon the 'two communities' perspective provide a more accurate picture of the political reality, particularly in controversial areas of policy (e.g. sexual health or commercial determinants of health) and have a number of implications for those who wish to increase the impact of research on policy:

1. Researchers should analyse the policy area politically to identify the advocacy coalitions and their core values and beliefs about the nature of the policy problem, its causes and potential solutions.
2. Researchers should engage directly with advocacy coalitions rather than focusing exclusively on managing the boundary between research and policy activities – in effect becoming quasi-embedded with a coalition.
3. Research evidence should be turned into arguments and advocacy rather than purportedly reveal uncontested 'truths'.
4. Researchers should seek to appeal to and influence values and beliefs, and produce compelling narratives, and more importantly counter narratives.

Rather than seeing the barriers to the use of evidence for policy as lying in the relationship between the research and policy communities, a political science perspective on the policy process locates the barriers and facilitators to the uptake of research for policy as lying in the relationships, conflicts and bargaining that take place in particular political contexts between groups each of which can involve both researchers, policy makers and others such as journalists and advocates closely involved in the policy process. The earlier example given in this chapter of pro- and anti-mask wearing in relation to COVID-19 is a good example this kind of process.

Summary

You have learned how evidence is only one among a wide variety of influences on policy processes. Yet, there is no doubt that the policy-making process is influenced by research and other sources of evidence: research can help define a phenomenon as a policy problem potentially worthy of attention and research provides 'enlightenment' through a process in which many ideas from research come to influence policy makers indirectly and over long periods of time. This is facilitated by the links between policy makers and researchers, the media, timing and how research is communicated. There are also many impediments to research being acted upon, including political (i.e. interests) and legitimate ideological differences, policy uncertainty, uncertainty about scientific findings, the perceived utility of research and how easy it is to communicate, as well as cultural and colonial legacies that shape the meanings and value attributed to different types of research (and biases of policy makers towards particular researchers or institutes).

The idea that researchers and policy makers comprise two distinct 'communities' is potentially misleading though it can be useful for identifying how their work differs and some practical actions to improve communication and interaction. However, neither group is politically homogeneous. Researchers and policy makers can be found together participating with a range of other interested actors in competing 'advocacy coalitions' or looser groupings around specific issues. This indicates that evidence enters the policy process as much through influencing political discourse and ideas as through the transmission of formal knowledge. This, in turn, indicates the value of wider systems perspectives and the limitations of positivist, rational models for increasing the odds of evidence being used in policy. Policy making, even at its best, remains the messy product of 'the interplay between institutions, interests and ideas' (John 1998).

Further reading

Boaz, A., Davies, H., Fraser, A. et al. (eds.) (2019) *What Works Now? Evidence-Informed Policy and Practice Revisited*. Bristol: Policy Press.

Parkhurst, J. (2017) *The Politics of Evidence: From Evidence-Based Policy to the Good Governance of Evidence*. London: Taylor & Francis. Available at: https://library.oapen.org/bitstream/handle/20.500.12657/31002/640550.pdf?sequence=1

Parkhurst, J., Ettelt, S. and Hawkins, B. (eds.) (2018) *Evidence Use in Health Policy Making: An International Public Policy Perspective*. Basingstoke: Palgrave MacMillan.

Smith, K. (2013) *Beyond Evidence-Based Policy in Public Health: The Interplay of Ideas*. London: Springer.

Walls, H., Liverani, M., Chheng, K. and Parkhurst, J. (2017) The many meanings of evidence: a comparative analysis of the forms and roles of evidence within three health policy processes in Cambodia, *Health Research Policy and Systems*, 15(1): 95. https://doi.org/10.1186/s12961-017-0260-2

Websites

Paul Cairney's website: https://paulcairney.wordpress.com

Transforming Evidence website: https://transforming-evidence.org

References

Andermann, A., Pang, T., Newton, J.N. et al. (2016) Evidence for health II: overcoming barriers to using evidence in policy and practice, *Health Research Policy and Systems*, 14: 17. https://doi.org/10.1186/s12961-016-0086-3

Best, A. and Holmes, B. (2010) Systems thinking, knowledge and action: towards better models and methods, *Evidence & Policy*, 6(2): 145–59.

Bhakuni, H. and Abimbola, S. (2021) Epistemic injustice in academic global health, *Lancet Global Health*, 9(10): e1465–70.

Boaz, A., Davies, H., Fraser, A. et al. (eds.) (2019) *What Works Now? Evidence-Informed Policy and Practice Revisited*. Bristol: Policy Press.

de Sousa Santos, B. (2015) *Epistemologies of the South: Justice Against Epistemicide*. London: Routledge.

Denis, J.L. and Lomas, J. (eds.) (2003) Researcher: decision-maker partnerships, *Journal of Health Services Research & Policy*, 8(suppl 2).

Fraser, A., Baeza, J.I. and Boaz, A. (2017) 'Holding the line': a qualitative study of the role of evidence in early phase decision-making in the reconfiguration of stroke services in London, *Health Research Policy and Systems*, 15(1): 1–9.

Gibson, B. (2003) Beyond 'two communities', in V. Lin and B. Gibson (eds.) *Evidence-Based Health Policy: Problems and Possibilities.* Melbourne: Oxford University Press, pp. 18–32.

Greenhalgh, T. (2020) Face coverings for the public: laying straw men to rest, *Journal of Evaluation in Clinical Practice*, 26(4): 1070–7.

Hart, J.T. (1971) The inverse care law, *Lancet*, 297(7696): 405–12.

Hawkes, S., Aulakh, B., Jadeja, N. et al. (2016) Strengthening capacity to apply health research evidence in policy making: experience from four countries, *Health Policy and Planning*, (2): 161–70.

Hyder, A.A., Corluka, A., Winch, P.J. et al. (2011) National policymakers speak out: are researchers giving them what they need?, *Health Policy and Planning*, 26: 73–82.

Innvaer, S., Vist, G., Trommald, M. et al. (2002) Health policy makers' perceptions of their use of evidence: a systematic review, *Journal of Health Services Research & Policy*, 7: 239–44.

John, P. (1998) *Analysing Public Policy.* London: Cassell.

King, L., Scheiring, G. and Nosrati, E. (2022) Deaths of despair in comparative perspective, *Annual Review of Sociology*, 48: 299–317.

Koum Besson, E.S. (2022) How to identify epistemic injustice in global health research funding practices: a decolonial guide, *BMJ Global Health*, 7: e008950.

Martin, G. P., Hanna, E., McCartney, M. et al. (2020) Science, society, and policy in the face of uncertainty: reflections on the debate around face coverings for the public during COVID-19, *Critical Public Health*, 30(5): 501–8.

Miguel, E. and Kremer, M. (2004) Worms: identifying impacts on education and health in the presence of treatment externalities, *Econometrica*, 72(1): 159–217.

Morris, S., Hunter, R.M., Ramsay, A.I. et al. (2014) Impact of centralising acute stroke services in English metropolitan areas on mortality and length of hospital stay difference-in-differences analysis, *British Medical Journal,* 349: g4757.

Naidu, T. (2021) Says who? Northern ventriloquism, or epistemic disobedience in global health scholarship, *Lancet Global Health*, 9(9): e1332–5.

Ndlovu-Gatsheni, S.J. (2014) Global coloniality and the challenges of creating African futures, *Strategic Review for Southern Africa*, 36(2): 181.

Parkhurst, J.O. and Abeysinghe, S. (2016) What constitutes 'good' evidence for public health and social policymaking? From hierarchies to appropriateness, *Social Epistemology*, 30(5–6): 665–79.

Rahman-Shepherd, A., Balasubramaniam, P., Gautham, M. et al. (2021) Conflicts of interest: an invisible force shaping health systems and policies, *Lancet Global Health*, 9: e1056.

Rossi, P. and Wright, S. (1979) Evaluation research: an assessment of theory, practice and politics, in C. Pollitt, L. Lewis, J. Negro an J. Pattern (eds.) *Public Policy in Theory and Practice*. London: Hodder and Stoughton.

Smith, K. (2013) *Beyond Evidence-Based Policy in Public Health: The Interplay of Ideas.* London: Springer.

Stewart, R. (2019) Using evidence in international development, in A. Boaz, H. Davies, A. Fraser, A. et al. (eds.) *What Works Now? Evidence-Informed Policy and Practice Revisited*. Bristol: Policy Press, pp. 171–89.

Supran, G. and Oreskes, N. (2017) Assessing ExxonMobil's climate change communications (1977–2014), *Environmental Research Letters*, 12(8): 084019.

Walls, H., Liverani, M., Chheng, K. et al. (2018) The many meanings of evidence: a comparative analysis of the forms and roles of evidence within three health policy processes in Cambodia, in J. Parkhurst, S. Ettelt and B. Hawkins (eds.) *Evidence Use in Health Policy Making: An International Public Policy Perspective*. London: Palgrave Macmillan, pp. 21–49.

Weiss, C.H. (1979) The many meanings of research utilization, *Public Administration Review*, 39(5): 426–31.

Weiss, C.H. (1991) Policy research: data, ideas, in P. Wagner, C. H. Weiss, B. Wittrock. et al. (eds.) *Social Sciences and Modern States: National Experiences and Theoretical Crossroads*. Cambridge, Cambridge University Press, pp. 307–332.

Yegros-Yegros, A., van de Klippe, W., Abad-Garcia, M.F. et al. (2020) Exploring why global health needs are unmet by research efforts: the potential influences of geography, industry and publication incentives, *Health Research Policy and Systems*, 18: 47. https://doi.org/10.1186/s12961-020-00560-6

Values in health policy

8

This chapter introduces you to the inescapable contribution of values and norms to health policy making. It discusses the reluctance of many health policy actors to acknowledge the values that underpin their commitment to particular positions in relation to health policies. It identifies some of the main value propositions at play in debates in the field of health policy at all levels from the global to the local.

Learning objectives

After working through this chapter, you will be better able to:

- define what is meant by values in health policy
- understand how values enter the policy process and why values matter in health policy making
- identify the main values that lie behind many health policy debates and processes, and the degree to which these values are universal or more culturally specific
- engage with contemporary debates as to whether 'facts' and 'values' are entirely separate forms of knowledge and as to whether normative statements cannot be derived from empirical data (the 'binary view')
- assess the 'quality' of health policy-making processes against a number of normative principles.

Key terms

Accountability The evaluative process by which an individual, group or organization provides an account of its behaviour and/or performance for which they are responsible to another, overseeing person, group or organization, or is held to account on the basis of performance reports provided by an independent body. Poor performance may lead to a range of sanctions of varying degrees of severity.

Autonomy Self-determination or the state of being or behaving in a self-governing way with the ability to make one's own decisions.

Beneficence   Acting for the good of the person or people served with a strong connotation of moral obligation (often applied to clinician behaviour).

Cognitive bias   A systematic error in reasoning arising from intrinsic limitations in the human brain's ability to process information and its tendency to simplify. For example, because our attention span is limited, we tend to be selective in what we pay attention to and tend to favour evidence that confirms our prior beliefs and values (confirmation bias).

Democracy   A system of societal governance in which the people elect their representatives to form a time-limited government through periodic elections (indirect democracy) or participate directly in decision making through mechanisms such as referenda.

Efficiency   A measure of the extent to which (health and health care) resources are being used to produce the greatest possible value. In health policy, efficiency typically focuses on the relationship between resource inputs, outputs (e.g. services delivered or reforms enacted in related policy fields such as education) and outcomes (e.g. health improvements in terms of reductions in mortality, reductions in morbidity or gains in quality-adjusted life years).

Equity   The absence of unfair, avoidable or remediable differences between groups of people defined socially, economically or in other ways (e.g. by gender, ethnicity, disability or sexual orientation).

Fairness   Fairness is an umbrella term that can refer to equality (equal treatment of all regardless of individual characteristics), equality of opportunity, justice and equity (unequal treatment of unequals, for instance, in relation to their needs). Fairness is one of the most contested but widely sought after features of policy and policy processes. This is because of the many definitions of fairness, and the value many actors accord to these ideas.

Nonmaleficence   The principle of ensuring that no harm is created by an action or omission (often applied to clinician behaviour).

Norms   The values accepted in a particular social group (a population or population sub-group) as the correct way to judge specific behaviour or policy decisions.

Public goods   Goods that are available to all and used by the individual but benefit the community as a whole such that the more people avail themselves of the good or service, the greater the social benefit.

Stigma   The shame, perceived disgrace or social disapproval associated with a particular social status or disease. Policies can amplify or counter stigma through the way they are labelled, designed or implemented (e.g. the 'dole' versus 'social security').

> **Transparency** A characteristic of a policy process in which the values, evidence, participants, method of deliberation, etc. are visible to those actors not directly involved, especially members of the public.
>
> **Values** The principles or norms people use to decide what, for them, is 'good' and important to pursue in relation to society or their own lives; that is, the basis on which they define 'the good society' or 'the good life' or 'being a good person'.

Introduction

There is a tendency in the field of health policy, especially among those who enter the field from the biomedical and natural sciences, to emphasize its foundations in the application of scientific methods and the evidence that flows from scientific enquiry to the mitigation of threats to population health. You may be familiar with the idea that health policy should be at least 'evidence-informed' if not, even more ambitiously, 'evidence-based'. Indeed, it might be commonly hoped that policy makers have access to and understand the latest and highest quality evidence relevant to the issues they are dealing with (see Chapter 7 for more on the role of evidence in health policy). However, if you think about any area of health policy that you are familiar with, you will realize that there is more to policy making than simply following the evidence. With some highly contested areas of health policy, this is particularly obvious.

Activity 8.1

It would be possible to supress community transmission of most infectious diseases by enforcing strict quarantine of all cases, suspected cases and their contacts. Can you identify the arguments against using such a policy except for a brief period of time during a public health emergency? When setting out the case against such a policy, also note down what you are basing your arguments on. Do your arguments take account of desirable goals that are not strictly related to population health?

Feedback

The principal argument likely to be advanced against such a policy is that it would represent an excessive interference in people's freedom to live their normal lives. Other arguments could include the way that such a policy disregards the consequences for other desirable goals such as educating students and maintaining the economy. Mention of the latter two goals indicates that people value things other than population health (at least directly) and that health policies often have to take account of these potentially competing goals. The former argument indicates an even more fundamental difference of view relating to when and to what extent it is legitimate for the state to intervene in the lives of the population in order to protect public health. This difference of view shows that people differ in what they value and the basis of their value judgements. In other words, people can disagree about what they consider to be 'the good society'.

Another empirical argument that could be made against such a policy is that it is likely to harm people's physical and mental health (e.g. by preventing physical and social activity and reducing access to health services for those with other existing health concerns). It may also impinge on the health of those who are unlikely to suffer much harm from the particular infection.

Defining 'values'

You can now see that people's and organizations' 'values' affect how they judge and support different policy choices. 'Values' in policy making can be defined as the: 'principles, or criteria, for selecting what are good (or better, or best) among objects, actions, ways of life, and social and political institutions and structures' (Schwartz 1990, page 8). Another way of describing these is to refer to 'normative principles' or simply 'norms'. A feature of norms is that they change over time and differ between societies. Sometimes, a change in values or a clash of different values leads to policy change, sometimes the opposite happens and a policy change can reset values by its example. One of the most striking examples of a change of norms relates to views about whether people should be free to express their sexual identities and preferences without legal restriction and sanction. In many, but by no means all countries, gay, bisexual, transgender and non-binary people are far freer to live their lives as they see fit than would have been the case even 30 years ago. Values also conflict and can differ between groups within societies. For example, not everyone agrees with the revolution in sexual freedom that has occurred in many parts of the world (e.g. on transgender people's rights or legal abortion). As a result, freedoms cannot be taken for granted once established. Social values do not always evolve in one direction.

How values enter the processes and outcomes of health policy making

Values and the preferences that flow from taking values into account in judging between policies enter the policy process at all stages. This is because policy making involves choices and these decisions cannot ultimately be made without taking values into account. For example, the evidence about the costs and benefits of implementing a particular policy is an important contribution to deciding whether to pursue a particular policy, but other factors are likely to enter into the judgement about the wisdom of pursuing it. The values people hold shape whether they see a specific 'framing' of a policy problem as entirely convincing. Their values also influence the range of policy goals and responses that they deem to be appropriate. Their values further influence whether they find a particular body of evidence in support of a policy to be convincing or not (see Chapter 7 for more on this).

The contribution of values to policy choices can be very obvious or much more obscure. For example, if there is a change of elected government within a democratic capitalist country from a broadly left of centre, social democratic administration to a more right of centre one, it is usually reasonably clear (e.g. by inspecting the parties' election manifestos) as to whether the ideological basis of the government (its underpinning values) has changed. By contrast, some societal values are far more deeply and widely held and thus can be more difficult to identify since they are taken for granted by the vast majority of the population and supported by powerful interest groups. For example, both the political parties contesting the above election are likely, in broad terms, to support the continuation of free market capitalism to the extent that this is not mentioned at all during the election campaign. They differ only in how they think a capitalist economy should be managed.

Rich and powerful organizations and nations as well as international organizations can impose their values on poorer and more dependent organizations and nations. This is visible in the way that external donors tend to attach conditions to their grants or loans consistent with their values. For example, the US administration under Republican President George W. Bush would only provide donor assistance under the President's Emergency Plan for AIDS Relief to countries for HIV prevention and treatment on condition that all their services promoted the 'ABC' principles of 'abstain, be faithful and use a condom'. Sometimes donors are unaware of the extent to which they are acting in this way and the extent to which their values differ from those they suppose they are assisting.

Ooms (2014, 2015) has commented on the tendency in the field of global health to ignore or downplay its value basis and how this affects attempts to change or defend policies. For example, he shows how researchers and advocates concerned with global health inequalities use terms such as 'inequity' without definition and without being clear what 'equity' as a desired state would look like. Similarly, those preoccupied with notions of *efficiency* focus on the comparative cost-effectiveness of different interventions without acknowledging that the size of the available budget is determined by a prior value-based decision. The threshold of what is deemed cost-effective varies from country to country depending on its wealth and also its own and donors' willingness to devote resources to health.

Ooms attributes the reluctance to acknowledge the normative (i.e. value) basis of the field of global health to the dominance in the field of researchers and practitioners trained in biomedicine and their discomfort with the proposition generally held in philosophy that normative statements cannot be derived directly from empirical data (see below for more on this strictly binary view of the distinction between facts and values). Another reason is that dealing with values and the trade-offs between them is difficult. It is much easier to take for granted that values such as *equity* (*fairness*) are 'a good thing'. Another more challenging explanation for this reticence is provided by Kim (2021), who argues that the *explicit* commitment of global health practitioners and researchers to improving health and improving health equity has the *implicit* function of reproducing the existing unequal power structure globally. He argues that the field of global health has always fulfilled an implicit ideological function, initially to protect the economic interests of colonizing nations and latterly to legitimize 'the hegemony of neoliberal values in its tendency to individualize and depoliticize causes of and solutions to ill health and health inequities' (Kim, 2021, page 2). He goes on to contend that global health programmes provide 'a sense of relief or redemption for (mostly European and North American, but really global) elites through acting out of "charitable" impulses or fulfilling a sense of "moral duty"'. See more on this in Chapter 9 on bilateral assistance.

Why values matter in health policy making

Policy making is inherently normative in that values shape the goals of policy. Giving priority to different values leads to different policy choices relating to both ends (goals or objectives) and means (types of policy instruments or interventions). This is most observable in the field of public health when balancing fairness and individual liberty, as shown in Activity 8.1.

✎ Activity 8.2

'Global health' often involves countries from wealthier regions of the world seeking to influence and improve the health systems of countries in a poorer region of the world. Why should the people and government of one country bother to help another country to improve its health? List the possible reasons you can think of and the principles underlying them.

Feedback

There are many possible reasons for intervening in the health of another country. Such intervention may be led by public opinion, the Third Sector, government or business interests. For example, there may be wide public sympathy for people less fortunate than themselves (i.e. a notion of charity), especially if those affected such as children or war refugees are not regarded as responsible for their suffering. The public may simply find it distressing to see suffering and would prefer it be stopped. Some people might be concerned because they see the situation as the result of past extractive colonialism or present capitalism. By contrast, governments may intervene because they are concerned to protect their populations from the spread of an infectious disease. This is similar to the original impulse behind most colonial health services. In contrast, intervention may be justified by a belief that everyone should have the right to experience a minimum level of good health or life expectancy. Another motivation for intervening could be to build ties with another country, for example, to avoid future conflicts or enable investment opportunities. As Ooms (2015) points out, none of these normative positions can be entirely proved to be superior to any other on empirical grounds (though they have empirical consequences), but all can be legitimately debated between people with different sets of values and each lead to different policy options. The principles that underlie these reasons include those of fairness, justice and enlightened self-interest.

Vélez et al. (2020) reviewed studies of the health policy process in Latin America in order to explain how and under what conditions different social values entered into decision making about health system financing. They characterized the values that were taken into account in four ways:

(1) goal-related values (i.e. guiding principles of the health system); (2) technical values (those incorporated into the instruments adopted by policy-makers to ensure a sustainable and efficient health system); (3) governance values (those applied in the policy process to ensure a transparent, representative and accountable process of decision-making); and (4) situational values (a broad category of values that represent competing strategies to make decisions in the health systems). (Vélez et al. 2020: 1)

The last category comprised things such as political history, changes in the relative power and self-interest of important groups, changes in national mood and international trends. The combination of these different sets of values begins to explain how and why decision makers can still arrive at different decisions in different institutional contexts, when faced with the same body of scientific evidence (see Chapter 7 for more on this).

The main values that underpin health policy goals and debates

The different values or norms defined in this section are not exhaustive of all the values at play in health policy but are included because they frequently shape health policy debates and can be seen at work at all levels of health policy making from the global to the local. However, the way that they play out will vary at the different levels. For example, it is likely that inhabitants of a rich country in one part of the world will be less willing to support policies in a faraway, poor country designed to improve the living standards of the poor than they would support policies to improve the lot of poor people in their own country.

Fairness

Strongly held notions of fairness are entwined in many decision-making processes in health policy at country and global levels. Frequently voiced arguments in favour of human rights to health are ultimately based on notions of fairness and justice.

Indeed, fairness can be seen as perhaps the fundamental normative criterion against which public policies are judged. As Peters (2021: 161) argues at the country level:

> Citizens may be willing to accept some deprivations, such as higher taxes or loss of services in times of crisis, provided they believe the policy treats all citizens equally, and is being implemented fairly. For example, rates of tax evasion appear lessened if citizens believe that the taxes and their enforcement is fair ... governments are responsible in the mind of most people for maintaining individual rights and fairness among individuals through law, and doing so through equal enforcement.

This insight explains why there was such public disapproval of the behaviour of former UK Prime Minister Boris Johnson when it was discovered that, along with his staff, he had taken part in numerous parties when the rest of the country was required by law to limit almost all forms of social gathering during the COVID-19 pandemic in 2020 and 2021.

Despite the importance of fairness in policy, there is no single, agreed definition of fairness or equity on which to base people's rights or entitlement to a particular level of health. Judgements about what is 'fair' can be very personal, context-specific and subjective. They can often hinge on judgements about things which are difficult to assess such as whether people are entitled to a particular standard of living on the basis of fundamental human needs versus the view that everyone has to earn their standard of living through their 'own efforts' – or indeed whether it is fair that some people can afford to pay accountants to avoid taxes and to lobby policy makers

to ensure ever more tax loopholes. 'Inequity' likewise is disputed though there is wider acceptance that inequity refers to a distribution of opportunities or resources which is unnecessary and avoidable but also unjustified (Whitehead 1992). For example, there are differences between the health of individuals and groups in all populations. These could be described simply as 'variations', which would tend to imply that they arise at random and are of no wider societal concern. Yet, it is well known that health differences are strongly patterned within populations (e.g. poorer people generally have poorer health), and the extent of disparity and who is most affected (e.g. poorer women within particular ethnic groups) are influenced by social and economic policy choices. Discussing differences in health within a country's population, the King's Fund health think tank defines health 'inequalities' in contrast to health 'variations' as 'avoidable, unfair and systematic differences in health between different groups of people' (Williams et al. 2022). It might be more accurate to describe these as health 'inequities'.

Philosophers have devoted great effort to try to produce theories or standards of fairness that most people would find reasonable. In the late twentieth century and still today, the ideas of John Rawls (1999) have probably been the most discussed in liberal democratic states, especially his conception of a just or fair society based on the distribution of benefits and costs that individuals would select behind the 'Veil of Ignorance'; that is, before they would have any knowledge of the actual distribution of goods that they would experience in life, whether as a result of government or market action (what Rawls calls 'the Original Position'). Faced with no information on the probabilities of ending up at the top, middle or bottom of any societal distribution of money, other resources, rights and freedoms, Rawls argues that individuals are likely to choose distributions that are more equal than those usually generated solely by the economic market in order to minimize the risk that they find themselves in the most disadvantaged position in society. Rawls argues that rational people would maximize the minimum that they could be sure to get. He calls this approach 'Maximin'. In societal terms, this would indicate the pursuit of policies that ensure that the worst-off do as well as possible.

Behind the 'Veil of Ignorance,' Rawls argues that two principles would arise to guide judgements about what constitutes a fair distribution of the resources necessary for a good life:

- *First principle* – each person should be given the same basic liberties and be treated as morally equal.
- *Second principle* – there can be some inequality in society but all positions that have the potential to generate unequal rewards must be open to everyone with equal talents and equal willingness to use their talents on an equal basis (i.e. there should be fair equality of opportunity) and any inequalities must also be to the greatest benefit of the least well off in society (the 'difference principle').

Although Rawls' use of ideas such as the Original Position and the 'Veil of Ignorance' are abstract and not to be found in the real world, they do help provide a basis for identifying what a fair policy might look like. For example, adopting the difference principle leads to preferring policies that minimize social and economic differences within society over ones that risk increasing inequalities. As it happens, this preference is a pretty good approximation of the principles underlying most global health policy statements such as the SDGs. Policy advocates influenced by Rawls' theory of justice or fairness would tend to develop policy proposals designed to ensure equal basic liberties for all, to bring equality of opportunity for all and to benefit the worst off as much as possible.

However, Rawls' approach to justice and fairness has been extensively criticized both for giving too much and too little weight to preserving individual freedom versus equality.

Activity 8.3

Can you think of any criticisms that could be made of Rawls' theory? Are all the assumptions he makes behind the 'Veil of Ignorance' entirely justifiable?

Feedback

There is no need to worry if you found it difficult to critique the most famous work of an influential philosopher. Three main criticisms have been levelled at Rawls' theory:

1. Having identified what a just distribution of goods would look like behind the 'Veil of Ignorance,' the theory would indicate that society should be reformed to move towards such a distribution. However, as Robert Nozick (1974) points out, many of these goods are already owned and many were worked for fairly (debatable, but Nozick's position), including those inherited. People have ownership rights that cannot simply be overridden. Just because redistribution would benefit someone else is no justification for the state forcibly removing goods from one person to give to another, for instance, via taxation (again debatable but not according to Nozick). Nozick overlooks the fact that someone's ability to work and obtain goods is likely to depend not just on their own efforts but also their education, health, living in a stable society, etc. Nozick's position represents an extreme libertarian definition of what is fair. Policies based on it would prioritize protecting property rights, limit or

reduce the scope of government action and lower taxes in the name of freedom (Nozick 1974).

2. Rawls aspires to a universal theory of justice which deliberately ignores the fact that people live in particular cultures and have connections to specific communities. Some critics have argued that what is regarded as a just policy may depend in part on the values of the specific society in a particular period of history, and that a rational person would not wish to ignore these values entirely.

3. The third criticism, like the second, focuses on the real-world implications of Rawls' theory. The abstract nature of the 'Veil of Ignorance' means that what happens behind it provides little practical guidance as to how to remedy existing injustices such as those caused by racism and sexism. For example, can Rawls' principles be used to identify whether restitution should be paid to colonized countries and peoples, or to the descendants of slaves for unjust acts committed in the past, or to women who have been paid less than men for the same work because of the gender pay gap?

The three criticisms above focus on the idealized nature of Rawls' theory of justice and question its applicability in practice. However, its great strength is the way it highlights the fact that what people judge to be just and fair is often influenced by their perceived self-interest, which is an inadequate basis for public policy.

From a more egalitarian standpoint, the main criticism of Rawls' approach is that it would go no further than ensuring that the opportunities for living a healthy life are distributed fairly rather than ensuring that the final outcomes are achieved. Daniels (2006) argues that the state should not only ensure equality of opportunity (e.g. to access health care) but also act to minimize structural barriers to good health that disproportionately affect particular groups (e.g. occupational exposure to hazards which disproportionately affect poorer manual workers). This would include policies to ensure that universal health care coverage benefits people from different socio-economic and minority backgrounds equally.

The Indian economist, Amartya Sen, goes further than both Rawls and Daniels since he regards good health as intrinsically valuable, not just a means to other ends, and argues that the focus of equitable policy should be not so much on the distribution of opportunities and resources as on ensuring that all individuals have the same ability to use their resources to attain the goals that they value. Sen (1999) thus focuses on equality of 'capabilities' rather than a fair distribution of opportunity. This means that people who differ by gender, disability, ethnicity, sexual orientation, etc., should be treated differently to ensure that the constraints on their flourishing are identified and removed, and their individual capabilities are developed as much as possible. 'Capabilities' are the things that people can attain if they choose to from the basic such as being properly fed through raising a family to things like getting an education and travelling. Unlike Daniels, who considers being healthy as a prerequisite for full participation in any society, Sen argues that individuals and communities should decide for themselves which capabilities they wish to prioritize.

Autonomy and personal responsibility

Rawls' emphasis on people being treated equally and given equality of opportunity indicates that he would regard it as fair, as a general rule, to allow individuals to reach their own decisions about the things that affect their own lives without state interference. However, there will inevitably be situations where this is not possible or desirable. Some of these are fairly straightforward to justify, at least in principle, such as intervening to protect the interests of vulnerable individuals, for example children, against abuse and exploitation. In such cases, the issue tends to be the extent of intervention or regulation rather than the principle. Others are much more intrinsically complicated and controversial. For example, should parents have the right to exempt their children from all forms of school sex education on the grounds that certain expressions of sexual identity and behaviour included in the curriculum are against their beliefs?

A perennial issue in public health where individual choices and collective benefit can come into conflict is that of vaccination. Vaccination is a classic example of a '*public good*' which should ideally be undertaken by as many members of society as possible since by becoming vaccinated the individual benefits not only themselves but also those around them. If a person refuses to be vaccinated or refuses to allow their children to be vaccinated, how should the state respond?

This is particularly pertinent during a pandemic and when that person is a celebrity. The case of the tennis player Novak Djokovik exemplifies many of the issues associated with personal *autonomy*, choice and responsibility to others. Djokovik refused all COVID-19 vaccines on the grounds that he alone should have the right to decide what to put into his body. This appeared, at least in part, to be an extension of his rigorous fitness, diet and health regime as a top athlete, since he claimed not to be opposed to vaccination on principle. As a result, he was prevented from playing in the Australian tennis open in February 2022 and deported from the country on the grounds that he could not be granted an immigration visa at that time of tight border controls without proof of vaccination. An alternative approach, but one which would have exposed the Australian government to the criticism of unfairly giving a super-star special treatment, would have been to require Djokovik to avoid physical contact with others and test daily for COVID-19. In other situations, individuals have been given exemptions from a prevailing requirement to be vaccinated if their objections have been on religious grounds.

Since the mid-1980s, there have been efforts in many countries to introduce more individual choice into public services such as health (see Chapter 6). Although such policies have usually been justified in terms of improving the quality or efficiency of care by putting providers under competitive pressure, they have also been justified according to the intrinsic value of choice. From the latter perspective, these policy instruments can be seen as an attempt to reconcile fair access to health services with individual autonomy. For example, the English NHS, which is tax-financed, universal and free at the point of use, offers patients a choice of hospital for elective (non-urgent) care. The issue of patient choice raises wider questions about how much people should be expected to take personal responsibility for their own health. Critics of these policies argue that not all patients have the knowledge or opportunity to make such choices effectively such that choice policies are highly likely to increase health inequalities. Strictly speaking, such a criticism is irrelevant to the question of whether or not the availability of choice is intrinsically valuable even if not exercised or not exercised well. An extreme libertarian such as Nozick (1974) would argue that individual choice is necessary for the operation of markets for goods and services, including for health, and that markets based on choice and the distributions of income and wealth that they generate are intrinsically fair.

Preservation of life

The preservation of life is clearly a value central to much health and related policy. The Australian philosopher Peter Singer (2010) invites people to imagine a scenario whereby they are walking to a business meeting and see a child drowning in a pond. He asks whether a person in this imaginary scenario ought to save the child even if it meant ruining their own smart clothes. The answer from most people is of course, 'Yes' – the morally right thing to do would be to save the child regardless of the damage to their clothes. Singer then invites people to apply the same principle to the problem of children dying of preventable diseases elsewhere in the world and argues from a utilitarian perspective that those with the means to do so should support charities delivering life-saving interventions to those who require them wherever they are located in the world, and that not to do so is as morally problematic as walking past the imaginary child drowning in the pond. It is common to hear people declaring that life is invaluable, yet policy makers, like individuals, have to decide how much to spend to save lives as against other uses for the same resources. As well as goals of efficiency, the preservation of life can conflict with other values such as autonomy and choice.

✎ **Activity 8.4**

Can you think of situations in health policy making where the values of autonomy and the preservation of life can conflict?

Feedback

There are many such situations. You will most likely have thought of others, but here are some of the most commonly discussed:

- Where the state on behalf of society either outlaws or takes steps to minimize the likelihood of suicide (e.g. by reformulating the household gas supply) in the name of preserving life. Libertarians would argue that individuals should be free to end their own lives in a manner and time of their choosing and should not be constrained or dictated to by law or regulation.
- Where the state on behalf of society requires that everyone takes the same safety precautions, regardless of their personal risk appetite (e.g. requiring seat belts or helmets to be worn). Governments may argue that it takes these measures in order to protect other members of society from the costs of treating injuries and family members from suffering.
- Where the state on behalf of society either bans or limits women's access to legal abortion in the name of preserving the right to life of the unborn child.
- Where the state on behalf of society requires a clear expression of intent or formal consent registered in life before any organs or tissue may be removed from the person in death even if more life-saving organs could be retrieved without these processes. Some countries have moved in the opposite direction, adopting a law of presumed consent to deceased organ donation (unless a person has explicitly opted out) in order to increase the supply of organs. However, they then have to deal with the possibility that family members may object to organ removal despite what the law says.

Efficiency

The intellectually dominant approach to assessing the 'value' of a policy both before and after deciding whether to pursue it relies on quantifying the costs and benefits to the widest possible extent using tools such as cost–benefit or cost–utility analysis. This approach rests on the assumption that policies should strive to produce the maximum benefit at least cost. This type of thinking is so deeply embedded and widespread that it is rarely if ever seen as a normative proposition. It is taken for granted as the correct way to assess policies.

 Activity 8.5

Can you identify any limitations of the cost–benefit approach to assessing health policies?

Feedback

You may have reflected on whether any of the other values already discussed in this chapter can be accommodated alongside the cost–benefit approach to policy analysis. Most importantly, this form of policy analysis takes no account of the distribution of costs and benefits, for example, between different socio-economic or ethnic groups in a society. Thus it treats concerns about fairness as either irrelevant (in that efficient solutions are intrinsically fair) or strictly secondary to efficiency (i.e. that equity can only be pursued to the extent that it does not interfere with efficiency). It also dismisses the impacts of policies that cannot be measured.

Stigma

While wishing to respond appropriately to the different needs of subgroups of the population in the name of fairness, policy makers also have to be aware of the risk that this could be stigmatizing. This is because in some societies and in some periods of history, people are or were stigmatized (i.e. regarded as less capable and less fully members of society) on grounds of race, religion, sexual orientation, physical deformity or mental illness, for example. In policy terms, *stigma* is generally defined as the shame, perceived disgrace or social disapproval associated with claiming or receiving particular types of public service. There is a long history in society of wishing to differentiate between the 'deserving' and 'undeserving' poor. Older people and children are typically seen as 'deserving' of assistance in all periods, whereas adults of working age in need of support from the state are often seen as 'undeserving'. Likewise, unmarried women in countries such as Nepal and Bangladesh are reluctant to come forward for family planning or sexual health services because of stigma. Similarly, men who have sex with men have been deterred from getting vaccinated against monkeypox for fear of identifying themselves to a generally hostile community in some countries.

Although there may be some sacrifice in efficiency of targeting of services to those in need, universal services (i.e. those open to all without having to self-identify as 'in need') are generally preferred to selective services if the goal is to reduce the risk of stigma. For example, in a capitalist society where being poor can be perceived as being a failure, a scrounger and a drain on the charity of others, claiming a means-tested benefit can be a stigmatizing experience. One solution is for the state to pay everyone a universal basic income thereby removing the requirement to self-identify as poor. Another is to make as much use as possible of the tax system to redistribute income and wealth rather than requiring citizens to apply more publicly for a cash benefit. Yet another is to provide opportunities for people receiving financial assistance to contribute to society in kind in return in ways that match their skills and opportunities, thereby emphasizing reciprocity.

Democracy and participation

A widely, if not universally held value relating to how policy is made relates to the nature of, and extent to which, the general public is involved in the making of policies that affect their lives. Democrats believe that ordinary people should at the very least be indirectly involved by being able to vote to replace their elected representatives periodically at elections. Free and fair elections depend on other values such as freedom of expression and freedom to protest against government policies. Proponents of more participatory forms of *democracy* believe that the public should also be able to become involved in policy making more directly, for example, through petitions, referenda, citizen's juries and the like. These can be advisory or binding on the government of the day.

Are values and value conflicts universal? The contribution of non-Western value systems

There are numerous 'non-Western' and indigenous value systems in different parts of the world relevant to health policy making such as Ubuntu in Southern Africa and Islamic Zakat thinking. While it would be ignorant and harmful to generalize about these systems, there are some similarities between them, at least compared with the range of Western value systems. In comparison with typical Western values, individuals tend to be seen as both more inter-connected and more dependent on , and respectful of, the natural world. For example, Maori concepts of health (*hauora*) and how to promote better health are very broad to this day, incorporating the inter-dependence of physical health, spiritual health, family and community health, mental health and the health of the natural environment. As a result, health promotion campaigns such as stop smoking have sometimes appealed less to the individual's self-interest and more to the effect of their (ill) health on their family (*whanau*) or grandchildren (*mokopuna*).

It can be argued that such values, especially the appreciation of human-kind's dependence on, and responsibility for, the natural world, especially for its climate, have grown in prominence in the West, partly as a result of engagement with these other ways of being and knowing, many of which had been marginalized or eradicated by colonialism. For example, Loewenson et al. (2021) show how traditional views of a 'healthy society' in India, Latin America and East and Southern Africa included strong features of reciprocity and harmony with nature. They argue that 'These were suppressed by biomedical, allopathic models during colonialism and by postcolonial neoliberal economic reforms promoting selective, biomedical interventions for highest-burden diseases.'

Should the same values guide health policy at the global level as domestically?

While there is a social consensus in most countries, if not unanimity, that the state has some obligation to act to secure good health for all so that people can participate fully in society, there is far less agreement on the scope of obligation of people in one country to those in other countries. Brown and Paremoer (2014) identify broadly *statist* and *cosmopolitan* positions on this issue. The statists argue that while the nation state has some responsibility for people beyond its borders, for example, on humanitarian grounds, this is legitimately secondary to its responsibility to its own people. The extent of international responsibility is dependent on contextual factors such as social ties, cultural affinity and distance. This position limits international state action beyond humanitarianism exclusively to countering threats to national (health) security. This tends to narrow the target to health problems such as the immediate threat of infectious diseases rather than their underlying causes such as climate change. It also tends to lead to underestimating the need for and effectiveness of collective action between states.

By contrast, the cosmopolitans argue that limiting the pursuit of justice and fairness to the nation state is arbitrary and that the same principles should apply at national and international levels. For example, the country where a person happens to have been born is outside their control. They should be able to enjoy at least a minimum level of health wherever they live. This has some echoes of Rawls' use of the idea of the 'Veil of Ignorance' behind which each individual is ignorant of their fate in life and thus tends towards an equitable distribution of opportunities and resources. The cosmopolitan or global normative position emphasizes the equal worth of all people and thus their right to fulfil their human potential. The cosmopolitans also emphasize the inter-dependence of peoples and argue that the notion of a fair distribution of opportunities and resources should be extended beyond the confines of a specific community (the nation state). This perspective can perhaps be encapsulated in the phrase 'citizen of the world'. It is also influenced by the recognition that many of the determinants of population health act across borders. It also recognizes that the current pattern of nation states is not static and should not be treated as such.

The cosmopolitan position on equity and justice clearly lies behind global initiatives such as the Millennium Development Goals (MDGs) and the SDGs. In turn, some of the limited progress towards realizing these goals can be attributed to the tenacity of the statist perspective on global health and its impact on the amount of resources devoted to responding to global health problems.

How can 'values' as well as 'facts' be handled in the policy process?

It is widely accepted in philosophy that a 'should' statement can never be derived from an 'is' statement; in other words, that there is a fundamental difference between normative and empirical claims: factual claims can be proved or disproved whereas normative ones can neither be verified nor falsified. This 'binary view' is very widely taught and accords with much personal experience of debating controversial policy issues with those who have very different values (e.g. over whether mask wearing during a pandemic should be compulsory or not). Yet, if accepted, the 'binary view' has the unfortunate effect, crucial to the policy process, of shifting value claims, however extreme, outside the scope of critical debate and questioning. An alternative approach is to interrogate factual and normative claims in much the same way. Ryan (2022) justifies this on the grounds that a 'should' (normative) claim is usually an incompletely formulated 'if–then' (empirical) claim. For example, a normative claim that abortion should be permitted because women should have the right to control their own bodies can be seen more completely as a claim that abortion should be permitted as a women's rights issue on the grounds that it will protect women's health better than the alternative. Ryan (2022) also argues that an 'if–then' claim is usually an incompletely formulated 'should' claim on the basis that, while there is an objective world beyond our individual consciousness, how we see that world and how we judge what is true in it depends on our values. This is the territory of *cognitive bias* for the psychologist. We tend to see and take notice of what we are primed to see. Sociologists call this the 'social construction' of reality (Berger and Luckmann 1967). Challenging the 'binary view' allows for a continuous process of policy questioning and discussion, the goal of which is to clarify both the factual and normative positions people hold and the basis on which they hold them.

This position has considerable significance for the way in which we look at the motivation and role of evidence producers in society, and how we judge what they produce (see Chapter 7). For example, according to this position, a researcher would not enter a field such as planetary health unless they already had a strong value commitment to the welfare of future generations. In this case, their value commitment drives their science and cannot ultimately be separated from their science but, crucially, this does not invalidate their scientific work. The same applies to policy advocates and even to the career choices of policy advisers such as civil servants. Everyone involved in the policy process comes with their values. They can be faced with difficult choices in which facts and values are intertwined. For example, should expensive third line chemotherapy drugs that may add a few very valuable months to the lives of a small number of lung cancer patients be preferred to allocating the same amount of funding to smoking cessation programmes that will benefit a larger number of individuals over a longer period of time? This is an example of a 'wicked problem', and any proposed solution to it cannot be objectively 'correct' – but will inevitably be normative and open to debate. There are many similar complex, wicked policy problems such as averting the climate crisis (Head 2022).

Normative principles for assessing health policies and health policy making

Values often enter into deciding whether we think that a policy and/or the process that led to a policy is a good one or not. It is clear that people care about how decisions are made on their behalf as well as the outcomes of these decisions. Not surprisingly, people tend to be more worried about the quality of the policy process when they dislike the result than when the result is in line with their values. This is similar to the phenomenon observed in relation to the use of evidence in policy making: that evidence that contradicts the direction of government policy will be subject to far more methodological critique than supportive evidence. Following Ryan (2022), people may also have legitimate grounds to judge that policies formulated and implemented in ways that contradict widely held values such as fairness and honesty will ultimately be less effective and sustainable than those that emerge from 'good' processes.

✎ **Activity 8.6**

Given the range of different values that enter into health policy making discussed earlier in this chapter, please list some principles of what you would regard as 'good' health policy making processes. To do this, you can think about activities at all levels of health systems from negotiations with international bodies to the management of local clinics. It is likely that many of the same principles apply.

Feedback

Your list is likely to have contained values related to things like consulting the people likely to be affected by a policy, dealing fairly with people with different interests and needs, making informed decisions and so on.

A large number of normative schemes have been developed to judge the quality of policy making. In general, 'good' policy making is seen as well informed, inclusive, fair, responsible and accountable. There will be some differences across the globe in terms of which principles are seen as the most important, and sometimes principles are taken for granted in some settings while being explicitly stated in others. For example, democratic *accountability*, government truth telling and adherence to the rule of law may be taken for granted in some parts of the world though need buttressing everywhere.

How to deal with differences in values between groups and societies in the policy process

There are a number of potential complementary approaches (Pielke 2012; Ooms, 2014, 2015), such as:

- 'objectivizing' values – that is, treating them as facts ('this is how people feel, in fact, about "right" and "wrong"'), without taking a position;
- referring to norms that are widely accepted such as statements of human rights, the SDGs;
- being explicit about your values as a policy adviser or decision maker;
- acting as an 'honest broker' between different value sets along the lines of:
  - if society is willing to contribute a lot of money and give up considerable individual freedom: for example, do A + B + C;
  - if society is unwilling to contribute a lot of money: for example, do A + B (lower cost options);
  - if society is unwilling to give up individual freedom: do A (lower cost) + C (higher cost but less restrictive) + F (freedom enhancing, low/no direct cost).

The criteria for 'good' policy making overlap with the wider values associated with the notion of 'good governance'. A relevant framework that has been extensively used as a benchmark for health system governance in many regions of the world was developed by Siddiqi and colleagues (2009), based on analysing frameworks previously used by the World Health Organization, Pan-American Health Organization, World Bank and United Nations Development Programme (UNDP). The framework comprises ten principles:

1. *Strategic vision* – system leaders take a wide-ranging, long-term view of health and human development.
2. *Participation and consensus orientation* – everyone should be able to be heard either directly or via organizations that represent their interests, and health system decision makers should strive to reach a broad consensus that accommodates these differing interests.
3. *Rule of law* – the law relating to health should be fair and enforced impartially, especially where this relates to human rights to health.
4. *Transparency* – there should be a free flow of information on health issues with enough information for the population to understand and monitor health policies.
5. *Responsiveness* – policies and programmes should be responsive to the health and non-health needs of users.
6. *Equity and inclusiveness* – everyone should have the opportunity to improve or maintain their health.
7. *Effectiveness and efficiency* – policies and programmes should influence health outcomes as well as make the best use of resources.
8. *Accountability* – public, private and civil society decision makers should be accountable not just to those with a direct interest in their activities (e.g. funders) but also to the public.
9. *Intelligence and information* – health systems should have the necessary evidence available to inform their decision making.
10. *Ethics* – health systems should act in line with the commonly accepted ethical principles of health care such as respect for autonomy, *nonmaleficence*, *beneficence* and justice.

The list mentions seeking consensus. To do so involves managing value conflicts and disagreements. The boxed text above provides some tips on this process. Taken together, these principles are extremely demanding for any health policy system to maintain consistently throughout all activities but represent a standard to which system leaders can aspire and which societies can use to assess whether their system lives up to its values.

The issue of how to achieve 'distributive justice' ('who gets what and how much') has attracted particular attention in relation to the principles of good policy making because of its normative and practical complexities, some of which are outlined in this chapter. In 1999, NICE was established to assess the clinical and cost-effectiveness of health technologies and treatments for potential provision in the NHS in England and Wales. There will never be agreement about the fairest way to distribute limited health care funds – with different lobby groups championing their own interests. Daniels and Sabin (2002) set out four principles to encourage distributive justice in the health care rationing decisions that NICE strives to respect.

The first is *relevance* – the rationale and evidence used to inform priority setting decisions must be seen to be relevant and valid by all interested parties. Second, *publicity* is important – these decisions and their rationales should be published and open to scrutiny. Third, there must be scope for *revisions* to all decisions if challenged on reasonable grounds. Fourth, *enforcement* is crucial – leaders must ensure the first three principles are always followed.

Trade-offs between values in real-world policy making

While the ten principles of 'good' policy making listed above would have few detractors, they can be difficult to respect equally in practice. Values can and do conflict in public policy and health is no different. Most conflicts about values in health policy tend not to centre on whether people are in favour of, or indifferent to, a particular value such as equity but rather between actors who prioritize equity over other values and to varying degrees, and those who prioritize other values more than equity. There can also be arguments between those who are guided by different concepts of equity such as egalitarians who focus on final outcomes versus Rawlsians who emphasize ensuring equality of opportunity and who tolerate some inequality as a result (see Vélez et al. 2020). Others would go further and object to any policies that redistribute resources to the extent that the best-off lose out.

One area of extensive debate relates to what a general commitment to truth telling and transparency should mean in practice, especially in the early stages of the policy process. For example, is it legitimate for an elected official to ask their civil servants to investigate the potential pros and cons of a particular response to an already contentious issue without disclosing this publicly or sharing the analysis more widely? Is it conducive to the provision of rigorous policy making if all policy advice is routinely published in real time? Will this reduce the odds of advisers 'speaking truth to power' and lead to unsatisfactory advice? On what basis can such advice be withheld and for how long before it becomes a matter of deliberately misleading the public?

It has long been argued that a full commitment to openness and truth telling cannot be sustained in all situations, and particularly not in the realm of foreign and security policy. For example, faced with a potential aggressor, a country's diplomats may be given the task of deliberately misleading the potential aggressor as to the extent of the country's military preparedness in the hope of delaying or deterring a war. Such behaviour is generally justified on the grounds of trying to preserve the lives of citizens. Thus one value in policy making – truthfulness – conflicts with another – preservation of life. While most people would probably have few qualms about diplomats exaggerating or lying on behalf of their country in such a situation, their calculus would most likely be different in relation to other issues such as pandemics or climate change.

Summary

This chapter has described the way that personal and social values (norms) are inescapable when health policy is being made. This insight can be uncomfortable for those who approach policy making as a purely technical activity. The chapter has summarized some of the main value positions that underlie debates and trade-offs in health policy making. You have seen how different notions of fairness and justice are central to many of these debates. The case has been made that there is no intrinsic reason why the principles of social justice accepted within countries should not apply between countries. While 'facts' and 'values' offer distinct considerations for policy making, the chapter has further argued that the two have more in common in practice than is usually acknowledged by philosophers. Both can be interrogated and clarified in the policy process. Finally, the chapter has engaged with discussions about how to manage value conflicts and trade-offs in the practice of health policy making, including providing some frameworks for assessing the quality of policy-making processes.

Further reading

Capano, G. and Malandrino, A. (2022) Mapping the use of knowledge in policymaking: barriers and facilitators from a subjectivist perspective (1990–2020), *Policy Sciences*, 55: 399–428. https://doi.org/10.1007/s11077-022-09468-0

Daniels, N. and Sabin, J.E. (2008) Accountability for reasonableness: an update, *British Medical Journal*, 337: a1850. https://doi.org/10.1136/bmj.a1850

Ooms, G. (2015) Navigating between stealth advocacy and unconscious dogmatism: the challenge of researching the norms, politics and power of global health, *International Journal of Health Policy and Management*, 4: 641–44. https://doi.org/10.15171/ijhpm.2015.116

Stewart, J. (2009) *Public Policy Values*. Basingstoke: Palgrave Macmillan, Chapters 1–6 and 11.

Stone, D. (2002) *Policy Paradox: The Art of Political Decision Making*, revised edition. New York: W.W. Norton, Part II (Chapters 2–5).

References

Berger, P.L. and Luckmann, T. (1967) The social construction of reality: a treatise in the sociology of knowledge. Harmondsworth: Allen Lane, Penguin Press.

Brown, G.W. and Paremoer, L. (2014) Global health justice and the right to health, in G.W. Brown, G. Yamey and S. Wamala (eds.) *The Handbook of Global Health Policy*. Oxford: Wiley Blackwell, pp. 77–95.

Daniels, N. (2006) Equity and population health: toward a broader bioethics agenda, *Hastings Center Report*, 36(4): 22–35.

Daniels, N. and Sabin, J. (2002) *Setting Limits Fairly: Can We Learn to Share Medical Resources?* New York: Oxford University Press.

Head, B.W. (2022) *Wicked Problems in Public Policy: Understanding and Responding to Complex Challenges*. London: Palgrave Macmillan. Available at: https://link.springer.com/book/10.1007/978-3-030-94580-0 (accessed 24 April 2023).

Kim, H. (2021) The implicit ideological function of the global health field and its role in maintaining relations of power, *BMJ Global Health*, 6: e005620 https://doi.org/10.1136/bmjgh-2021-005620.

Loewenson, R., Villar, E., Baru, R. and Marten, R. (2021) Engaging globally with how to achieve healthy
   societies: insights from India, Latin America and East and Southern Africa, *BMJ Global Health*, 6:
   e005257. https://doi.org/10.1136/bmjgh-2021-005257

Nozick, R. (1974) *Anarchy, State, and Utopia*. Oxford: Blackwell.

Ooms, G. (2014) From international health to global health: how to foster a better dialogue between
   empirical and normative disciplines, *BMC International Health and Human Rights*, 14(1): 36.

Ooms, G. (2015) Navigating between stealth advocacy and unconscious dogmatism: the challenge of
   researching the norms, politics and power of global health, *International Journal of Health Policy
   and Management*, 4(10): 641–44. https://doi.org/10.15171/ijhpm.2015.116

Peters, B.G. (2021) *Advanced Introduction to Public Policy*, 2nd edn. Cheltenham: Edward Elgar.

Pielke, R.A. (2012) *The Honest Broker: Making Sense of Science, Policy and Politics*. Boulder, CO: University of Colorado Press.

Rawls, J. (1999) *A Theory of Justice*, revised edn. Harvard, MA: Harvard University Press.

Ryan, P. (2022) *Facts, Values and the Policy World*. Bristol: The Policy Press.

Schwartz, B. (1990) The creation and destruction of value, *American Psychologist*, 45(1): 7–15.

Sen, A. (1999) *Development as Freedom*. Oxford: Oxford University Press.

Siddiqi, S., Masud, T.I., Nishtar, S. et al. (2009) Framework for assessing governance of the health
   system in developing countries: gateway to good governance, *Health Policy*, 90: 13–25.

Singer, P. (2010) *The Life You Can Save: How to Play Your Part in Ending World Poverty*. London: Pan
   Macmillan.

Vélez, C.M., Wilson M.G., Lavis, J.N. et al. (2020) A framework for explaining the role of values in health
   policy decision-making in Latin America: a critical interpretive synthesis, *Health Research Policy
   and Systems*, 18: 100. https://doi.org/10.1186/s12961-020-00584-y

Whitehead, M. (1992) The concepts and principles of equity and health, *International Journal of Health
   Services*, 22(3): 429–45. https://doi.org/10.2190/986L-LHQ6-2VTE-YRRN

Williams, E., Buck, D., Babaloa, G. and Maguire, D. (2022) *What are Health Inequalities?* London:
   The King's Fund. Available at: www.kingsfund.org.uk/publications/what-are-health-inequalities
   (accessed 24 April 2023).

Globalizing health policy: co-operation and constraints

9

In this chapter you will learn about why and how a range of actors, both state and non-state, engage with one another to influence and make 'global' health policy. First you will consider why these actors seek to pursue their interests through global and collective means, before considering the policy instruments and processes they use. You will be introduced to a selection of the actors with examples of the interests they pursue and the roles they play in these global processes, processes which can influence national health policy. You will also learn about the limits of global health policy in shaping the decisions of national governments, including the formal limits on supranational authority. This theme continues in the next chapter.

Learning objectives

After working through this chapter, you will be better able to:

- understand why states co-operate to address health problems, and why such co-operation has intensified with increased globalization
- identify a range of actors who operate globally to influence health policy and how they do so
- appreciate the range of mechanisms and instruments through which global co-operation takes place – and how conflicts are addressed and resolved
- appreciate the significant limits on the ability of global health policy to influence domestic policy making.

Key terms

Conflicts of interest A set of circumstances that create a risk that an individual's ability to apply professional judgement is, or could be, or could be perceived to be, impaired or influenced by a secondary interest (such as a financial one).

Global civil society Civil society groups which are global in their aims, advocacy or organization.

Global public goods   Goods which are undersupplied by private markets, inefficiently produced by individual states, and have universal benefits.

Global social movements   Networks of individuals and organizations that collaborate across borders to advance similar policy agendas and in doing so have become powerful actors in global governance and policy making.

Globalization   The interdependence of the world's economies, cultures and populations, brought about by cross-border trade in goods and services, technology, and flows of investment, people and information.

Multilateralism   The practice of co-operation and co-ordination among three or more states to pursue common interests as well as the more recent phenomenon of formal institutions (which may or may not include non-state actors) to support such co-operation (e.g. UNICEF or the Global Fund).

Public–private partnership   A contract between a private sector organization and a public body (e.g. government agency) to provide a public asset (e.g. a hospital building) or service, in which the private organization bears significant risk and management responsibility, with its remuneration linked to its performance.

Transnational advocacy networks   Actors, who share common values or policy objectives, collaborate internationally on an issue by sharing complementary resources, to frame and advance specific problems and policy solutions (typically more structured than global social movements).

Transnational corporations   For-profit enterprises operating across multiple countries comprising parent enterprises and their foreign affiliates.

Introduction

Most of this book addresses policy making within countries. Apart from the set of contextual factors highlighted in Chapter 1 that were described as 'international' or 'global', as well as examples throughout the text, international or global factors were treated as external ('exogenous') to domestic policy making. Recent history reminds us, however, that many health challenges are global in nature. The COVID-19 pandemic revealed how easily the virus could cross national borders. It also demonstrated how policies in one country affect the trajectories of the pandemic in other countries, from the stringency of public health measures to intellectual property regimes that impeded the development of a COVID-19 'People's Vaccine'. The vaccine issue also showed the strict limits on global health policy making in that calls for equitable distribution were made, sometimes even agreed to in principle by wealthy governments and then largely ignored. The same cross-border nature of health risks and policy impact is true of climate-related health risks or the challenges facing One Health strategies designed to combat AMR (i.e. those that try to consider human, animal and environmental influences on AMR). With the intensification of global integration, these transnational factors have played an increasingly prominent role in shaping national policy making.

Few countries or health policies are immune from global influences. You have seen in other chapters that health policies, even in high-income countries, are subject to pressures from *transnational corporations* (see Chapters 4 and 5). For example, multibillion-dollar food and beverage firms work across multiple national jurisdictions to resist graphic warnings being placed on their products which contain high levels of unhealthy ingredients such as sugar, salt and transfats. National health policies can also be subject to international trade rules. High-income countries also voluntarily adopt policies to co-ordinate to address global health threats, for example, efforts between some countries to harmonize their border controls to combat the spread of the COVID-19 pandemic.

Similarly, and arguably to a much greater extent, health policies in LMICs are subject to such external forces. Policy conditions may be set by rich countries on ministries of health in return for access to loans or grants. Policies may also be established in response to pressure from *global social movements*, as in South Africa's decision to provide treatment for people living with HIV. Moreover, implementation of policies, such as childhood immunization programmes, may be dependent on external support from global *public–private partnerships* such as the GAVI Alliance.

Health Ministers of both the G7 (club of rich nations) and the G20 (a platform connecting the world's major 'developed' and 'emerging' economies) have convened since 2006 and 2017 respectively to address shared health agendas and to harmonize policy. Reflecting shifts in the global geopolitical realm, the health ministers of the BRICS nations (Brazil, Russia, India, China and South Africa) met for the first time in Beijing in July 2011 to co-ordinate policy and, as an emerging economic and political bloc, to influence the global health agenda. A comparison of the health agendas of the BRICS, G7 and G20 found overlaps, differences and gaps which reflect the increasing complexity of global health policy making and changing power dynamics between countries over time.

How do these manifestations of the *globalization* of health policy making affect national policy making? This can be broken down into three further questions. First, how do global interactions facilitate the transfer of policies among countries and organizations? Second, who influences the transfer of policies? Third, how has globalization shaped the content of health policy? This chapter addresses these questions – but doing so requires that you first have some background knowledge of the process of globalization more widely and an overview of how governments have traditionally co-operated in health.

Globalization

The term *globalization* remains ubiquitous and has been used at least five ways over time. First, globalization is associated with the increasing volume, intensity and extent of cross-border movement of goods, people, ideas, finance or infectious pathogens (internationalization). Second, globalization refers to the removal of barriers to trade which have made greater movement of goods and services possible (liberalization). Third, some associate globalization with the trend towards a homogenization of cultures (universalization), or fourth of a convergence around Western, 'modern' and particularly US values and policies (McDonaldization).

Jan Scholte (2000) argued that the key development associated with globalization over the past two or three decades was the reconfiguration of 'social space' and specifically the emergence of 'supraterritorial' or 'transworld' geography. This is the fifth form of globalization. While 'territorial' space (villages and countries) remains important to people and policy makers, people and organizations have increasing connections to others that transcend territorial boundaries. For example, people can have loyalties, identities and interests that go beyond an allegiance to the nation state, linked to values, religion, ethnicity or sexual identity – of course these traits are not entirely new but have become more pronounced. Moreover, technologies seemingly compress both time and space. Not only do people and things travel much further, much faster and much more frequently, at times they do so in ways that defy territorial boundaries. Problems can occur everywhere and nowhere. For example, a virus can almost simultaneously infect millions of computers irrespective of their physical location. On any one day, hundreds of millions of people will connect on different global social networking sites. Hundreds of millions of currency transactions take place in 'cyberspace' daily.

Globalization has spatial, temporal and cognitive dimensions (Lee et al. 2002). The spatial dimensions have already been alluded to (distance is increasingly being 'overcome') as have the temporal ones (through telecommunications and transport the world has speeded up). The cognitive element concerns the thought processes that shape perceptions of events and phenomena. The spread of communication technologies conditions how ideas, values, beliefs, identities and even interests are produced and reproduced. For some, globalization is producing a 'global village' in which all villagers share aspirations and interests whereas others see Western-inspired values, particularly consumerism and individualism, coming to dominate the 'village'. Yet others perceive an increasingly polarized world between those who benefit from globalization and those who merely serve it. Views are similarly polarized on whether different aspects of globalization are good or not.

Some commentators suggest that the peak of Western-led globalization linked to trade liberalization was reached in the first decade of this century, and that since the Global Banking Crash of 2008, the globalizing impulse has weakened. In its place, nationalist ideologies and ideologues, such as Donald Trump, Narendra Modi and Jair Bolsonaro, have sought to disengage from *multilateralism* and we have seen the reintroduction of trade barriers – typified by the actions of the UK government since leaving the European Union. In the place of the US as a leading globalizing force, recent years have seen an increase in Chinese influence across many LMICs. The increased influence on global health policy since the 1990s of non-governmental organization (NGO) donors is also notable. Despite these trends, globalizing forces remain strong, taking a slightly different form to those that dominated the second half of the twentieth century, and globalization remains an important influence on global health policy.

 Activity 9.1

Provide an example of each of the five meanings of globalization.

Feedback

- Internationalization – more people flying around the world; the ability to buy 'seasonal' fruits all year around.
- Liberalization – removal of protection for domestic production of cigarettes.
- Universalization – same shops and same brands found around the world or the same words used on signs (Internet, STOP).
- McDonaldization – IKEA stores in India and Latvia.
- Super-territoriality – buying products over the Internet from a third country.

To fully appreciate the health policy implications of globalization, it is necessary to understand some of the ways that globalization impacts on health.

Globalization and health

The impact of globalization on health is most evident around infectious diseases. Microbes can now find their way to multiple destinations across the world in less than 24 hours. The most recent example is the COVID-19 virus, which, like severe acute respiratory syndrome (SARS), started in China and spread rapidly around the globe from late 2019. Acute COVID-19 led to millions of deaths and chronic, or 'long-covid', has led to significant morbidity for millions of people world-wide. The indirect health impacts of COVID-19 are also stark. Overwhelmed health services across the globe had to respond rapidly to the pandemic, often refashioning services to prioritize COVID-19 patients. This led to cancellations of elective procedures and exacerbation of pre-existing challenges. The 'lockdowns' instigated in most countries in response to the virus meant that many people could not access primary care services – thus delaying diagnosis and treatment for non-COVID-19 illnesses. The lengthy 'lockdowns' themselves had wider impacts upon populations – with increases in mental and psychological stress. The pandemic also carried significant social and economic ramification for all nations across the globe.

It is not only infectious diseases that benefit from globalization. The global production, distribution and marketing of foods high in sugar, salt and transfats, for example, are linked to rising rates of noncommunicable diseases. Globalization also promotes and enables activities such as smoking, misuse of alcohol, the sex trade and so on which impact health. Globalization can also affect the ability of health care systems to respond to health threats. One pressing example relates to health workers. WHO estimates a projected shortfall of 15 million health workers by 2030, mostly in low- and lower-middle-income countries. However, demand for health workers in rich countries has resulted in significant recruitment from poorer countries.

🖉 Activity 9.2

Most health issues and problems are affected in one way or another, often both positively and negatively, by forces associated with globalization. Select a health issue or problem with which you are familiar and attempt to identify the transnational dimensions of the determinants of the problem.

Feedback

You will have first identified the determinants of the health issue. Subsequently, you would need to think about how globalization (in its many guises) may have affected its determinants. Take, for example, the incidence of sexually transmitted infections (STIs) in Bangladesh. Arguably, the most important determinants are the position of women, access to treatment for infected people, and human mobility. Globalization is likely to have affected each of these determinants in different ways.

> For example, trade liberalization and other factors, such as entry permit relaxation have resulted in large movements of workers to and from the Gulf States as well as busy overland trucking routes between India, Bangladesh, Nepal and Myanmar. This has facilitated a booming sex industry with attendant consequences for STI rates. Trade liberalization and increased foreign investment have resulted in the rapid development of a ready-made garment industry which now accounts for one of the country's largest industrial sectors and over 80 per cent of export earnings. The industry employs largely young women – an estimated 3 million. This has improved the bargaining position of the women in the industry, in general terms, though from a very poor previous situation and perhaps in relation to their sexual relationships. For example, it has also delayed sexual debut. All of these changes may help slow the spread of STIs.

Not all countries, peoples and problems are equally integrated. Some countries in sub-Saharan Africa are not as well integrated into the global economy, as are, for example, China and India. Nonetheless, because of globalization, even these less integrated countries will not be able directly to control all the determinants of ill health of their populations and will therefore have to co-operate with other actors outside their borders to protect the health of those within them. In a highly connected world, this is increasing evident in relation to low-paid migrant workers. Both WHO and the International Labour Organization (ILO) have recognized that both sending and receiving countries have important roles to play in relation to the determinants of the health of this growing population group in relation to living and working conditions, pay and access to educational opportunities and other services, such as food and nutrition, housing, access to safe and potable water and adequate sanitation, safe and healthy working conditions and so on.

Formal global policy mechanisms and instruments

Traditional inter-state co-operation for health

States have always been concerned about the spread of disease over their borders. For example, as early as the fourteenth century, the city-state of Venice forcibly quarantined ships which were suspected of carrying plague-infected rats. The practice spread to other ports. These early initiatives paved the way for more formal international agreements in the nineteenth century which aimed to control the spread of infectious disease through restrictions on trade. These, in turn, resulted in the International Health

Regulations (IHR), which were accepted by all members of WHO in 1969. The regulations provide norms, standards and best practice to prevent the international spread of disease, but equally importantly require states to report on six diseases. The regulations provide a useful illustration of how states have co-operated to address common problems. The IHR also illustrate the limits of such co-operation. In particular, many states failed to report to WHO, and there was nothing that WHO could do about the lack of compliance. In consideration of the effects of globalization on the spread of disease and the emergence or re-emergence of a wider range of communicable diseases and public health threats, the regulations were revised and re-negotiated over a ten-year period. The revised regulations of 2005 require member states to report to WHO on 'events that constitute a public health emergency of international concern' and provide the Organization, for the first time, with authorization to take into consideration 'unofficial reports'. This provided WHO with an ability to better monitor outbreaks and marks an evolution in international co-operation to broader forms of public-private interaction that we will return to later in the Chapter.

However, the advent of COVID-19 revealed that there were limitations to the Regulations, namely in relation to: (1) compliance and empowerment; (2) early alert notification and response; and (3) financing and political commitment. During the pandemic, the functioning of the IHR was reviewed leading to recommendations to strengthen all three of these identified weaknesses and a commitment to fully implement the IHR without the need for years of political negotiations that might result in further failures next time the world faces a threat similar to COVD-19 (WHO 2021). Nonetheless, it remains the case that there is no formal mechanism for monitoring the implementation of critical provisions in the IHR and hence no accountability mechanism for their enforcement. They can only keep people safe if governments work together and with WHO, which would require further transparency and trust.

States may co-operate in many ways, both formally and informally. You will now learn about the other formal arrangements that have been established to facilitate co-operation, focusing particularly on multilateral organizations.

The United Nations

The United Nations (UN) system was established at the end of the Second World War to maintain peace and security and to save further generations from the scourge of war. At the heart of the system was the sovereign nation state, which could take up membership in the various UN organizations (such as WHO, UNICEF). These organizations were established to promote exchange and contact among member states and to provide platforms to co-operate to resolve common problems. Member states dictated the policies of the organizations with little interaction with non-governmental bodies. Thus, through the UN system, as you will see later in this chapter, governments, particularly those of high-income countries, were able to influence international health policy. At the same time, UN organizations themselves were also, to varying degrees, able to influence national policies.

WHO was founded in 1948 as the UN's specialized health agency with a mandate to lead and co-ordinate international health activities. Currently, most nation states (194) belong to WHO and another 220 non-state actors are in 'official relations' with WHO allowing them to participate in the governance of the organization (e.g. the International Federation of Pharmaceutical Manufacturers and Associations and the World Obesity Federation). WHO is governed through the WHA. Delegations of member states, typically led by their ministers of health, convene at the WHA annually to approve the Organization's programme and budget, and to make international health policy decisions. WHO's constitution grants the WHA the authority 'to adopt conventions or agreements with respect to any matter within the competence of the Organization'. Decisions are made on the basis of one vote per member and are binding on all members unless they opt out in writing. Most resolutions are agreed by consensus without recourse to a vote (although at the Assembly in 2022, around two thirds of the delegations abstained or absented themselves from a vote on the global HIV, viral hepatitis and sexually transmitted infections strategies which had contentious sexual health provisions). The constitution does not provide for sanctions for failure to comply with resolutions. In practice, most of the decisions of the WHA are expressed as non-binding recommendations, in particular, as technical guidelines or strategies, which states may adopt, adapt or dismiss depending on their perceived relevance and national politics. As this book went to print there was disagreement among member states as to whether the pandemic treaty under negotiation should be binding or non-binding.

The WHA is advised by an Executive Board which facilitates the work of the Assembly and gives effect to its decisions and policies. The WHO Secretariat is led by an elected Director-General, who is supported by over 7,000 staff working at headquarters in Geneva, in six regional offices and in nearly 150 country offices. Collectively, they attempt to fulfil the following very ambitious functions:

- articulating consistent, ethical and evidence-based policy and advocacy positions;
- managing information by assessing trends and comparing performance;
- setting the agenda for, and stimulating research and development;
- catalysing change through technical and policy support in ways that stimulate co-operation and action and help to build sustainable national and inter-country capacity;

- setting, validating, monitoring and pursuing the proper implementation of norms and standards. For example, in response to the health workforce crisis, in 2010, WHO used its constitutional authority to develop a code – the WHO Global Code of Practice on the International Recruitment of Health Personnel;
- stimulating the development and testing of new technologies, tools and guidelines for disease control, risk reduction, health care management, and service delivery;
- negotiating and sustaining national and global partnerships.

WHO is also the most important global co-ordination mechanism for preparing for and responding to pandemics and other health threats, providing a vital public good that serves all countries.

Among its functions, WHO is best respected for the technical norms and standards developed by its extensive networks of experts and its technical advice to member states. However, while WHO may provide the technical basis for health policies around the world, it has virtually no ability to 'impose' these policies on sovereign states – its influence rests on its technical authority. Again, this was all too obvious in the country responses to COVID-19.

Like other UN organizations, WHO has been the subject of much criticism. Some of this criticism has been fair, and some has been motivated by the move away from multilateralism of populist nationalist leaders. The Organization is constrained in what it can do and say and cannot do as a function of its political principals (i.e. member states), who do not always agree with one another, as well as by its funding model. The latter includes not simply a relatively small budget (for 2022 and 2023, this was set at US$6.12 billion) but also the structure of that budget – less than 20 per cent of which comes from regular assessed contributions paid by member states. The bulk of its budget comes from voluntary contributions by governments and other bodies, which not only hampers its ability to work on its core mandate but also skews its priorities in line with the preferences of individual sponsors' interests. The biggest contributors being the US and the Bill and Melinda Gates Foundation. Fortunately, at the 2022 meeting of the WHA, member states agreed to work towards a target of 50 per cent of the core budget coming from assessed contributions by the 2030–2031 budget cycle to improve predictability and independence.

Other organizations within the UN system also have some responsibility for health. These include the World Bank, the United Nations Children's Fund (UNICEF), the United Nations Fund for Population (UNFPA), the United Nations Joint Programme on HIV/AIDS (UNAIDS), the UNDP, the Food and Agricultural Organization of the United Nations (FAO), the World Food Programme (WFP) and the UN Office on Drugs and Crime (UNODC).

Unsurprisingly, as these organizations matured and grew in size, they began not only to serve their members' needs (i.e. to provide a platform for information sharing and collaboration), but to pursue their own organizational interests in policy debates at both the national and international levels. In this process, UN organizations became actors in their own right; often competing and pursuing different health policy alternatives. For example, the 1980s were marked by a major conflict between WHO and UNICEF over the interpretation of primary health care policy. WHO took the position that a multi-sectoral and preventive approach that improved water and sanitation, literacy and nutrition, based on community participation was required to improve health and health equity in poor countries (i.e. a social determinants approach). In contrast, UNICEF advocated focusing on a selected set of health care interventions that had proved cost-effective and implementing them through specialized programmes separate from the rest of the health system (e.g. childhood immunization). Although this public quarrel was short-lived, it points to differences between UN organizations over policies which they promote to member states.

Partly as a response to the challenge of overlapping mandates, itself a natural reflection of the range of socio-economic determinants of most health conditions, and the need for improved co-ordination among UN agencies, UNAIDS was established in 1996. Twenty-five years on, it remains an innovative partnership that aspires to lead the world to achieve universal access to HIV prevention, treatment, care and support – co-ordinating the eleven co-sponsoring UN agencies. It is distinctive for having a joint budget and accountability mechanism and is also unique within the UN system for including representatives of civil society as full members of its governing body. In addition to co-ordinating the efforts of the UN system on HIV, the Joint Programme serves additional functions. First, it serves as a platform for setting the global agenda on the response to HIV. It does so by co-ordinating a complex process of consultation with state and non-state actors on global AIDS strategy every five years. This process is ultimately approved by the UNAIDS governing body. That text then serves as the basis for political negotiations leading to a United Nations General Assembly declaration on HIV and AIDS shortly thereafter. The declaration is a mixture of best practice as well as commitments made by the international community to support efforts to be made by countries and collectively to address the disease. The declaration is not binding on countries. But the global strategy and the declaration serve as a reference point for country strategies and targets. UNAIDS also co-ordinates processes at global and country levels to monitor, report and hold countries to account for achievement of targets set. Second, it provides a platform to convene governments and civil society at the country level to promote evidence informed national responses. Third, it seeks to ensure that people living with, and affected by, HIV are part of policy-making processes. Yet as another UN body, UNAIDS adds the complexity of the global health landscape and the scope for international disagreement.

One UN organization with significant influence on health policy is the World Bank. The Bank has a mandate to provide financial capital to assist in the reconstruction and development of member states. Unlike other UN organizations, which make decisions on the basis of one country–one vote, voting rights in the World Bank are linked to capital subscriptions of its members. As a result, the Bank has often been perceived as a tool of high-income countries since they make the largest contributions. The Bank entered the health field through lending for 'population control' programmes in the 1960s, before beginning lending for health services in the 1980s and leading international policy on health system financing reforms for several decades. In 2000, it was the largest external financier of health development in LMICs. Its influence derived not just from the loans it disbursed but also from the perceived objectivity and authority of its economic analysis (at least as seen by donors if not its critics) and its relationships with finance ministries in borrowing countries. In effect, acceptance of policy conditions associated with health sector loans could be required in return for Bank support to projects in energy or industrial sectors which other ministries cared deeply about. Although the Bank's policies have been contested, particularly for advocating for its promotion of privatization of services, most donors, industry and governments have supported them in general terms. Since the late 2000s, the Bank has not always been the largest multilateral financier of health development – with the Global Fund and GAVI Alliance at times eclipsing it – although the Bank's influence remains significant.

While UNAIDS represents an exemplar co-ordination instrument in the multilateral system, its singular disease focus has raised longstanding questions about whether it could possibly serve as a model for the plethora of other diseases facing humanity. An alternative approach to co-ordination across the many multilateral organizations with a health-related mandate can be found in the Global Action Plan for Healthy Lives and Wellbeing for All (SDG3 GAP) to support country priorities to accelerate progress towards the SDG (Sustainable Development Goal) health targets. Developed in 2019, at the request of several member states and led by WHO, the SDG3 GAP brings together 13 multilateral agencies (both UN, such UNDP and UNICEF, and non-UN, such as GAVI Alliance, the Global Financing Facility and the Global Fund). Instead of setting up a large, dedicated entity with ensuing staff, and bricks and mortar, this mechanism supported by a small team at WHO aspires to better align and harmonize their ways of working to reduce the burden and transaction costs for governments and provide more streamlined technical and financial support to countries. Through the SDG 3 GAP, the agencies provide joint, co-ordinated support to countries under seven 'accelerator themes' (e.g. financing, research and development, determinants of health, engaging civil society). The GAP is also involved in the joint development of global policy and guidance, for example in relation to research and development and gender equality in the health sector. One of the strengths of the process has been establishing incentives for collaboration, such as new funding instruments to enable co-ordinated support to governments in LMICs. Under the terms of the GAP, the WHO Director-General welcomes countries to hold GAP signatories to account for how well they collaborate to support countries.

The World Trade Organization

A significant addition to the international architecture since the founding of the UN emerged in 1995 with the establishment of the WTO to replace the series of multilateral trade negotiations that took place from 1948 under the auspices of the General Agreement on Tariffs and Trade (GATT). The WTO administers and enforces a series of international agreements with the goal of facilitating trade by reducing both tariff and non-tariff barriers. These global rules can impact on health directly through access to medicines, trade in health services or flows of health workers, and indirectly through consumption of unhealthy products and exposure to environmental risks that arise from trade. Domestic policies addressing many of these issues have become more constrained as a result of the WTO agreements because, by joining the organization, states commit themselves (with no reservations allowed) to alter their policies and statutes to conform with the principles and procedures established in all the WTO agreements.

The WTO Trade Policy Review Body conducts periodic surveys of member governments' policies to ensure that they are WTO-consistent. Alleged violations can also be notified to the WTO by other member states. Panels of experts review the alleged violations and their decisions, including the need to amend laws to make them WTO-compliant, are binding on member states.

A number of WTO agreements have implications for health policy. The Agreement on Technical Barriers to Trade, the Agreement on the Application of Sanitary and Phytosanitary Measures and the General Agreement on Trade in Services have all been invoked to challenge the health policies of member states when other governments fear that they serve to protect domestic industries instead of protecting health. TRIPS, or the Agreement on Trade Related Intellectual Property Rights, has had the highest profile of such agreements because of its impact on policies concerned with generic drug production and trade – and thus access to and the costs of medicines. The interests behind the TRIPS agreement are revealed in the example below.

The implementation of TRIPS has led to bitter and ongoing diplomatic rows between countries whose pharmaceutical companies are the major holders of intellectual property over drugs (EU, UK, Japan and Switzerland) and poorer countries which cannot afford patented drugs and wish to procure or produce generic ones. In 2001, an attempt was made to bridge the differences with an agreement reached in Doha, Qatar called the Doha declaration on TRIPS and Public Health. It stresses the importance of implementing and interpreting the TRIPS agreement in a way that supports public health – by promoting both access to existing medicines and the creation of new medicines. In particular, it states that the TRIPS agreement does not and should not prevent members from taking measures to protect public health. The agreement strengthened countries' ability to use the flexibilities in the TRIPS agreement, including compulsory licensing and parallel importing, to obtain supplies of generic versions of new medicines.

The COVID-19 pandemic revealed that despite these provisions to override intellectual property rights, in the case of public health emergencies, this would in no way guarantee access to medicines for the bulk of humanity living in poorer countries. Although TRIPS was not the only barrier, it was a substantial one. As a result, in October 2020, South Africa and India proposed a broad three-year waiver of the TRIPS agreement covering intellectual property rights related to COVID-19 tests, vaccines and treatments. The European Union, Switzerland and the UK opposed the proposal. The US only supported an intellectual property waiver for vaccines. The final text, agreed as late as June 2022, when the worst of the pandemic had passed, was a much watered-down waiver of one clause of the TRIPS agreement relating to exports of vaccines (and doesn't cover diagnostics of therapeutics). This clash of national interests reveals the limitations of the international system to put the health needs of global citizens before national economic interests.

Bilateral co-operation

Bilateral relationships (that is, government to government) including co-operation and assistance, are as old as the notion of nation states. Currently, there are many bilateral organizations, including the United States Agency for International Development (USAID), the UK's Foreign, Commonwealth and Development Office, and the Swedish International Development Agency (Sida), that play roles at the international, regional and national levels. They are often major financiers of health programmes in LMICs and of health programmes of UN organizations. Bilateral co-operation often involves a political dimension, and these organizations may use their bilateral support and relationships to pursue a variety of objectives (diplomatic, commercial, strategic) within the UN system and recipient countries. For example, UK bilateral support often favours Britain's former colonies, while a large proportion of US bilateral assistance is earmarked for Egypt and Israel, and that of Japan for South-East Asian countries.

While most bilateral donors profess to adhere to the principle of national sovereignty and national 'ownership' over the health policy agenda and pledge to align their support with countries' priorities, in practice, these 'external partners' are often intimately involved in setting the health policy agenda (through, for example, influencing priorities by their engagement in policy co-ordination forums or by stipulating which programmes and services they will fund) and in policy formulation – through, for example, the technical support they provide to ministries of health.

In 2000, the bulk of all aid was provided by 15 or so rich countries. That has been changing as Western donors are increasingly joined by new donors from the Gulf States and increasingly powerful economies such as China. For example, India, which had over its history been the largest recipient of aid, had by 2010 become a significant donor. China has also moved from being a net recipient to donor, complementing the medical teams that it has been sending to African countries since the 1960s, with significant loans and grants for the construction of hospitals and roads. China published two White Papers on foreign aid in 2010 and 2014. Both stress the principle of equality and mutual benefit through south–south co-operation, although questions have been raised about the extent to which Chinese aid activities are commercial ventures or ways of drawing countries into alliance rather than traditional development assistance. It remains difficult to estimate the extent of Chinese state funding for foreign health and development as China does not publish data through the OECD (Organisation for Economic Co-operation and Development) unlike the other major funders (McDade and Mao 2020). However, it is clear that the bilateral role played by China is significant and challenges the Western dominance of bilateral assistance over the past 50 years.

Development assistance for health as a foreign policy instrument

Overall, reported development assistance for health has increased dramatically from about US $5.6 billion in 1990 to around US$40 billion just before the COVID-19 pandemic and an estimated US$54 billion in 2020. There are many difficulties in defining and measuring such development assistance and differences of opinion as to what is appropriate to include – should countries, for example, include the value of about-to-expire vaccines and how should they be valued?

The proportion of development assistance for health channelled through the United Nations and development banks has declined as the proportion channelled through global health partnerships and NGOs has increased. What is striking, however, is the explicitness with which support for aid, including health assistance, has come to be seen as a foreign policy instrument by governments in the last decade. The 2022 development assistance strategy of the UK provides a good example. It more or less halved allocations to the UN and identified aid as an adjunct of trade (i.e. using aid to ensure access to foreign markets for UK goods and services). The policy was explicit that aid was to be part of foreign policy and be used to further the UK's geopolitical ends. For example, a focus on Africa is justified in part due to 'geostrategic competition'. The health section of the strategy names three global health organizations that it will invest in: WHO, GAVI Alliance and the Global Fund.

International co-operation on health has been advocated increasingly in the twenty-first century as a 'security issue'. Health as a security issue was given a political boost by the SARS threat in 2003 and later by avian influenza. For a period, international public health enjoyed the 'high politics' status of defence and the economy, and the term 'health diplomacy' was coined. One manifestation was the Oslo Declaration in 2007 – issued by Ministers of Foreign Affairs of Brazil, France, Indonesia, Norway, Senegal, South Africa, and Thailand – which proclaimed global health as a pressing, neglected foreign policy issue. A recent manifestation of health as a foreign policy instrument can be seen in relation to what became known as COVID-19 vaccine diplomacy. China began to supply vaccines across the world before Western COVID-19 vaccine manufacturing countries. It was more or less the only provider until the spring of 2021, particularly since India took the decision to ban exports to focus on its domestic needs. At their summit in June 2021, leaders pledged to donate one billion doses to LMICs through COVAX, a multilateral vaccine sharing instrument, over the following year (i.e. enough to immunize about 5 per cent of that population if commitments were met). Subsequently, these rich countries and the EU pledged the donation of additional doses under considerable domestic and international pressure, particularly since they were blocking efforts through the WTO to enable countries to manufacture their own vaccines. Nonetheless, despite efforts to deflect criticism of vaccine hoarding, by summer 2022, less than half of the commitments had been fulfilled, resulting in an estimated 600,000 preventable deaths.

✎ Activity 9.3

List up to ten examples of multilateral and bilateral organizations that operate in a country with which you are familiar.

Feedback

Clearly your list will depend on the country chosen but is likely to include several of the UN organizations discussed above as well as multilaterals, such as GAVI, and bilaterals, such as USAID or the Norwegian Agency for Development Cooperation (Norad).

You have learned that states have a long history of collaboration in relation to health and that they have established a variety of mechanisms and instruments to this end. The impetus for such collaboration has been varied. Some states have clubbed together so as to create *global public goods*, which are goods that markets will not produce and governments cannot efficiently produce on their own but have universal benefits (e.g. eradicating polio, developing an AIDS vaccine). At times, co-operation has been predominantly altruistic – perhaps because of shortcomings or lack of resources in other states (e.g. through humanitarian or development co-operation arrangements). Co-operation has, however, also arisen for reasons of enlightened or naked self-interest (e.g. improving disease surveillance in LICs to reduce the threat of bio-terrorism in high-income ones). At times, 'co-operation' resulting in policy change, has been achieved through threats or coercion, for example, during 'mopping up' campaigns to achieve universal immunization coverage in a country or as a result of trade sanctions imposed through the WTO regime. Whatever the impetus for interaction, domestic policy processes are not hermetically sealed from international processes; international actors are often actively engaged in national policy making.

Informal and non-state global policy mechanisms and instruments

So far, collaboration has been discussed in terms of formal interaction among states, and between states and the international system. Yet, two of the features of the contemporary global health landscape are the emergence of many non-state actors and of policy making through informal mechanisms. Both of these developments will now be considered. Particular emphasis is placed on the activities of global civil society, transnational corporations and global public–private partnerships. The aim is to demonstrate that these actors actively participate in international and national health policy processes.

Global civil society

There has been a spectacular proliferation of *global civil society* groups over the past 50 years. Global civil society encompasses a diverse set of actors targeting a diverse set of issues (see also 'Civil society groups' in Chapter 4). For example, there are global civil society organizations active in:

- planetary health – such as the Global Climate and Health Alliance, which is presently advocating for a Fossil Fuel Non-Proliferation Treaty;
- reproductive health – such as the International Women's Health Coalition;
- access to medicines – such as Health Action International or MSF;
- rights of people living with HIV – for example, the 15,000 members of the International Community of Women Living with HIV/AIDS who live in 120 countries representing 17 million women living with HIV;

- ethical standards in humanitarian relief – for example, the Sphere Project, launched by a group of humanitarian NGOs, the Red Cross and Red Crescent movement, which defines and uphold standards of response to the plight of people affected by disasters;
- landmines – for example, the International Campaign to Ban Landmines is co-ordinated by a committee of 13 organizations bringing together over 1,300 groups from over 90 countries;
- health policy and systems research – the Alliance for Health Systems and Policy research hosts a Hive which brings together researchers, advocates and policy makers with an interest in this area.

Global civil society is heterogeneous comprising everything from a group of people linked together via the Internet to communicate a shared vision across national frontiers to organizations which have vast amounts of political assets. For example, the People's Health Movement offers an alternative global health agenda, an alternative to the World Health Assembly by way of its own Assembly and it publishes an occasional *Global Health Watch*, which provides critical analysis of health policy.

One civil society organization has in some important respects eclipsed UN agencies as the epicentre of global health policy. The Bill & Melinda Gates Foundation was established in 2000 and is now a central actor in international health. The Foundation announced in 2022 that it would increase its endowment from US$50 billion to US$70 billion. It also plans to increase its annual disbursements from approximately US$6 billion currently to US$9 billion by 2026. This is far larger than the current annual budget of the World Health Organization.

The Foundation is led by Bill and Melinda Gates and run by a relatively small secretariat. The Foundation wields considerable influence over health policy and priority setting in international health as a result of the magnitude of resources at its disposal and hence who and what it supports. Whereas the other major financier of health development, the World Bank, largely provides loans to governments, the Foundation has mainly supported NGOs, particularly public–private partnerships with grants. Indeed, one of the most striking features of the Foundation is the number of global public–private partnerships and alliances that it has engineered, incubated and supported financially as well as providing staff to sit on many of their governing bodies. For example, the Foundation played a central role in conceiving the GAVI Alliance, the Foundation for Innovative New Diagnostics, and the Global Alliance for Improved Nutrition, among others. More recently it has financed and co-financed major initiatives in the areas of pandemic preparedness and response – such as the Pandemic Antiviral Discovery (PAD), an initiative to catalyse discovery and early development of antiviral medicines for future pandemics. While the Foundation's support has been critical in financing research (e.g. trebling the amount spent on malaria research during the 2000s), and development and product access for a range of neglected conditions, equally important has been its success in getting public and private sector actors to collaborate on policy projects.

The Foundation has been involved in health policy in other ways as well. Universities, think tanks and policy research institutes, academies of science as well as public awareness and advocacy organizations have all been major recipients of Gates grants. Funding provided by the Foundation acts to set public priorities in a wide range of countries as well as national and international health organizations by default as governments, NGOs and international organizations gravitate to where the resources are to be found. Moreover, as a result of large investments in international health activities, the Foundation has easy access to influential decision makers at all levels. Over the years a number of criticisms have been levelled at the Foundation, including its support for 'magic bullet' technological solutions to complex social problems and its lack of accountability (which stands in contrast to, for example, the United Nations agencies). The Foundation has been joined in recent years by several other large philanthropic donors who support global health such as Open Philanthropy.

Like their national counterparts, international or global civil society organizations play a range of roles in the policy process – either influencing formal international organizations (such as the Global Fund to Fight AIDS, TB and Malaria) or influencing debates at the national level. They adopt different strategies: some as 'insider' groups, through accreditation to the United Nations, for example, or through global policy communities and issue networks as in the case of MSF, which works on principles for humanitarian interventions in conflict zones; others as 'outsider' groups which use confrontational tactics, such as the Extinction Rebellion groups in various cities of the world using non-violent civil disobedience to protest against climate breakdown; and some act as thresholder groups which shift between the two positions. For example, MSF was part of a wider issue network working with WHO, UNAIDS and other groups to increase access to AIDS drugs but was also a member of a network of activist groups using confrontational tactics to lower AIDS drug prices, among other demands.

Civil society often performs critical roles in the policy process, including enabling public participation, representation and political education, and individual civil society organizations can motivate (draw attention to new issues), mobilize (build pressure and support) and monitor (assess the behaviour of states and corporations and ensure policies are implemented). Partially as a result of improved global communications, global civil society plays the same roles at the sub-national, national and international levels.

✏️ **Activity 9.4**

As you read the following account by Jeff Collin and colleagues (2002) of the role of global civil society in a high-profile health policy process, make notes and draw a two- or three-sentence conclusion on the functions it performs at different political levels.

The role of transnational civil society advocacy networks in influencing intergovernmental health policy processes

In May 2003, the text of the Framework Convention on Tobacco Control (FCTC) was agreed after almost four years of negotiation by the member states of the WHO. The process was highly contested and often polarized with industry pitted against public health activists and scientists, and both sides seeking to influence the negotiating positions of member states. While the text provides the basis for national legislation among ratifying countries, the process highlights the important role that global civil society can play in international health forums and its limits as well. First, interested NGOs with 'consultative status' at WHO participated formally, but in a circumscribed manner (i.e. not voting), in the negotiation process – but were able to use this status to lobby official delegations. Moreover, many NGOs pressed WHO to accelerate the process by which international NGOs enter into official relations with the Organization – and a decision was made to provide official relations for the purposes of the FCTC process. Second, WHO hosted public hearings in relation to the Convention at which many civil society organizations provided testimony and written statements. Third, civil society groups, such as Campaign for Tobacco Free Kids and Action on Smoking and Health (ASH), provided an educative function – organizing seminars, preparing briefings for delegates on diverse technical aspects of the Convention, publishing reports on technical issues and publishing a daily news bulletin on the proceedings. A fourth, and perhaps unique, role involved acting as the public health conscience during the negotiations. For example, some NGOs drew attention to the obstructionist positions of some member states and industry tactics – often in a colourful manner such as issuing an Orchid Award to the delegation that they deemed had made the most positive contribution on the previous day and the Dirty Ashtray award to the most destructive. Fifth, individuals working for civil society organizations were, on some occasions, able to participate directly in the negotiations through their inclusion in national delegations. Over the course of the negotiations, global civil society organizations became a more powerful lobbying force through the formation of a Framework Convention Alliance, which sought to improve communication between groups directly involved in systematically building alliances with smaller groups in developing countries. By the end of the negotiations, over 180 NGOs from over 70 countries were members of this *transnational advocacy network*. The Alliance thus provided a bridge to national level actions, which involved lobbying, letter writing, policy discussions, advocacy campaigns and press conferences before and after meetings.

Source: adapted from Collin et al. (2002)

Feedback

> There is general agreement that civil society provided critical inputs to the FCTC process which influenced the content of the Agreement in a variety of ways. Yet there were limits to its influence. For example, the final negotiations were restricted to member states – thus, effectively restricting the direct contribution of civil society.

Keck and Sikkink (1998) have drawn attention to the advocacy role that global civil society networks and coalitions play in world politics in diverse areas such as policies on breast milk substitutes and female genital mutilation. Such coalitions aim to change the procedures, policies and behaviour of states and international organizations through persuasion and asserting new norms – by engaging with and becoming members of a larger policy community on specific issues. Keck and Sikkink (page 16) argue that the power of such networks and coalitions stems from their information, ideas and strategies to 'alter the information and value contexts within which states make policies'. In Chapter 4 you learned about the role of cause groups in altering perceptions of interests through discursive and other tactics in relation to HIV. Groups such as the Treatment Action Campaign (largely national) and ACTUP (global) have redefined the agenda and altered the perspectives of corporations (e.g. persuading them to lower the cost of drugs, drop lawsuits against governments wanting to implement TRIPS flexibilities, etc.) and successfully invoked policy responses at the national and international levels (Seckinelgin 2003).

The growth and growing influence of global civil society has been welcomed by many diverse groups. For some it is welcomed due to the declining capacity of some states to manage policy domains – such as health. For others, it is a means to improve the policy process – by bringing new ideas and expertise into the process, by reducing conflict, improving communication or transparency. For others, civil society involvement provides the means to democratize the international system – to give voice to those affected by policy decisions thereby making these policies more responsive. Civil society is also thought to engage people as global citizens and to 'globalize from below'. Others equate civil society with pursuing humane forms of governance; providing a counterweight to the influence of the commercial sector. Despite these promises, there are others who are less sanguine.

🖋 **Activity 9.5**

> You have read some of the positive reasons for welcoming the growth of global civil society. What criticisms do you think have been made of global civil society groups?

Feedback

Your list may include:

- *Legitimacy of 'global' groups* may be questioned as a result of Northern domination – most funds and members come from the North and the agenda is set accordingly. Only approximately one third of the NGOs accredited to the UN Economic and Social Council (ECOSOC) are based in the South (the much more populous part of the globe).
- *Concerns about elitism* – while global civil society is often thought to represent the grass roots, in practice, some organizations are described as 'astroturf' in that they draw their membership from, or are funded by, southern elites.
- *Lack of democratic credentials* – many organizations have not considered the extent to which they involve and truly represent the individuals and groups that they claim to advocate for, and how to do so better.
- *Lack of transparency* – many groups fail to identify clearly who they are, what their objectives are, where their funds originate and how they make decisions. Some are fronts for industry and would be better described as being market actors.
- *'Uncivil' civil society* – global civil society is a catch-all phrase for a diverse group of entities. Transborder criminal syndicates and pro-racist groups both have a place in this sector.

Transnational corporations

In Chapter 4 you learned about the heterogeneous character of the commercial sector and the ways that the sector wields influence in domestic health policy debates. The commercial sector, particularly transnational corporations (TNCs), commercial associations and peak associations, also pursue their interests through the international system. In 1998, the Secretary General of the International Chamber of Commerce (ICC) wrote that 'Business believes that the rules of the game for the market economy, previously laid down almost exclusively by national governments, must be applied globally if they are to be effective. For that global framework of rules, business looks to the United Nations and its agencies' (Cattaui 1998). The ICC was particularly interested in the WTO fostering rules for business 'with the proviso that they must pay closer attention to the contribution of business'. The then ICC President made clear that 'We want neither to be the secret girlfriend of the WTO nor should the ICC have to enter the World Trade Organization through the servants' entrance' (Maucher 1998). As a result, the ICC embarked on a systematic dialogue with the UN and a multi-pronged strategy to influence UN decision making – including an attempt to agree a framework for such input. The activities resulted in a joint UN–ICC statement on common interests as well as a 'Global Compact' of shared values and principles which linked large TNCs with the UN without the shackles of formal prescriptive rules or a binding legal framework. The ICC sets its sights on the epicentre of the UN seeking observer status to the General Assembly. Although initially unsuccessful, it was granted that status in 2017.

While the Global Compact is a highly visible, tangible and controversial expression of the interaction of the commercial sector with the international system, other avenues have also been utilized. One analysis of corporate lobbying on US positions in relation to WHO (Russ et al. 2022) found that members of the Engaging American Global Leadership coalition and the associated National Association of Manufactures sought to influence the US stance on, among others, the following:

- WHO Guidance on Promotion of Food for Infants and Children;
- WHO Prequalification of medicinal products;
- WHO Guidance on diagnostics;
- WHO Cancer Resolution – pricing and intellectual property language;
- WHO Global Alcohol Strategy;
- proposed classification for video games;
- resolution of infant and young child feeding.

The following case study provides an in-depth look at industry involvement in the development of global trade rules.

✎ Activity 9.6

As you read through the case study on intellectual property rights (IPR) consider the following questions, making notes as you go.

1. Why does industry want binding as opposed to voluntary rules governing IPR?
2. Why does industry seek global rules?
3. Why did the American administration support the Intellectual Property Committee?
4. Why are these trade rules important for public health?

Commercial sector influence on global health policy making

Sell (2003) provides a fascinating account of industry influence on the development of an inter-governmental agreement on IPRs that is virtually global in scope. The impetus for global rules arose from the concern among certain industries that weak intellectual property protection outside the US was 'piracy' and represented a huge loss and threat to further investment in knowledge creation. As a result, the Chief Executive Officers of 12 US-based TNCs (in chemicals, information, entertainment and pharmaceuticals) established the Intellectual Property Committee (IPC) to pursue stronger and world-wide protection of IPR. The Committee was formed in 1986, just before the launch of the Uruguay Round of trade negotiations which culminated in the establishment of the WTO.

The Committee worked as an informal network. Its goals were to protect IPR through trade law. The Committee began by framing the issue – linking inadequate protection to the US balance of payments deficit. Based on these economic arguments, its considerable technical expertise and links to officials, it was able to win the support of the US administration. The IPC then set about convincing its industry counterparts in Canada, Europe and Japan of the logic of its strategy (linking IPR to trade law) and gained their support to put the issue on the agenda of the Uruguay negotiations. The IPC commissioned a trade lawyer to draft a treaty which would protect industry interests. This draft was adopted by the US administration as 'reflecting its views' and came to serve as the negotiating document in Uruguay. The IPC was able to position one of its members, the chief executive of Pfizer, as an adviser to the US delegation. Although India and Brazil attempted to stall negotiations and to drop IPR from the round due to their interests in domestic generic drug manufacturing, economic sanctions brought them into line. As a result, the TRIPS agreement emerged and according to industry, 'The IPC got 95% of what it wanted.'

As a WTO agreement, TRIPS has a particularly powerful enforcement mechanism and as you learned above has profound implications for public health. The Agreement obliged countries that had hitherto failed to protect product or process patents to make provisions for doing so and in particular to set the patent period at 20 years. Industry argues that monopoly protection is required to encourage investment in research and development. Critics are concerned that this will place unnecessary restrictions on the use of generic products, inevitably increase drug costs and erect barriers to scientific innovation.

Feedback

1. Industry wanted binding rules so that all firms would have to comply. Voluntary schemes often result in piecemeal compliance.
2. Industry wanted global rules as they did not want countries to be allowed to opt out.
3. The US administration is thought to have supported the IPC for a number of reasons. First, the administration accepted the framing

of the problem and the magnitude of the problem as estimated by industry. Second, industry provided unique expertise in the area which the US government did not have. Third, these industries provided a great deal of campaign finance and invest heavily in lobbying the governing party.

4. The public health impact might be positive and negative. There will likely be more private investment in health research and development. Yet, the availability of these advances might be limited to those able to pay.

As you learned in Chapter 4, the commercial sector influences domestic health policy in a variety of ways and can be a force for positive or negative change in health terms. You will recall that the commercial sector also develops private health policy initiatives without the involvement of the public sector. For example, it has developed numerous codes of conduct that are global in scope.

Global public–private health partnerships

One of the features of the globalizing world is the tendency of actors from distinct sectors and levels to work collectively as policy communities and issue networks on policy projects as described in Chapter 4. One of the most visible forms of collaborative efforts (albeit at the formalized end of the spectrum) in the health sector is the multitude of global public–private health partnerships (GHPs) which have been launched since the mid-1990s. While the GHP label has been applied to a wide range of co-operative endeavours, most bring together disparate actors from public, commercial and civil society organizations who agree on shared goals and objectives and commit their organizations (sometimes numbering in the hundreds as is the case with the Stop TB Partnership) to working together to achieve them. Some partnerships develop independent legal identities, such as the International AIDS Vaccine Alliance or the GAVI Alliance, whereas others are housed in existing multilateral or nongovernmental organizations, such as the Partnership for Maternal, Newborn and Child Health in WHO.

GHPs assume a range of functions. Some undertake research and development for health products, for example, the Medicines for Malaria Venture raises funds from the public sector and foundations which it uses to involve pharmaceutical and biotechnology companies to focus on producing malaria vaccines for use in LMICs. Others aim to increase access to existing products among populations which could otherwise not afford them. The International Trachoma Initiative, for example, channels an antibiotic donated by Pfizer to countries which use it as part of a public health approach to controlling trachoma. A small number of GHPs mobilize and channel funds for specific diseases or interventions. The most prominent is the Global Fund to Fight AIDS, TB and Malaria, which since its launch in 2002 has approved funding of over US$50 billion in 150 countries. During the COVID-19 pandemic was given a mandate to provide grant support to LMICs for tests, treatments (including medical oxygen) and personal protective equipment. Some GHPs operate primarily in advocacy mode, such as the International Partnership for Microbicides. In the course of their work, many GHPs develop policies, norms and standards that might have been developed by governments or inter-governmental organizations in a previous period, and most actively seek to influence the priority given to health issues, set policy agendas and become involved in policy formulation or implementation by national governments and international organizations.

From a policy perspective, what makes GHPs noteworthy is the fact that they have come to represent important actors in the global and national health policy arenas. Even partnerships hosted by other organizations (e.g. the Stop TB Partnership, which was hosted by WHO and later United Nations Office for Public Services UNOPS) assume distinct identities and pursue specific objectives in the health policy arena. Their influence often stems from the range of political resources at their disposal, which gives them an edge over organizations working independently. Resources range from political access, multiple sources of knowledge and perspectives relating to many facets of a policy process, as well as breadth and depth of skills in research capacity, product distribution or marketing techniques. Their power is also a function of their ability to unite a number of important policy actors behind a particular position; actors who may have pursued competing policy alternatives or who may have not been mobilized at all. Consequently, GHPs have become powerful advocates for particular health issues and policy responses (Buse and Tanaka 2011).

✎ Activity 9.7

Closer relationships between public and private sectors, including through partnerships, while welcomed by most have drawn criticism from some quarters. Write down four or five reasons which may explain critics' misgivings of GHPs as they relate to health policy making.

Feedback

Your response may have included any of the following points, most of which are valid at least some of the time:

- GHPs may further fragment the international health architecture and make policy co-ordination among organizations even more difficult.

- GHPs increase the influence of the private sector in public policy-making processes, which may result in policies which are beneficial to private interests at the expense of public health interests.
- Decision making in GHPs may reflect embedded *conflicts of interest*. Although many GHPs develop technical norms and standards, few have mechanisms for managing real, apparent or potential conflicts of this nature.
- Through association with public sector actors, GHPs may enhance the legitimacy of socially irresponsible companies (what critics term 'blue wash').
- Private involvement may skew priority setting in global health towards issues and interventions, which may, from a public health perspective, be questionable. GHPs have tended to be product-focused (often curative) and deal with communicable as opposed to NCDs. Addressing NCDs is both more difficult and may directly affect the interests of commercial lobbies (e.g. food, beverage and alcohol).
- GHPs may distort policy agendas at the national level. They behave as other international actors in that they pursue particular policy objectives.
- Decision making in GHPs is dominated by a northern elite which stands in contrast to decision making in many UN organizations (i.e. one country–one vote). Moreover, representatives from the South tend also to be members of elites.

Although critics have raised valid concerns about public–private partnerships, in an increasingly integrated world it is natural that policy is increasingly made through policy communities and issue networks. These open up new sites for actors to develop partnerships to pursue particular policy goals and in so doing add further complexity to the health policy arena.

Globalizing the policy process

In Chapter 4, the concept of an 'iron triangle' was introduced – the idea that three broad sets of actors are active in the policy process at the national level (i.e. elected officials, bureaucrats and non-governmental interest groups – particularly the commercial sector). The changes described in this chapter suggest that policy making has an increasing global dimension and specifically that global and international actors often play important roles. Cerny (2001) coined the term 'golden pentangles' to reflect these changes to the policy process. While domestic bureaucrats, elected officials and interest groups remain influential, they have been joined on the one hand by formal and institutionalized activities of international organizations (e.g. the World Bank, the WTO, the G20, etc.) – the fourth side of the pentagle – and less formal, often networked, entities (e.g. public–private partnerships) and transnational civil society and market activities on the other – the fifth side. Depending on the issue, any or all five categories of actors may be involved and one or more sets may dominate. The image of the pentagle is useful to policy analysts in that it draws attention to the range of interests that may be active and the complexity of any policy process. For governments, particularly those in LMICs, managing this cacophony of inputs in the political system is a difficult business.

Ministries of health in LMICs face an increasing number of actors in the policy process in addition to managing numerous bilateral relationships with diverse donor organizations – often in the context of discrete projects (see Chapter 10 for more on this dynamic). One unidentified minister has been quoted as follows:

> When I was appointed minister, I thought I was the minister of health and responsible for the health of the country. Instead, I found I was the minister for health projects ... run by foreigners.

By the early 1990s it was increasingly clear that the demands placed on many ministries by donors who pursued different priorities and demanded separate and parallel project accounting mechanisms were overwhelming, undermining limited capacity and making it a challenge to formulate coherent and consistent policy in the sector. As a result, a broad consensus emerged on the need for improved co-ordination, and efforts were placed on establishing 'sector-wide approaches' (SWAPs). These involved articulating an agreed policy framework and medium-term expenditure plan. All external donors were expected to operate within the framework, only to finance activities contained in the plan (preferably through a common pool and ideally intermingled with domestic funds) and to accept consolidated government reports.

Given the politics of development co-operation, success with SWAPs was mixed; many donors continued to fund off-plan externally designed projects which were poorly harmonized and subject to burdensome and complex reporting and accounting practices – often for purposes of attribution. In countries where progress was made, these gains were often threatened by the arrival of new global public–private partnerships. By 2010, many countries hosted over 25 health GHPs, which often operated as vertical programmes with parallel systems – thus pulling the MoH in differing directions as they competed for attention and priority. As a result, there were renewed and high-profile pleas for coherence at the country level. Similarly, it was recognized that country-level co-ordination needed to be supported by global-level co-ordination. One prominent attempt to do so were the manifestation of this are the Millennium Development Goals (MDGs) agreed in 2000 by 189 countries, Three of the eight MDGs were health related and served to given greater focus and coherence to global health. These were replaced by the SDGs in 2015.

✎ **Activity 9.8**

Why has it been so challenging to co-ordinate efforts to support government health policies at the country level? Give two or three reasons.

Feedback

Your answer should have discussed the fact that different actors pursue different interests. Often these interests are difficult to reconcile. Bilateral donor organizations may pursue diplomatic or commercial interests in addition to health and humanitarian objectives through development co-operation. These may be at odds with priorities established through a consultative process within the recipient country. As you learned above, international organizations can pursue distinct and multiple objectives as well. All organizations, including global health partnerships, will compete to get their issues onto the policy agenda and to see that they receive attention. External agencies may, for example, prefer the use of their own countries' commodities and equipment, may advocate for transparency, value-for-money, decentralization or resource re-allocation which may adversely affect the interests of the recipient country. Hence, there will always be a political as well as a technical dimension to co-ordination with external agencies attempting to set agendas and get national counterparts to implement their preferred policy alternatives.

The pentangle model raises questions of whether or not the addition of new categories of actors leads to greater pluralism and whether or not increased interaction leads to the consideration of a wider range of policy alternatives. There is no one answer to these questions as they depend on the policy and context. Studies of health policy making suggest that although some areas have included a greater range of groups, decisions tend still to be dominated by members of policy elites, often representing a narrow range of organizations, albeit from public, civil society and for-profit sectors (i.e. elite pluralism).

As for the question of whether or not globalization increases the range of policy options under consideration, it would appear that policy agenda setting and formulation are marked by increasing convergence – particularly in relation to the health sector reforms. Yet the transfer of policies from country to country – often through international intermediaries (such as global partnerships or international organizations) – which results in convergence is not a straightforward process. Explicit cross-border and cross-sector lesson learning (e.g. through study tours) or the provisions of incentives (e.g. loans, grants) does not automatically lead to policy transfer and change. Often the processes are long drawn out, and involve different organizations and networks at various stages. This is covered in greater detail in the next Chapter.

Summary

In this chapter you have learned that globalization is a multifaceted set of processes that increases integration and inter-dependence among countries. Integration and inter-dependence have given rise to the need for multi-layered and multi-sector policy making (above and below the state as well as between public and private sectors). As a result, state sovereignty over health has generally, albeit differentially, diminished. Yet the state retains a central regulatory role even if it has to pursue policy through conflict and collaboration with an increasing number of other actors.

Further reading

Khan, M.S., Meghani, A., Liverani, M. et al. (2018) How do external donors influence national health policy processes? Experiences of domestic policy actors in Cambodia and Pakistan, *Health Policy and Planning*, 1; 33(2): 215–23.

Labonté, R. (2019) Trade, investment and public health: compiling the evidence, assembling the arguments, *Global Health*, 15(1). https://doi.org/10.1186/s12992-018-0425-y

McBride, B., Hawkes, S. and Buse, K. (2019) Soft power and global health: the sustainable development goals (SDGs) era health agendas of the G7, G20 and BRICS, *BMC Public Health*, 19: 815.

Shiffman, J., Quissell, K., Schmitz, H.P. et al. (2016) A framework on the emergence and effectiveness of global health networks, *Health Policy and Planning*, 31 (suppl 1): i3–16.

Smith, S.L and Rodriguez, M.A. (2016) Agenda setting for maternal survival: the power of global health networks and norms, *Health Policy and Planning*, 31(suppl 1): i48–59.

References

Buse, K. and Tanaka, S. (2011) Global public-private health partnerships: lessons learned from ten years of experience, *International Dental Journal*, 61(suppl 2): 2–10.

Cattaui, M.S. (1998) *Business Partnership Forged on a Global Economy*. ICC Press Release. Paris: International Chambers of Commerce.

Cerny, P. (2001) From 'iron triangles' to 'golden pentangles'? Globalizing the policy process, *Global Governance*, 7(4): 397–410.

Collin, J., Lee, K., Bissell, K. (2002) The Framework Convention on Tobacco Control: the politics of global health governance, *Third World Quarterly*, 23(2): 265–82.

Keck, M.E. and Sikkink, K.I. (1998) *Activists Beyond Borders*. Ithaca, NY: Cornell University Press.

Lee, K., Fustukian, S. and Buse, K. (2002) An introduction to global health policy, in K. Lee, K. Buse and S. Fustukian (eds.) *Health Policy in a Globalizing World*. Cambridge: Cambridge University Press, pp. 3–17.

Maucher, H.O. (1998) *The Geneva Business Declaration*. Geneva: ICC.

McBride B, Hawkes S, Buse K. (2019) "Soft power and global health: the SDG era health agendas of the G7, G20 and BRICS." *BMC Public Health*. 19:815. https://doi.org/10.1186/s12889-019-7114-5

McDade, K.K. and Mao, W. (2020) Making sense of estimates of health aid from China, *BMJ Global Health*, 5: e002261.

Russ, K.N., Baker, P., Kang, M., McCoy, D. (2022) Corporate lobbying on US positions toward the World Health Organization: evidence of intensification and cross-industry coordination, *Global Health Governance*, XVII(1): 4–83.

Scholte, J.A. (2000) *Globalisation: A Critical Introduction*. Houndsmill: Palgrave.

Seckinelgin, H. (2003) Time to stop and think: HIV/AIDS, global civil society and peoples' politics, in M. Kaldor, H.K. Anheier, and M. Glasius (eds) *Global Civil Society Yearbook 2003*, Oxford: Oxford University Press, pp. 114–27.

Sell, S. (2003) *Private Power, Public Law: The Globalisation of Intellectual Property*. Cambridge: Cambridge University Press.

WHO (2021) *Report of the Review Committee on the Functioning of the International Health Regulations (2005) During the COVID-19 Response*. Available at: www.who.int/publications/m/item/a74-9-who-s-work-in-health-emergencies (accessed on 3 October 2022).

10

The relationships between national, regional and global health policy making

In this chapter you will learn about the relationships between national, regional and global health policy making. First, you will consider these multi-level policy processes and the interconnections between them including in the context of globalization. Then, you will consider how global corporations and donor agencies influence these processes and relationships, the limitations of global policy making and importance of local context. Finally, you will consider policy transfer between the global and national levels.

Learning objectives

After working through this chapter, you will be better able to:

- understand the roles of global, national and regional policy, the changing relationships between them including in the context of globalization
- appreciate the importance of local realities and local 'ownership' of policy, and tensions between this and global policies
- consider the influence of global corporations and external donors on national health policy
- understand policy transfer between global and local levels, and its limitations and challenges.

Key terms

Coloniality The legacy of systems and practices, including particularly 'ways of thinking', resulting from the imposition of the will of one people on another and the use of the resources of the subordinated people for the benefit of the imposer, as in the case of European colonialism.

Donor agency A foreign government or philanthropic organization that provides resources for social welfare, health and social services or development.

Downstream interventions Policies or programmes focused on behaviour change at the individual level, not addressing the structural influences on individual behaviour.

Globalization   The interdependence of the world's economies, cultures and populations, brought about by cross-border trade in goods and services, technology, and flows of investment, people and information.

Global constitutionalism   Attempts to institutionalize and order governance processes 'above' the level of the state through mechanisms similar to those at state level.

Multilateral   Having members or participation from several groups, especially the governments of different countries.

Multilateralism   The practice of co-operation and co-ordination between three or more states to pursue common interests, as well as the more recent phenomenon of formal institutions and organizations (which may or may not include non-state actors) to support such co-operation (e.g. UNICEF or the Global Fund).

Multinational corporation   Business which operates in at least one country other than its home country.

Nationalism   Identification with one's own nation and support for its interests, especially to the exclusion or detriment of the interests of other nations.

Neoliberalism   An ideology and policy model that emphasizes the value of free market competition and reducing, especially through privatization and austerity, state influence in the economy. It has been described as a hyper-form of capitalism and/or a means for wealthy elites to intensify their capital accumulation.

Policy transfer   A process in which knowledge and ideas about policies (broadly defined) in one political setting (past or present) are used in the development of policies in another political setting.

Populism   An approach to politics that is difficult to define since it is not intellectually coherent but usually includes leaders and potential leaders who define themselves as the champions of the ordinary people, purport to be anti-elitist and who brand any opponents as disloyal to the country. Populism particularly appeals to those who are concerned to protect the security and cultural integrity of their country against outsiders ('others') but who are also sceptical of the ability of democratically elected government to do so.

Saviourism   A belief in a saviour; also used to describe, critically, a white person or tendency for countries of the Global North to engage in activities that they see as or are as perceived as undertaken with an intention to liberate or rescue non-white people or countries of the Global South.

Introduction

In the previous chapter you learnt about why and how a range of actors can influence and make health policy at the global level. In this chapter, we focus on the differences and connections between national, regional and global health policy making. National and sub-national policies are those policies designed to affect conditions in a particular country; national policy is made at the state or federal level, with sub-national policy being made at more local levels of government within a country. At times, we also use the word 'local' to refer to policy making at a level closer to citizens, typically at the national or sub-national level. Regional and global policy refer to policy beyond the sovereign state, targeting multiple countries and with global policy, multiple regions.

At all of these levels, policy can include that of both state and non-state actors (both for-profit and not-for-profit). The multiple actors at these different levels of health policy making wield different types of power and authority – an issue which links well to Chapter 2. The previous chapter also discusses these actors, which include commercial actors and civil society actors and – for regional and global policy – intergovernmental organizations.

Most of this book has considered policy making in either the global or national context, and many of the examples were of national contexts. At the beginning of the textbook, in Chapter 1, there were factors described as 'international' or 'global' and explanation of how these are sometimes treated as 'exogenous' to domestic policy making. However, global factors such as contextual issues associated with international conflict, or the recommendations of global organizations such as WHO, play a prominent role in national policy making, and policy making at different levels – national and sub-national, regional and global. All of these levels of policy making – national, regional and global health policy making – are interconnected.

The health policy arena has in recent decades become a much more crowded space, and whilst individual states do still have the responsibility for making public policy and law for their citizens, non-state organizations have been gaining considerable influence in global, national and sub-national, as well as regional policy making. The pathways for this influence are numerous. Furthermore, in recent decades there has been a move by many governments away from *multilateral* policy processes, towards more regional and bilateral approaches. For example, moves away from multilateral trade and investment policy processes through WTO to regional and bilateral processes, and to different forms of international trade and investment agreements with lower risk of multinational corporate influence on domestic policy making. There has also been a recent rise in *populist* and *nationalist* views in many countries. These changes may represent a response to global integration which has led to growing inequities, and the disenfranchisement felt by significant sections of society.

Global policy

Global policy is a term often used to designate activities aimed at the governance of issues that transcend national borders, and sometimes emanating from a diverse group of public and private, state and non-state actors. As with the other levels of policy, global policy can be conceptualized as a process, but also as sets of rules, norms and practices.

A high-profile example of global policy are the SDGs. They are a collection of 17 interlinked global goals designed to be a 'blueprint to achieve a better and more sustainable future for all' (United Nations 2022). The third goal (SDG3) specifically addresses health: 'Ensure healthy lives and promote wellbeing at all ages', but all of the goals address health, broadly defined. The SDGs were set up in 2015 by the United Nations General Assembly and are intended to be achieved by the year 2030. The SDGs were developed as the global development framework to succeed the Millennium Development Goals, another example of global policy, which ended in 2016 (United Nations 2022).

Global policy is considered to have an important normative role in creating and strengthening global norms, monitoring implementation, and holding states to account. But whose values and goals shape global policy? (For more information of values in policy making, refer to Chapter 8.) Whose agenda is being promoted? The *proliferation* of non-state, private actors working in the area of global health governance, as discussed in Chapter 9, raises many issues including in regard to leadership and decision making.

As Gostin et al. (2015) describe, the normative powers of the WHO, for example, 'are impressive, obliging sovereign states to submit agreements or conventions to a national political process and informing the Organization of the result. Its regulatory powers are even more far reaching' (Gostin et al. 2015). However, all UN agencies including WHO depend on the consent of member states for their activities and they therefore do not have the ability to compel a sovereign state to undertake or implement any particular activity or policy. In its history, the WHO has developed only two treaties considered legally binding: the FCTC and the IHR, with the latter having no clear route of penalizing non-compliance. In a world with a proliferation of non-state actors working in the area of global health, increasingly diverse actors shaping global health outcomes, complex and interdependent law regimes make it difficult for the WHO to gain international agreement in the World Health Assembly, and with the challenges faced by WHO in catalysing state implementation, soft law instruments (quasi-legal instruments like recommendations or guidelines, which do not have legally binding force or whose binding force is weaker than that of traditional law) containing specific, clear provisions are sometimes considered a better approach by which WHO can facilitate improved policy making at national levels (Sekalala and Masud 2021). Furthermore, while the WHO is nominally the leading organization in global health governance, it is funded by contributions from states and in significant part by the Bill & Melinda Gates Foundation (currently the WHO's second biggest donor, and accounting for over 88 per cent of philanthropic donations to the WHO). There are several other large funders of health programmes including the World Bank and IMF. The challenges to global health from a diverse set of actors with vastly different interests and resources have been described in the previous chapter. However, what this diverse and proliferating set of actors in global policy with different interests and resources points to is the challenge to developing a complete general understanding, both amongst analysts and the actors themselves. This is in regard to how the system of global health governance operates, how actors relate to one another and how they independently and collectively influence this system, including how policy and decisions are made. This complexity leads to significant gaps in understanding of the following: political dynamics and patterns of interaction at the level of global policy; the (dis)connection between identified health needs, policy; and the influence of private, non-state actors on policy making.

Recent trends shaping global policy

Alongside a proliferation of actors in the health space have been other important changes to the political landscape affecting health policy. After a long period of neoliberal reforms (led by the Global North) since the 1980s, hand in hand with increasing *globalization* and the opening up of new markets, has been a movement from around 2010 away from multilateral governance to a retrenchment and return to nationalist populism. Some political science scholars have emphasized the role in catalysing this change of the Global Financial Crisis – the name given to the severe world-wide economic crisis of 2008 and crash of the stock market. The changes since this time have been exemplified by: a return of the term 'America First' during Donald Trump's 2016 presidential campaigns and presidency (2017–2021), which was accompanied by US withdrawal from international treaties and organizations including the WHO (Gostin et al. 2020); the UK's vote in 2016 to leave the European Union (Brexit; completed in 2021) (Clarke et al. 2017); entrenchment of the political belief that India is fundamentally 'for and of the majority Hindu community' under Narendra Modi (Kaul 2019); and moves away from multilateral processes for example in trade with a corresponding rise in bilateralism (Walls and Smith 2015). Many scholars have also described the increased nationalist populism of this post-2008 era as also reflecting a response to the previous era of increasing global integration, which, within a neoliberal paradigm characterized by growing income and wealth inequities, has led to a disenfranchisement felt by significant sections of society (Cox 2020). At the same time, non-governmental organization (NGO) donors have since the 1990s been flexing their muscles as NGOs both in the Global North and

Global South become increasingly prominent in public service delivery, yet often without concomitant legislation to establish accountability mechanisms (Mayhew 2005). China has moved into a more dominant position, for example through its Go Out policy initiated in 1999 that has encouraged its enterprises to invest overseas, and has seen its increased presence in a number of African, Asian and South American countries (Keane and Wu 2018). Overall, this period is characterized by complexity, confrontation, and a waxing and waning of national/global initiatives and foci.

Trade and investment policy has important health implications and changes at the global level have included moves by many governments away from multilateral processes to regional and bilateral processes, and to different forms of international trade and investment agreements which have lower risk of multinational corporate influence on domestic policy making. Although *multinational corporations* cannot themselves initiate a dispute through WTO processes, they can however encourage and support states to do so on their behalf. For example, in 2012 after considerable lobbying by tobacco corporations, five LMIC WTO member-states initiated a WTO dispute against Australia for their proposed cigarette plain packaging legislation (Milsom et al. 2021). Many of the changes to the trade and investment regime have been made with the intention of lowering the risk from multinational corporate influence on domestic policy making. However, a large number of trade and investment agreements that are situated outside of WTO frameworks contain an investor-state dispute settlement (ISDS) mechanism, which allows foreign companies to directly sue host governments for compensation when policy changes threaten the company's ability to generate earnings from their investments (Walls and Smith 2015).

Corporate influence on domestic policy making through regional and bilateral trade and investment agreements

Two well-known investor-state disputes through trade and investment agreements relevant to public health have been the cases of Philip Morris Asia vs Australia and Phillip Morris International vs Uruguay for their tobacco plain packaging and graphic warning labelling policies, respectively (Milsom et al. 2021). In response to such disputes, a number of countries (South American countries, South Africa and Indonesia) have in recent years either refused to include the ISDS mechanism in new trade and investment agreements, or have cancelled or let lapse existing agreements containing the ISDS mechanism (Peinhardt and Wellhausen 2016). Brazil has concluded several Co-operation and Facilitation Investment Agreements that completely exclude the ISDS (Muniz et al. 2017). Twenty-eight EU states have agreed to terminate ISDS arrangements between themselves, committed to exclude ISDS from any current negotiations, proposed replacing ISDS provisions with an Investment Court System modelled after the WTO dispute resolution system with appointed permanent judges and proposed an appellate mechanism (European Union 2015). These developments highlight that many governments of particularly middle-income countries (MICs) have been rethinking and undertaking steps to lower the risk of multinational corporate influence on their domestic policy making through trade and investment agreements.

Global policy has many strengths, including, and as described above, having an important normative role in creating and strengthening global norms, monitoring implementation, and holding states to account. Despite the advantages and strengths of global policy, there are limitations and constraints, which are described below.

Limitations and constraints of global policy

The limitations and constraints of global policy relate to a range of issues including the inability to obtain enforceable consensus across countries, significant power inequities associated with the influence of funders and powerful corporate actors as well as the colonial nature of global policy making (which also contributes to the inability to obtain enforceable consensus across countries); the limited focus that global policy often takes for many reasons that can mask considerable issue complexity; and statistics compiled at a more macro level (national/global) masking health/social inequities in particular demographics or at more local (national/subnational) levels. Also, global policy is by its nature unsuited to addressing health issues in a context-specific manner that is most relevant to particular populations defined for example by geography and culture. This underlines the importance of policy making at more local levels, as we describe in more detail in the next section.

✐ Activity 10.1

Global policy and lack of contextual consideration

Choose a global policy that interests you – perhaps a written policy recommendation from a UN agency such as the FAO, UNICEF or WHO.

Your policy might relate to an issue such as improving maternal and child health, reducing hazardous alcohol consumption, addressing the spread of an infectious disease, or enhancing biodiversity within agricultural systems. Consider how such a global level policy may be too broad-brush, with its lack of contextual specificity affecting its relevance to a country or local region with which you are familiar.

Feedback

Examples of a lack of contextual specificity may include issues such as:

- Policies to improve maternal health by removing the financial burden of accessing maternal health care services that do not adequately address socio-cultural and gender norms affecting access to care. This may include issues such lack of mobility for some women; or women's limited independence and power resulting in them needing permission from husbands or in-laws to access care.
- Alcohol reduction policies to address bar and pub culture that do not adequately address hazardous drinking in contexts where drinking in informal community environments, rather than bars and pubs, is more common.
- 'Lockdown' pandemic response strategies (e.g. in regard to movement restriction to control COVID-19) not adequately considering the significant social and economic burdens on individuals and societies, particularly in countries without social protection schemes and paid sick leave.
- Policies to enhance biodiversity in agricultural systems through converting natural habitats into croplands and pastures may have unintended consequences for a region (and for other regions) such as of shifts to increased food imports from countries with less regulation to protect biodiversity.

An example of the limited focus often taken by global policy is WHO's five-target '25 × 25' strategy for tackling NCDs globally. As described by Pearce et al. (2014), this 25 × 25 strategy focuses on four diseases (cardiovascular disease (CVD), diabetes, cancer and chronic respiratory disease), four risk factors (tobacco, diet and physical activity, dietary salt, and alcohol), and one cardiovascular preventive drug treatment. The goal is to decrease mortality from NCDs by 25 per cent by the year 2025. This standard approach to the 25 × 25 strategy has the benefit of simplicity, but also has significant weaknesses – importantly, it overlooks the major causes of morbidity. Considering morbidity and disability measured by Years Lived with Disability, the top four NCD conditions globally are in fact entirely different to those emphasized by the 25×25 strategy. Instead, the top NCD conditions are musculoskeletal conditions, mental health disorders, neurological conditions and diabetes (Pearce et al. 2014). The 25 $\times$ 25 strategy is based on the top causes of mortality, but not morbidity. This focus at the level of global policy poses significant limitations to addressing NCDs at least in terms of those posing the greatest levels of morbidity. Furthermore, local realities and local ownership are very important to the success of policy implementation, as addressed in greater detail below, and those NCDs that resonate strongly in particular local contexts may in fact be those prioritized by alternative measures, for example measures of morbidity.

 Activity 10.2

Strengths and weaknesses of the World Health Organization

What do you consider one strength and one weakness of the World Health Organization in setting global policy during the COVID-19 pandemic?

Feedback

Strengths:

- its formal role as a scientific advisory body;
- scope to achieve high-level policy co-ordination;
- providing an 'objective' counterpoint to national government information;
- communicating information that shaped public understandings of the pandemic and its policy solution.

Weaknesses:

- WHO not equipped with the authority to effectively hold states accountable for their policy decisions, for example in regard to the implementation of travel bans during the pandemic which contradicted WHO advice, or HICs such as the UK ignoring test, trace, isolate guidance in the early days.
- WHO's inadequate funding in relation to the range of its task including in regard to pandemic preparedness and response.
- WHO unable to challenge unequal vaccine availability.

Limitations and constraints of global policy related to power inequities can be found throughout all aspects of global health, with hugely significant consequences and implications. Such power inequities – whether between the wealth and influence of different countries, the resources of multi-national corporations and small/medium-sized countries, or the budgets of intergovernmental organizations – shape the functioning of organiza-tions, act to further institutionalize the influence of dominant countries and other actors, and shape policy decision making including in regard to which issues are prioritized on (and excluded from) political agendas. Some global health scholars argue that these contemporary power inequities in global health – resulting in what has been described as the exploitation and marginalization of the global majority, pathologization of some world regions and 'saviourism' in the Global North (which in turn enable further exploitation and marginalization) – can be traced back to nineteenth-century colonial relationships (Buyum et al. 2020).

Many issues in global health cannot be well understood without exploring their history, including of power inequity and *coloniality*, and consideration of the tension between global, regional and national forces. Historically, global (formerly international) health has prioritized certain infectious dis-eases, often those perceived as an immediate threat to the Global North, and arising from the Global South. This attention has often been at the expense of important shared challenges – such as the growing prevalence of NCD, and threats posed by climate change and ecological degradation, as well as weak health systems, and the pervasive effects of the social, economic and political determinants of health. See Chapter 7 for discus-sion of disparities in research focus and funding between HICs and LMICs.

The COVID-19 pandemic emphasized a range of issues relevant to this discussion:

- the interconnectedness of countries as well as health issues and their solutions;
- the weak and under-resourced nature of health care systems in many countries;
- the politicized nature of pandemic responses and their poor co-ordination and implementation in many HICs of Europe and North America previ-ously considered to be in a strong position in a pandemic;
- the inequities in who is affected with an over-representation of mar-ginalized and economically disadvantaged populations including ethnic minorities – many of whom are also more vulnerable to other hazards such as ecological degradation, pollution, food and economic insecu-rity, and inadequate access to health care services;
- the need to sustainably address the important 'upstream' social, eco-nomic and political determinants of health rather than an over-focus on biomedical and technical solutions at the 'downstream', more individual, level.

The approaches taken to address health issues, and how these issues are framed for policy makers, are often more appropriate for high-income settings rather than low-income settings. Finally, as the COVID-19 pandemic also highlighted, lessons in regard to how best to respond to health issues are not confined to low-income settings – HICs also have a lot to learn from LIC responses and country responses from the Global South.

National policy – and 'local realities'

The role and attention given to global policy should not distract from considering the importance of local realities and local/national 'ownership' of policy making. Ultimately, it is the state that holds sovereignty over its territory and (over and with) its people, and historically, the health and well-being of citizens has been considered a key responsibility of sovereign states. This creates tensions between the aspirations of global policy and what is implemented at national level. Although differing in type, domestic political systems have established government and bureaucratic structures that shape authority, decision making, accountability and distribution of political power. Governments and the associated bureaucracy are responsible for making public policy and law (national policy) applicable to all individuals and legal entities within the territory of the particular country. This is reflected in the focus of studies on the role of governments, working with other actors, for example in the provision of primary health care (Saif-Ur-Rahman et al. 2019), or in achieving the multisectoral action needed to address health challenges in LMICs with opportunities to learn from countries such as Australia and Canada (Ssennyonjo et al. 2021). Even within the European Union, the focus of health policy remains at the national level – with health not included as an EU-level competence. In the UK, health is largely an issue that is devolved to the governments of Scotland, Wales and Northern Ireland. (Note that there are some international aspects of health policy which are not devolved and remain with the Westminster Parliament, e.g. who can enter the country on health grounds, quarantine, etc.) See the case study below for an example of the devolution of the United Kingdom's NHS to Scotland, Wales and Northern Ireland. Further information on domestic governance and political systems can be accessed in Chapter 3.

Devolution of the UK's NHS to Scotland, Wales and Northern Ireland

Historically, the UK has a largely unitary system in which local government derives its powers from central government. Scotland, Wales and Northern Ireland were granted their own powers over most of their domestic affairs, including health, under legislation passed by the national parliament in London in 1999. Bevan (2014) terms the UK health policy devolution as being 'asymmetric' as England is so much larger than Scotland, Wales and Northern Ireland. A significant governance issue is that whilst the smaller countries have local directly elected assemblies to make health and other policy decisions, England does not; it relies on the UK Parliament in London to do this. This raises questions about non-English members of Parliament and whether they should or should not vote on English health policy issues. Health policy devolution has led to some important divergences between the UK nations. Most notably, many of the NPM reforms of the 1980s and 1990s (see Chapter 6), including the 'purchaser–provider split', were abolished in Wales and Scotland, and the ethos of competition, which was favoured in the English NHS, is downplayed in the other UK nations. Significant too is the integration of health and social care services in Scotland and access to greater free support than in England where health and social care services are less integrated and more expensive for individuals – raising important questions about equity across the UK.

Along with considerations of sovereignty, it is worth reflecting on other key concerns about the importance of national and sub-national policy. First, it is national and sub-national policy, rather than global and even regional policy, that is best equipped to address the complexity and unique nature of local contexts. Second, local 'ownership' of policy by people directly affected by the health problem is important for achieving intended health outcomes – as well as achieving sustainable change.

People's lives and health are to a significant extent, with the increased levels of global integration over the past fifty years, influenced by big-picture structural factors – political, economic and social. These structural factors operate at national as well as regional and global levels, and their history also shapes current settings and power relations. However, the impact of these structural determinants of health is highly context-specific, as they interact with local context to shape outcomes including health-related behaviour. For an example of social outcomes of this with health consequences, think about how liberalized labour markets for health care professionals can have very different consequences in different country contexts, with migration of health workers from LMICs to HICs contributing to issues of inadequate workforce and 'brain drain', an issue facing many LMICs. Consequently, it is critical for improving health outcomes that policy and programme interventions consider and are relevant to the local context (political, economic, and socio-cultural) of countries and regions – taking into account the priorities, processes and practices that influence social factors and behaviour. Local understanding of the barriers and protective factors/facilitators within a specific context is vital in designing effective behaviour change interventions that would resonate with the targeted populations (Essue and Kapiriri 2018). Public health practitioners have described the importance of understanding culture and its relationship to health and well-being for Aboriginal and Torres Strait Islander people, for example (Salmon et al. 2019; Finlay et al. 2021), with implications for how to shape culturally appropriate policy and programme interventions (Vallesi et al. 2018).

Furthermore, rather than public health being unique to Western biomedicine, people and cultures everywhere have their own models of supporting health and well-being that are shaped by the local context. Some scholars describe how much of the discourse in global and public health reinforces the powerlessness of local people, ignoring unique local knowledge and practices, especially of indigenous people (Nichter 2008; Reid et al. 2019). You can read more about neo-colonial influences on knowledge and evidence for health policy in Chapter 7. Effective policy and programme interventions need to fit local contexts, and are thus often best designed and implemented locally, and they need to be supported by the people in that context. 'Ownership' of health policy by the people directly affected by a particular health issue itself alters the policy process in a way more likely to lead to impact (see Chapter 6 on implementation). Donor-driven policies, for example, are sometimes reported as not being appropriate for particular local contexts, and therefore lack support from recipient country governments (Adams et al. 2014). Vanyoro et al. (2019) posit that this ownership also extends to the research shaping the evidence base for policy change, with embedded and participatory research shown to 'help facilitate the use of evidence by making data more relevant to real-word (contextual) challenges' (Vanyoro et al. 2019). Important for addressing these issues including cutting through the challenge of global or national-led policies versus locally led-policies, is co-creation or co-production (also discussed in Chapter 7). This involves the key actors involved in an issue – including local NGOs and communities as well as researchers and decision makers – working collaboratively to generate knowledge and support policy change (Turk et al. 2021).

Many questions remain about how health can be best governed at a local (national, sub-national) level – questions that also relate to some of the theory presented in the Chapter 6. Whilst bottom-up policy making starting from the local level may be ideal for some health issues, how realistic is this in many settings, particularly where an emergency response is needed, for example in the case of Ebola, or where institutions may be weak (for reasons related to power and coloniality)? Sierra Leone's response to the 2014–2015 Ebola outbreak and the Democratic Republic of Congo's response to the 2018–2020 outbreak encapsulate many of these issues. Both countries' health sectors had been weakened by civil war and periods of colonial and neo-colonial exploitation (Mayhew et al. 2021). When Ebola broke out in these countries their health sectors could not cope with the rapidity and scale of the outbreaks and communities were thrown back on their own resources to isolate and care for the sick. In Sierra Leone, this approach met with considerable success despite the limited resources possessed. Had the national and international responders attempted to learn from local efforts (including identifying the particular symptoms manifest in Sierra Leone that were different from other outbreaks; accepting the role of locally constituted and trusted burial teams to enhance compliance with testing, reporting and quarantine; and siting of treatment centres close to communities instead of in isolated sites that were distrusted) the outbreak in that country could have been more quickly curtailed (Richards et al. 2019). A key challenge is how national and international decision makers can rapidly engage with frontline responders and whether and how hierarchical systems of emergency response can become flexible enough to give voice and power to local wisdom (Mayhew et al. 2021).

There are a number of issues that you may want to consider in regard to how health can best be governed at a local level. These include whether regional governance, through creating 'nodes of excellence' or areas in which the development of particular regional capacity is prioritized (Walls et al. 2015), is a way forward to help mitigate the challenges facing some LMICs with resourcing and shortages of expertise including in relation to skilled worker migration; and the (dis)connections between the different levels of policy making, particularly in the context of local social institutions often functioning very differently to government institutions, with different goals, values and cultures. Furthermore, as described in more detail in Chapter 6, policy is itself adapted during its implementation. However, there are in many settings poor channels of communication from the grass-roots to higher levels of policy making, creating disconnects between top-level policy makers and those policy makers on the ground as well as those targeted by the policy. An example of this was provided in Chapter 6, exploring agricultural policy to address nutrition in Malawi (see the case study 'Agricultural policy and malnutrition in Malawi'). You may wish to refer back to this example, which relates to understandings of policy implementation but also to the importance of local context and the co-production of knowledge and policy.

Influence of non-state actors

Individual states do still have the responsibility for making public policy and law for their citizens, but non-state organizations have in recent years been recognized as gaining considerable influence in global, national and regional policy making. The pathways for this influence are numerous, and include via direct influence on countries through for example shaping national policies, indirect influence on countries through for example shaping trade rules and issue discourse, and through shaping the rules of the game, for example in regard to *global constitutionalism* (i.e. attempts to institutionalize and order governance processes 'above' the level of the state through mechanisms similar to those at state level (Hawkins and

Holden 2016) and *neoliberalism* (Milsom et al. 2020). Refer to Chapter 2 to explore the different ways of using power and influence.

Direct influence of non-state actors on countries is the most intuitive to understand, and includes the sometimes misguided efforts of international NGOs to respond to the Ebola crises in West Africa and the Democratic Republic of the Congo (the DRC). For example, MSF (Médecins Sans Frontières, or Doctors Without Borders in English) was the leading emergency responder to the pandemic and a key member of the national Ebola Response Committee in Sierra Leone during the 2014–2016 pandemic. When MSF first went into Sierra Leone their policy – and that followed by the national government – was to isolate people infected with Ebola in treatment centres but not to rehydrate them with drips once they became too weak to drink, saying it was too dangerous for their staff. This led to death rates of around 70 per cent. It was not until a Ugandan doctor, who was helping with the response, told them it was possible to rehydrate patients safely that MSF – and the Sierra Leone government – changed their policy. Consequently, death rates were transformed, dropping to around 30 per cent. MSF is one of the more reflective international NGOs in public health and learned from their West Africa experience to take local perspectives seriously. When their policies of maintaining Ebola-specific isolation and treatment centres in the 2018-20 DR Congo outbreak did not appear to be working they transformed one of their clinics into a facility that 'normalized' Ebola treatment as part of routine services in clinics that also treated other health issues (Mayhew et al. 2021). In the DR Congo Ebola response context, however, the WHO was the more powerful actor – often in direct conflict with MSF – and MSF was unable to entirely transform the response.

The indirect influence on countries through, for example, shaping trade rules and issue discourse is being increasingly recognized. Milsom et al. (2021) have described the influence that corporate actors have had on NCD policy making globally, through the use of trade rules to delay the implementation of food labelling and plain-package tobacco regulation, for example.

The influence of non-state actors is also becoming increasingly pervasive – as well as recognized. Some scholars have identified how corporate entities (and a small group of private international lawyers who benefit financially from this process) are using their power and influence to establish laws and judicial systems 'above' the level of the state through mechanisms equivalent to state-level constitutions (Hawkins and Holden 2016). These processes, also described previously as 'global constitutionalism', have been reflected in the international trade and investment regime, through the formation of legally binding agreements and dispute resolution systems, some of which are arguably very favourable to corporate interests and restrict the ability of national governments to legislate for their own social, health and environmental goals (Walls and Smith 2015). An example is the ISDS mechanism, described in more detail on page 261. Recent analyses indicate an ongoing trend towards progressive empowerment of corporate actors via the international trade and investment system to influence domestic health policy-making processes (Labonte et al. 2016; Médecins Sans Frontières 2016). For more information on the power tactics corporate actors use to further their interests, refer back to Chapter 2. Here, we will focus instead on another important player: *donor agencies*.

Influence of external donors on national policies

External donors – a group of actors also discussed in Chapter 9 – conduct activities with the aim of improving health in LMICs, and often influence the policy agendas, policy decisions and governance arrangements of recipient countries. One route of external influence on national policy decisions or priorities is through the control of financial resources. This influence can be most pronounced when there is substantial reliance of recipient countries on external funding (Okuonzi and Macrae 1995), and has been found to impact on agenda setting and policy implementation (Khan et al. 2018). However, in several countries, donor influence has been prominent even in the absence of substantial funding flows though alternative routes of power and influence (Sridhar and Gomez 2011). These routes include greater (perceived) technical expertise of representatives from external agencies and intersectoral leverage. Technical expertise has its influence through the ability to produce, interpret and disseminate knowledge and information to policy actors (what the political scientist Jeremy Shiffman has termed 'epistemic power' in global health) (Shiffman 2014); it can play an important role particularly in policy formulation. Intersectoral leverage refers to means of influence operating outside of the health sector, such as tapping into national policy makers' concerns about maintaining a good international reputation to avoid harms to non-health areas of concern (e.g. tourism or trade). For example, policy makers in Pakistan indicated that the threat of travel and trade restrictions being introduced by international organizations if polio was not controlled was important in placing polio high on the national agenda (Khan et al. 2018).

In terms of how external influence on national policy processes manifests, development scholars have emphasized how deeply external agencies have shaped the functioning of policy-making institutions of lower-income countries (Mamdani 1997). Others concerns have also been raised including: the dominance of foreign trade and industrial interests; the emphasis on technological solutions; strengths and absorptive capacities of national health systems being overlooked; and sustainability and ownership of health policies and programmes being reduced (Khan et al. 2018). On the other hand, external donors can support health ministries in putting forward the case for investing in health broadly or raising specific health issues higher on the domestic political agenda; for example, the attention to antimicrobial resistance from funding agencies in Europe and the US has pushed forward national action plans (World Health Organization 2019).

Reductions in external funding can often result in shifts in power dynamics and priorities between global, national and regional policy actors. Studies have shown that external and domestic decision makers may have different views about what health impacts they would like to sustain through their investments, the timelines they want to work to and how focused they are on measurable impacts (Moucheraud et al. 2017; Khan et al. 2019). The different participants may well have divergent goals. For example, when external donors are reducing investments in a country, they may seek to reduce the scope of specific health programmes, whereas health programme managers may be most concerned about maintaining their jobs, while beneficiaries may think mainly about continuation or expansion of services.

 Activity 10.3

Routes of donor influence on country health policy

Reflecting upon the three routes of donor influence described above (financial resources, technical expertise and intersectoral leverage), make notes on which strategies you have observed to shape health policy in a country with which you are familiar.

Feedback

Financial resources:

- making funding available only for specific health interventions, such as certain contraceptive methods rather than reproductive health more broadly;
- cutting funding from some programmes if 'rules' or targets are not met.

Technical expertise:

- domination of policy formulation toward biomedical approaches based on the notion of better public health expertise.

Intersectoral leverage:

- restrictions related to specific infectious diseases in humans or animals;
- lack of vaccine coverage linked to travel restrictions or requirement of certification of travellers (e.g. polio).

Policy and knowledge transfer

Policy can be transferred in many different ways – within a country, between countries possibly in a region, and from a global setting to a local setting as well as potentially the reverse. Chua et al. (2021), for example, describe how lessons from previous epidemics applied by African and Asian nations helped these countries implement successful responses to COVID-19 (Chua et al. 2021). *Policy transfer* and translation is a concept inherent in the concept of global policy and in the practices of organizations operating at the global level.

Policy and knowledge transfer relates to the process by which policies and evidence used in one place and time are applied to another. Scholars have developed a range of models and theories of policy and knowledge transfer, some of which have been critiqued for their positivist approach and focus on policy makers as rational actors, ignoring the social and institutional contexts in which the transfer takes place (Peck 2011).

Chapters 6 and 7 on policy implementation and evidence have further discussion of models and ideas relevant to understanding policy and knowledge transfer. Here, in Table 10.1, we present a spectrum of policy transfer models, developed by Rose (1991), from copying and emulation, to hybridization and synthesis, to providing inspiration.

The main reasons given for policy 'failure', in which there is a delivery failure or negative consequences of the policy transfer, include: uninformed policies, where the policy adopter has little or inadequate knowledge about the policy and its operations; incomplete policies, when the policy is not transferred in its entirety, that is, the adopter transfers part of the policy and leaves out some parts; and inappropriate policies, when the differing contexts have not been taken into account (Cockerham and Cockerham 2010).

This concept of policy failure raises several important questions. Failure by whose definition? And, who defines what should be sustained? These

Table 10.1 The policy transfer spectrum

Models of transfer	Description
Copying	Adopting policy used in other contexts without making any changes.
Emulation	Not copying all the details of the policy but acknowledging that the policy provides the best standard for designing own policy.
Hybridization and synthesis	Combining policies or policy elements from more than one country and designing a policy 'best suited to the emulator'.
Inspiration	Policy in another area used to inspire policy change for the emulator.

Source: adapted from Rose (1991).

questions raise issues of different actor interests and power including at a national versus international level. Policy transfer failures also raise issues in regard to the use of evidence in policy making and how and where local context, knowledge and practices are positioned. Global policies and recommendations are often developed in HICs and thus compete with other evidence types, ideas, institutions and local knowledge in LMIC settings. This brings us back to the issue of local policy making and the importance of more effective and inclusive bottom-up policy-making approaches that embed programmes within the local context. Local interest in, and responses to, public health interventions are dependent on perceptions of importance/relevance to the local population. Thus, many examples of policy transfer 'failure', in which there is a delivery failure or negative consequences of the policy transfer, relate to the constraints and limitations of global policy and the importance of local policy and local 'ownership'.

Summary

After considering the different levels at which policies operate (global, regional, national and subnational), this chapter has discussed the strengths, limitations and constraints of broad global policies. It is clear that local (national, sub-national) and also regional 'ownership' in policy making is important; examples from diverse contexts are provided to illustrate this and the importance of local realities. Despite the importance of national/sub-national involvement, external influence on this stemming from unequal power relations and resourcing continues to be salient. It is also clear that policy and knowledge can be transferred in many different ways, and that this idea of policy transfer raises a number of issues including the constraints and limitations of global policy and the importance of local policy and local ownership.

Further reading

Hawkins, B. and Holden, C. (2016) A corporate veto on health policy? Global constitutionalism and investor-state dispute settlement, *Journal of Health Politics, Policy & Law*, 41(5): 969–95.

Khan, M.S., Meghani, A., Liverani, M. et al. (2018) How do external donors influence national health policy processes? Experiences of domestic policy actors in Cambodia and Pakistan, *Health Policy and Planning*, 33(2): 215–23.

Mayhew, S., Kyamusugulwa, P., Kihangi Bindu, K. et al. (2021) Responding to the 2018–2020 Ebola virus outbreak in the Democratic Republic of the Congo: rethinking humanitarian approaches, *Risk Management and Healthcare Policy*, 14: 1731–47.

Okuonzi, S. and Macrae, J. (1995) Whose policy is it anyway? International and national influences on health policy development in Uganda, *Health Policy and Planning*, 10(2): 122–32.

Rose R. (1991) What is lesson-drawing? *Journal of Public Policy*, 11(1): 3–30.

References

Adams, V., Burke. N. and Whitmarsh, I. (2014) Slow research: thoughts for a movement in global health, *Medical Anthropology*, 33: 179–97.

Bevan, G. (2014) The impacts of asymmetric devolution on health care in the four countries of the UK, *The Health Foundation and Nuffield Trust*.

Buyum, A., Kenney, C., Koris, A. et al. (2020) Decolonising global health: if not now, when?, *BMJ Global Health*, 5: e003394.

Chua, A., Al Knawy, B., Grant, B. et al. (2021) How the lessons of previous epidemics helped successful countries fight covid-19, *British Medical Journal*, 372: n486.

Clarke, H., Goodwin, M. and Whiteley, P. (2017) *Brexit: Why Britain Voted to Leave the European Union*. Cambridge: Cambridge University Press.

Cockerham, G. and Cockerham, W. (2010) *Health and Globalization*. Cambridge: Polity Press.

Cox, L. (2020) Nationalism and populism in the age of globalization, in L. Cox, *Nationalism: Themes, Theories, and Controversies*. Singapore: Palgrave Macmillan, pp. 97–131. https://doi.org/10.1007/978-981-15-9320-8_5

Essue, B.M. and Kapiriri, L. (2018) The unfunded priorities: an evaluation of priority setting for noncommunicable disease control in Uganda, *Globalization and Health*, 14(1): 22.

European Union (2015) Commission proposes new Investment Court System for TTIP and other EU trade and investment negotiations. Press release, 16 September. Brussels: European Union. Available at: https://ec.europa.eu/commission/presscorner/detail/en/IP_15_5651 (accessed 12 June 2023).

Finlay, S., Canuto, K., Canuto, K. et al. (2021) Aboriginal and Torres Strait Islander connection to culture: building stronger individual and collective wellbeing, *Medical Journal of Australia*, 214: S5–40.

Gostin, L., Hongju Koh, H., Williams, M. et al. (2020) US withdrawal from WHO is unlawful and threatens global and US health and security, *Lancet*, 396(10247): 293–5.

Gostin, L., Sridhar, D. and Hougendobler, D. (2015) The normative authority of the World Health Organization, *Public Health*, 129: 854–63.

Hawkins, B. and Holden, C. (2016) A corporate veto on health policy? Global constitutionalism and investor-state dispute settlement, *Journal of Health Politics, Policy and Law*, 41(5): 969–95.

Kaul, N. (2019) The political project of postcolonial neoliberal nationalism, *Indian Politics & Policy*, 2(1): 3–30.

Keane, M. and Wu, H. (2018) Lofty ambitions, new territories and turf battles: China's platforms 'go out', *Media Industries*, 5(1): 51–68.

Khan, M., Meghani, A., Liverani, M. et al. (2018) How do external donors influence national health policy processes? Experiences of domestic policy actors in Cambodia and Pakistan, *Health Policy and Planning*, 33(2): 215–23.

Khan, M., Pullan, R., Okello, G. et al. (2019) 'For how long are we going to take the tablets?' Kenyan stakeholders' views on priority investments to sustainably tackle soil-transmitted helminths, *Social Science & Medicine*, 228: 51–9.

Labonte, R., Schram, A. and Ruckert, A. (2016) The Trans-Pacific Partnership: is it everything we feared for health? *International Journal of Health Policy and Management*, 5(8): 487–96.

Mamdani, M. (1997) *Citizen and subject: Decentralised Despotism and the Legacy of Late Colonialism*. Delhi: Oxford University Press.

Mayhew, S. (2005) Hegemony, politics and ideology: the role of legislation in NGO–government relations in Asia, *The Journal of Development Studies*, 41(5): 727–8.

Mayhew, S., Kyamusugulwa, P., Kihangi Bindu, K. et al. (2021). Responding to the 2018–2020 Ebola virus outbreak in the Democratic Republic of the Congo: rethinking humanitarian approaches, *Risk Management and Healthcare Policy*, 14: 1731–47.

Milsom, P., Smith, R., Baker, P. and Walls, H. (2020) Corporate power and the international trade regime preventing progressive policy action on non-communicable diseases: a realist review, *Health Policy and Planning*, 36(4): 498–508.

Milsom, P., Smith, R., Modisenyane, S. and Walls H. (2021) Do international trade and investment agreements generate regulatory chill in public health policymaking? A case study of nutrition and alcohol policy in South Africa, *Globalization and Health*, 17: 104.

Moucheraud, C., Schwitters, A., Boudreaux, C. et al. (2017) Sustainability of health information systems: a three-country qualitative study in southern Africa, *BMC Health Services Research*, 17(1): 1–1.

Médecins Sans Frontières (2016) *MSF RCEP IP Chapter Technical Analysis: Regional Comprehensive Economic Partnership Intellectual Property Chapter and the Impact on Access to Medicines*. Geneva: Medecins Sans Frontieres.

Muniz, J.P., Duggal, K.A.N. and Peretti, L.A.S. (2017) The new Brazilian BIT on cooperation and facilitation of investments: a new approach in times of change, *ICSID Review – Foreign Investment Law Journal*, 32(2): 404–17.

Nichter, M. (2008) *Global Health: Why Cultural Perceptions, Social Representations, and Biopolitics Matter*. Tucson, AZ: University of Arizona Press.

Okuonzi, S. and Macrae, J. (1995) Whose policy is it anyway? International and national influences on health policy development in Uganda, *Health Policy and Planning*, 10(2): 122–32.

Pearce, N., Ebrahim, S., McKee, M. et al. (2014) The road to 25 x 25: how can the five-target strategy reach its goal?, *Lancet Global Health*, 2(3): e126–8.

Peck, J. (2011) Geographies of policy: from transfer-diffusion to mobility-mutation, *Progress in Human Geography*, 35: 773–97.

Peinhardt, C. and Wellhausen, R. (2016) Withdrawing from investment treaties but protecting investment, *Global Policy*, 7(4): 571–6.

Reid, P., Cormack, S. and Paine, J. (2019) Colonial histories, racism and health – the experience of Māori and Indigenous peoples, *Public Health*, 172: 119–24.

Richards, P., Mokuwa, E., Welmers, P. et al. (2019) Trust, and distrust, of Ebola treatment centers: a case-study from Sierra Leone, *PloS One*, 14(12): e0224511.

Rose, R. (1991) What is lesson-drawing?, *Journal of Public Policy*, 11(1): 3–30.

Saif-Ur-Rahman, K., Mamun, R., Nowrin, I. et al. (2019) Primary healthcare policy and governance in low-income and middle-income countries: an evidence gap map, *BMJ Global Health*, 4: e001453.

Salmon, M., Doery, K., Dance, P. et al. (2019) *Defining the Indefinable: Descriptors of Aboriginal and Torres Strait Islander Peoples' Cultures and Their Links to Health and Wellbeing*. Canberra: Aboriginal and Torres Strait Islander Health Team, Research School of Population Health, The Australian National University.

Sekalala, S. and Masud, H. (2021) Soft law possibilities in global health law, *Journal of Law, Medicine & Ethics*, 49: 152–5.

Shiffman, J. (2014) Knowledge, moral claims and the exercise of power in global health, *International Journal of Health Policy and Management*, 3: 297–9.

Sridhar, D. and Gomez, E. (2011) Health financing in Brazil, Russia and India: what role does the international community play?, *Health Policy and Planning*, 26: 12–24.

Ssennyonjo, A., Van Belle, S., Titeca, K. et al. (2021) Multisectoral action for health in low-income and middle-income settings: how can insights from social science theories inform intragovernmental coordination efforts?, *BMJ Global Health*, 6: e004064.

Turk, E., Durrance-Bagale, A., Han, E. et al. (2021) International experiences with co-production and people centredness offer lessons for covid-19 responses, *British Medical Journal*, 372: m4752.

United Nations (2022) *Take Action for the Sustainable Development Goals*. New York: United Nations. Available at: www.un.org/sustainabledevelopment/sustainable-development-goals (accessed 30 October 2022).

Vallesi, S., Wood, L., Dimer, L. and Zada, M. (2018) 'In their own voice' – incorporating underlying social determinants into Aboriginal health promotion programs, *International Journal of Environmental Research and Public Health*, 15(7): 1514.

Vanyoro, K., Hawkins, K., Greenall, M. et al. (2019) Local ownership of health policy and systems research in low-income and middle-income countries: a missing element in the uptake debate, *BMJ Global Health*, 4: e001523.

Walls, H. and Smith, R. (2015) Rethinking governance for trade and health, *British Medical Journal*, 351: h3652.

Walls, H., Smith, R. and Drahos, P. (2015) Improving regulatory capacity to manage risks associated with trade agreements, *Globalization and Health*, 11(14).

World Health Organization (2019) *Turning Plans into Action for Antimicrobial Resistance (AMR): Working Paper 2.0: Implementation and Coordination*. Geneva: World Health Organization.

11

Doing policy analysis

In this chapter you will be introduced to a political science-based approach to policy analysis and a range of tools for gathering, organizing and analysing health policy data. The aim is to assist you to analyse policy processes and to develop politically informed strategies that can be used to bring about health policy change.

Learning objectives

After working through this chapter, you will be better able to:

- gather and present data for policy analysis
- undertake retrospective and prospective policy analysis
- identify actors with an interest in a given policy issue, and assess their power, position and how they seek to alter the perceptions of relevant policy solutions
- develop politically informed strategies to attempt to influence policy change.

Key terms

Social media Software that uses web-based and mobile technologies for the creation, sharing and exchange of user-generated content in virtual networks and communities.

Social network analysis Methods used for mapping, measuring and analysing the social relationships between people, groups and organizations.

Stakeholder analysis Process through which those making policy or affected by it are identified and their likely position and levels of interest and influence are assessed.

Introduction

Having arrived at the final chapter of this book you will appreciate that policy change is political, dynamic and complicated. Policy change in the health sector is challenging because health systems are technically complex, and changing one part of the system invariably affects other parts and many different actors. Experience with health sector reform, for example, suggests that the costs of change often fall on powerful and well-organized groups (e.g. doctors and drug companies) while the benefits are often intended for widely dispersed and disadvantaged populations with little political clout (e.g. pregnant women). Achieving successful equity-enhancing policy reform is, therefore, often difficult. Moreover, addressing the social and structural determinants of health through policies in other sectors raises additional political challenges (de Leeuw 2017).

After reiterating the way that policy analysis can be used retrospectively and prospectively, this chapter introduces you to tools that are employed in policy analysis, both to assess and improve the prospects of successful policy change. These tools permit you to gather, use and apply knowledge in systematic ways. You will be introduced to *stakeholder analysis*. Actors are critical to policy change. They are placed at the centre of the 'policy triangle', and therefore considerable emphasis is placed on stakeholder analysis to identify the interests and preferences of affected actors. We then present an approach to developing politically informed strategies and guidance for gathering evidence for analysis, as well as some suggestions for using the 'policy triangle' to present the results of the analysis. The chapter concludes with some thoughts on the ethics of policy analysis. We do not cover rational-comprehensive approaches to policy analysis, such as applied economic techniques (e.g. cost–benefit analysis), because they do not incorporate analysis of the politics of decision making. These are well addressed elsewhere (Weimer and Vining 2010).

Retrospective and prospective policy analysis

In Chapter 1 you learned that there are two types of policy analysis; these were characterized as analysis *of* policy and analysis *for* policy. Analysis of policy tends to be retrospective, descriptive and explanatory. Analysis of policy looks back at why or how a policy made its way onto the agenda, its content, and whether or not and why it achieved its goals (e.g. a summative evaluation). For example, disappointing results with health sector reform in some countries have prompted the World Bank to undertake analysis of past reform processes to diagnose the political dimensions of the problem. Analysis *of* policy comprises the bulk of this book. In the following four sub-sections, we present a number of approaches to the analysis of policy, but note that some may also be applied to analysis for policy (i.e. prospectively).

Often both approaches are undertaken within one analysis – understanding why and how a particular policy content was agreed upon (analysis *of*) so as to better appreciate (and influence) the future trajectory of policy in the same space (analysis *for*). Many of the analytical and methodological tools introduced in this chapter can easily be applied to both analysis *of* and *for* policy. The Shiffman and Smith (2007) framework on priority setting, for example, has been used as a checklist and interview guide for analysing the factors which accounted for getting drowning prevention on the global policy agenda over the past decade; as well as, in the same study, making recommendations to inform the actions and agenda of the associated advocacy coalition to enhance prospects for policy adoption and implementation (Scarr et al. 2022).

Policy process-tracing

Process-tracing is a qualitative method that enables the analyst to unpack the causal processes and relationships between independent variables and the outcome of the dependent variable in relation to single case studies, or specific policies. There are three different approaches that the analyst might take to process-tracing. First, *theory testing process-tracing* deductively tests an existing theoretical approach from the wider literature by looking for evidence of a particular causal mechanism to explain why a particular policy arose (though other factors may have impacted the outcome). Stedman-Bryce (2013) provides an example in 'Health for all' in a Universal Healthcare Campaign in Ghana. A deeper commentary on the methods used can be found in Befani and Stedman-Bryce (2017). Second, *theory building process-tracing* inductively attempts to arrive at a generalizable theoretical explanation from a set of empirical data relating to policy. An example of this approach is Hacker's (1998) comparative work exploring health policy formulation in Canada, the UK and US. Third, *explaining outcome process-tracing* seeks to create a plausible explanation for the outcome of a particular policy rather than building or testing more generalized theories (Beach and Pedersen 2019).

Policy ethnography

Ethnography explores how people interact in real-life environments, and how meaning and value are established. Ethnographic approaches typically rely on immersive observation that can build rich interpretations of actor's views, practices and cultural context. Ethnography typically pursues depth over breadth, exploration beyond hypothesis testing, and unfolding the meaning and role of actors in a given setting. Ethnographic approaches – particularly participant observation – have been deployed in political research to understand institutions and their politics, political legitimacy, as well as power construction within and beyond health systems (Mishra and Nambiar 2018). These approaches offer tools to explore dimensions of political activity that are not necessarily recognizable as political, because they occur outside of the usual political arenas and in seemingly apolitical ways, offering new knowledge and new understandings of political phenomena. Yet such approaches can be challenging to deploy in organizations that lack transparency and are wary of outside researchers.

Policy discourse analysis

Discourse analysis is a qualitative approach that involves a rigorous analysis of the use of written (e.g. laws, policies, strategy documents, media articles, social media posts, etc.) and oral (e.g. interviews, debates, speeches) communication and of the reproduction of dominant ideologies (and belief systems) in such communication. Discourse analysis emphasizes the contextual meaning of language.

Examining how communication is used can offer insights into the interests and position of policy actors or the rhetoric that informs a policy argument. Discourse analysis can also help illuminate how language contributes to forming shared (and manufactured) understandings of dominant ideologies and framings (what is considered normal) and also of what is possible, legitimate or true within the sociocultural and political context in which communication takes place. This methodology enables the analyst to explore what is assumed or ignored, revealing hidden power asymmetries, dominant representations of a policy problem and solutions and social hierarchies existing within health policy making (Yazdannik et al. 2017). Discourse analysis extends beyond a simpler content analysis of what is written or said in policy communications, to examine the ideas, ideologies, power relations and contextual factors reflected in those statements.

The following are some steps to discourse analysis to help you answer your chosen policy question. First, identify the material (e.g. written policy documents, visual texts) that are likely relevant to the policy question. Second, gather information about the context in which the policy material and communication has been used to understand what conditions made it possible and appropriate to communicate it in that manner. Once you have finished collecting the data, you can start your analysis of the content of your policy material in order to identify emerging themes and patterns. The final step involves reflecting on the results to examine the meaning and purpose of the policy language used to draw conclusions to inform the answer to your policy question.

Policy cube approach

The 'policy cube' approach provides a heuristic to examine the content of policy along three axes: comprehensiveness; salience; and its equity orientation (Buse et al. 2020). Comprehensiveness refers to the extent any given policy covers the range of evidence-informed measures one would expect are needed to effectively address the problem under consideration. The policy cube approach was used to explore nutrition policies in a number of countries (Buse et al. 2020). In that context, comprehensiveness refers to the number of the World Health Organization's 'Best Buys' for diet-related NCDs that were reflected in relevant policies in those countries. The second axis concerning policy salience can be thought of in terms of the likelihood of implementation of the policy under consideration. Analysis is often based on several considerations: first, the perceived authoritativeness of the policy document (typically based on the place of the issuing authority in the political and bureaucratic hierarchy) and the priority that it places on the policy; second, whether an implementing agency and budget line item is associated with the policy; and third, whether an accountability mechanism is outlined in the policy document. In the above-mentioned analysis of diet-related policies the authors saw different levels of salience for these policies across the countries, but they were generally weak. Weakness also marked performance on the third axis of countries' nutrition policy cubes, which examined the text for commitments to equity consideration in terms of whether or not the needs of marginalized groups were recognized and whether or not rights-based approaches were proposed in the policies. The policy cube approach enables the analyst to better understand elements of policy content (e.g., its distributional intentions) and strengths and weaknesses as well as gauge why it might not have delivered what it could or should have in light of the likelihood that it would be implemented.

Prospective analysis

Analysis *for* policy tends to be prospective. It is usually carried out to inform the formulation of a policy (e.g. a formative evaluation) or anticipate how a policy might fare if introduced (e.g. how other actors might respond to the proposed changes). Typically, analysis for policy will be undertaken, or sponsored, by interested parties to assess the prospects and manage the politics of policy change in a way that meets their goals. At times, such analysis will result in the decision to adjust the policy or goals or even abandon a particular course of action due to its poor political feasibility.

Having read the preceding chapters, you will appreciate that an astute policy reformer will engage in prospective analysis at all stages of the policy cycle – from problem identification, through agenda setting, formulation and implementation – as each of these stages are subject to the flow of political events. Hence, successful policy change depends on continuous and systematic political analysis.

Analysis in the early stages of policy making, particularly in problem definition and agenda setting, is typically critical to achieving policy objectives. Chapter 7 explained why facts arising from research, whether epidemiological or economic, do not simply speak for themselves in setting priorities, but may be used strategically, ignored or not used at all depending on political processes. The role of the media, including social media, in agenda setting was highlighted as critical to raising and framing problems in public debates and in policy circles. Similarly, policy 'entrepreneurs' actively promote attention to particular problems and solutions and look for 'windows of opportunity' to get issues onto the agenda and ensure the formulation of a policy response that suits their interests or ideas (Kingdon 1995).

If you want to successfully influence policy outcomes, you will need to:

- engage in framing problems and solutions;
- understand how to shape political processes to encourage wider acceptance of your definition of a problem and proposed solution;
- understand how agendas are set and issues receive political prioritization;
- learn to recognize political windows of opportunity;
- understand the positions, interests and power of interested parties based on the potential distribution of costs and benefits of the proposed policy;
- adapt your solutions to make them more politically feasible.

Undertaking these tasks constitutes analysis *for* policy and will provide the basis for developing politically informed strategies to influence or even manage policy change. While such analyses may enhance your success in influencing policy outcomes, they cannot guarantee such outcomes – for success depends on many factors beyond the control of any one actor – including serendipity.

Stakeholder analysis

Irrespective of whether or not analysis is retrospective or prospective, it will be based on an analysis of those individuals and groups with an interest in an issue or policy, including those who might be affected by a policy and those who may play a role in relation to making or implementing the policy – in other words, actors in the policy process. Although a variety of approaches to stakeholder analysis have been described (Gilson et al. 2012), three distinct activities recur (Roberts et al. 2004): (1) identifying the policy actors; (2) assessing their power and political resources; and (3) understanding their interests and hence position with respect to the issue.

Identifying 'stakeholders'

A number of chapters in this book have focused on the range of actors in health policy – from those inside government to the spectrum of interest groups in civil society and the private sector. The relevant actors will be specific to the particular policy and the context within which it is being discussed. Identifying the actors who are, or might become, involved in a particular policy process, requires judgement. For example, it may be necessary to identify groups within organizations which may have different interests (e.g. a MoH would rarely be treated as one actor as there are likely to be different groups and programmes within any ministry pursuing differing interests). The idea is to discover independent actors who wield considerable influence while keeping the number sufficiently small to make the analysis manageable (for a greater number of actors, a social network analysis approach is more useful – see below). Identifying an initial set of actors can be conducted through a brainstorming session with knowledgeable informants.

To compile a list of relevant actors, you will need to think about the likely implications of the content of the proposed policy – in particular how it will affect the interests of different actors or groups. Relevant actors will include those who are likely to be impacted by the policy either positively or negatively and those who might act in support of or against the policy change or could be mobilized to do so. Particular importance needs to be devoted to individuals or organizations which can either block policy adoption (often leaders of political parties, heads of agencies, etc.) or implementation (often bureaucrats, service providers and users, but other groups as well depending on the policy).

Activity 11.1

Choose a health area with which you are familiar and consider a change you would like to see to a policy affecting that area (e.g. if you are concerned with excessive alcohol consumption the policy intervention might be concerned with minimum pricing, digital advertising, sport sponsorship, etc.). Using the above guidelines identify 15–20 individuals or groups who have an interest in the issue or a role to play in adopting or implementing the policy.

Feedback

Health sector reform often involves the following types of groups, some of which you may have identified as having a stake in the issue you are analysing (Reich 1996): consumer organizations (e.g. patient groups); producer groups (nurses, doctors, pharmaceutical companies); economic groups (workers who may be affected, industries, companies with health insurance schemes, donor agencies); and ideological groups (single-issue campaign organizations, political parties, researchers, media groups).

Assessing power

The second step in a stakeholder analysis consists of assessing the power of each actor. You learned in Chapters 2 and 4 that political resources take many forms. Tangible assets (e.g. votes, finance, infrastructure, members, social media following) can be distinguished from intangible assets (expertise and legitimacy in relation to the policy issue, access to the mass media, networks and political decision makers). Control over resources increases actors' influence in the policy process. For example, groups with a mature organization and infrastructure will often have more power than groups which have yet to organize themselves. Doctors, for example, often have health policy-relevant expertise and are, therefore, often viewed as legitimate; they are often organized into long-standing professional organizations, and, because they usually have high social status, frequently have access to financial resources and relationships with decision makers or policy influencers. As a result of these political resources, doctors are usually characterized as a group with considerable political power on most health policy issues. Pharmaceutical companies have great expertise, considerable finance and in some countries considerable influence over regulatory bodies, but often limited legitimacy – at least in so far as civil society and activist groups are concerned because of their propensity for price gouging, patent hoarding, free riding on public investment in research and development, and tax avoidance. The type of strategy any group will employ in wielding its power will depend on the nature of the political resources at its disposal (Gilson et al. 2012). The context will often determine the precise value of any particular resource. During a pandemic, an understanding of epidemiology and mathematical modelling can enable an expert to gain access to decision makers.

Some further considerations to aid stakeholder analysis in policy implementation have been elaborated by Balane and colleagues (2020). Topp and colleagues (2021) have elaborated a comprehensive framework to assist policy analysts link theories of power (in their words 'what we ask about power') to methods ('how we ask about it and interpret it') to sites (sources) of power.

Activity 11.2

Select ten of the participants you identified in Activity 11.1. For each, make an inventory of the major resources at their disposal. Differentiate between tangible and intangible resources. Given these political assets, characterize each of your actors as having high, medium or low power in relation to the health policy under consideration.

Feedback

Clearly your inventory will depend on the actors you select. For example, we use a patient group with medium power to illustrate:

- tangible resources – for example, large number of members, electoral votes, funding is often from pharmaceutical companies;
- intangible resources – for example, passion, first-hand experience, access to media, public sympathy and support, highly legitimate interest.

Assessing interests, position and commitment

Each actor's interests, position and level of commitment to a particular policy issue will determine how they will deploy their political resources. Assessing these attributes constitutes the third and final stage in a stakeholder analysis.

You learned about interest groups in Chapter 4 – here we are concerned not just with so-called cause and sectional interest groups, but the 'interests' of any relevant actor in a particular policy issue. Interests are those things which benefit an individual or group (as distinct from their wants or preferences). Often it is the expected economic effect of a policy on an actor's interests which plays an overriding role in determining their position on a policy. Having said that, in some instances, wants and preferences may also constitute the interests of actors, as is the case of groups such as Extinction Rebellion who seek to compel government action to prevent social and ecological collapse from fossil fuel use.

Determining what these interests are can be complex. At times, actors may conceal their real interests for tactical purposes, perhaps because they are illegal (e.g. illicit payment for referrals). At other times, interests may be difficult to discern because the policy content may be fuzzy or there may be a number of variants of the policy under discussion. For example, a minister of health may be committed to a policy of contracting out publicly funded service delivery to non-state organizations. Doctors employed in the public sector who practise privately may not be sure whether or not to support such a policy unless they have assurances that they will be eligible to compete for contracts with NGOs or private practitioners and/or have assurances that their employment in the public sector will not be compromised by the proposed policy. These may be details that the minister may not wish to elaborate upon until a stakeholder analysis has been undertaken.

Activity 11.3

Select any five of the participants you have identified in Activity 11.2 and list their interests in relation to your chosen policy. Seek to reveal what they would stand to gain or lose from the policy change you are considering.

Feedback

Often the financial or material impacts of policy change constitute central interests to individuals and groups. In the example of a policy to contract out publicly financed services, public sector doctors might perceive their interests at risk if they think that the policy's aim is to reduce their number (i.e. they could lose their jobs) or if they fear that one outcome of such a policy would be to increase the competition that they face in their private practices (i.e. limiting the amount they can earn by practising illegally). Yet other interests might also be perceived to be under threat. For example, the potential loss of a public sector position may not be compensated for by increased income in the private sector due to the credibility, prestige and symbolic value of a public sector post in many countries – as well as other perks, which might include housing, invitations to conferences, further education, etc.

The impact of policy change on participants' interests will determine their position with respect to the proposed policy – whether they are supportive, neutral or opposed. As with identifying interests, positions may not be easily determined as they may be concealed or because publicly aired positions may be different from privately held ones (the latter often determining how a group may actually react to a policy proposal). For example, a minister may publicly support a policy so as to win favour with voters or specific interest groups but may be quietly working against the policy within government on the grounds that it is unaffordable. At times, actors may not be certain of their position if they are not sure how a policy might affect their interests. This may happen if the policy content is vague, the context changing rapidly or if there are a number of policy options being discussed, each with different repercussions on the actor's interests.

✎ Activity 11.4

Identify the likely publicly stated and privately held positions of the five actors you analysed in Activity 11.3.

Feedback

An example will illustrate the difference in publicly aired and privately held positions an actor might have. Doctors in a publicly funded system might complain publicly about a lack of resources and patients having to wait for treatment. However, in private they might resist any attempt by policy makers to appoint extra doctors as this would jeopardize the size of their private practice and income.

In addition to assessing interests and positions, it is necessary to assess the importance of the issue to each participant in terms of other priorities they hold. What you want to uncover is the intensity of actors' commitments to the policy and how much of their political resources they are likely to devote to pursuing their interests through influencing or blocking the policy proposal. While a powerful actor may be opposed to a particular policy, the issue may be of marginal importance to them and they may do little to block policy adoption or implementation. For example, a former UK Secretary of State for Health expressed his view that the legal limit for abortion should be halved from 24 to 12 weeks but took no steps to amend the abortion law (Quinn 2012). One can gauge the level of commitment of an actor in several ways – by asking them, or from assessing how critical the issue is likely to be to the pursuit of the organization's mandate, or from the time that senior organizational figures devote to it, and so on.

It is important to attempt to determine each actor's real interests, position and level of commitment to a proposed policy. This knowledge will play a central part in understanding the likely success of the proposed policy and in designing politically oriented strategies and tactics to bring about policy change.

Activity 11.5

For each of the actors analysed in Activity 11.4, list the interests they hold (what they gain or lose from policy change), their position (opposed, supportive, neutral), and their level of commitment to the policy issue (high, medium, low). Construct a table with the data including position and power (from Activity 11.1) for each of the actors – this is commonly referred to as a position map or force field analysis. As for Activity 11.4, you may need to undertake some research.

Feedback

Each stakeholder analysis table or position map will look different depending on the policy content, actors and context. A position map of players in relation to health sector reform in the Dominican Republic in the mid-1990s is presented in Figure 11.1. Although there is bound to be a degree of uncertainty in relation to each of the variables, the position map provides a good starting point for thinking about who might form a coalition in favour of reform and which groups might try to undermine a reform.

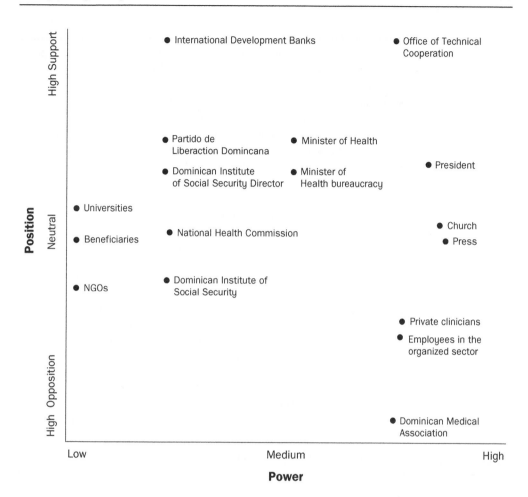

Figure 11.1: Position map for health sector reform in the Dominican Republic in 1995
Source: Glassman et al. (1999)

The next step in a more sophisticated stakeholder analysis would aim to model how each actor's commitment and position may shift with a modification to the content of the proposed policy. This issue will be returned to in the section on developing political strategies for policy change.

Social network analysis

Given the centrality of networks and advocacy coalitions in influencing policy, stakeholder analysis can be extended with a *social network analysis*. Such analysis maps, measures and analyses quantitatively and visually the social relationships between people, groups and organizations – typically to determine the position of actors within networks as this conditions their access to information and power. In particular, analysts use computer software to analyse network features including 'betweenness', centrality, density, distance and 'reachability' to characterize participants and their relationships in a network. Using a social network analysis approach, Blanchet and James (2013) examined the evolving network engaged in eye care policy implementation in Ghana between 2008 and 2010. They observed a shift in relations and power between managers, nurses and doctors and international organizations. Examining distance between actors and the centrality and reachability of actors through social network analysis can help to assess the cohesion of a network as well as identify the key individuals – the brokers and opinion leaders – and organizations at the centre of networks who can exchange information, forge common positions and alliances and thereby influence policy change.

Before we move on to thinking about how to use the results of stakeholder analysis to bring about policy change, it is useful to consider some of the limitations inherent in stakeholder analysis. It is obvious that any analysis is only as good as the analyst's attention, creativity, tenacity and access to information on the interests, positions, influence and commitment in relation to a particular policy change. On a related note, and as you will recall from Chapter 2 on power, the positionality of the researcher will influence the findings (see below). Moreover, the findings are by their nature time and issue-specific, and stakeholder analysis only provides data on actors and reveals little about the context and process of policy making, which, you will appreciate, play equally important roles in policy change.

Developing political strategies for policy change

Roberts et al. (2004, pages 66–67) suggest that the political feasibility of policy change is determined by 'position, power, players and perception'. The viability of a proposed policy change can be improved by developing strategies to influence the position of relevant actors, the power or political resources at the disposal of key actors, the number of players actively involved in the policy arena, and the perceptions held by participants of the problem and proposed policy solution. Based on their experience with health sector reform in numerous countries, Roberts and his colleagues provide useful guidance in terms of influencing positions, power, players and perceptions.

Activity 11.6

While reading through the following summary of Roberts et al.'s work, make notes on which strategies you have used in your past efforts to effect policy change and/or others which you think might be useful in the policy context where you operate.

Position, power, players and perception

Position strategies

Roberts and colleagues (2004) begin by presenting four types of bargains that can be used to shift the position of actors with respect to a particular policy proposal (e.g. from neutral to supportive). Deals can be made with actors who are opposed or neutral so as to make them more supportive or less opposed by *altering a particular component of the proposed policy*. For example, health centre managers may drop their opposition to a proposal to introduce user fees if they are allowed to retain a percentage of the revenue to improve quality or provide perks for their staff. Second, deals can be struck through which *support is sought for one issue in return for concessions on another*. For example, a medical association may drop its opposition to a MoH proposal to train paramedical staff to assume additional clinical functions, if the ministry agrees to drop its proposal to curb spending on teaching institutions – which is in the interests of the association's members. Third, *promises can be made*. If the medical association drops its opposition to the paramedic upgrading programme, the ministry can promise to consider the need to increase the number of specialists in particular areas in future policy developments. In contrast, *threats can be used to change the positions of actors*. In Bangladesh, development agencies threatened to suspend aid if the ministry did not proceed with agreed reforms while ministry staff threatened to strike if the reforms went ahead (Buse 1998).

In summary, a variety of deals can be made and compromises reached to change the position of actors without altering the balance of power in a given arena. These can involve seeking to change the content of policy so that it is more closely aligned to the interests of some of the players.

Power strategies

A range of strategies can be used to affect the distribution of political assets of the players involved to strengthen supportive groups and undermine opposition groups. These involve providing supportive actors with:

- funds, personnel and facilities;
- information to increase expertise;
- access to decision makers and the media;
- links to supportive networks;
- public relations material which highlights supportive actors' expertise, legitimacy, victim status or heroic nature.

Roberts and colleagues (2004) suggest that actions can also be taken to limit the political resources of opponents, for example by:

- challenging their legitimacy, expertise, integrity or motives, for example by characterizing them as self-interested and self-serving;
- seeking to fragment their coalition by appealing to or buying off some of their members;
- reducing their access to decision makers;
- refusing to co-operate or to share information with them.

Player strategies

Player strategies attempt to affect the number of actors actively involved in a policy arena, in particular to mobilize those that are neutral and to demobilize those groups who are opposed. Recruiting un-mobilized actors can be achieved at times by simply informing a group that an item is on the agenda and what their stake in the issue is likely to be. For example, an association of private providers may not be aware that a particular policy is being discussed which may have consequences for its members. Player strategies can, however, be difficult to execute if new organizations need to be formed or if they involve demobilizing a group which has already publicly taken a position on an issue. It may be possible to persuade the group that its stake or impact is different to that which it had previously calculated – but then efforts at face saving will also have to be made. Alternatively, it may be possible to undermine opponents by dividing them. For example, it may be possible to identify a sub-group within the larger group which might benefit from your proposal whom you might win to your side. Roberts et al. (2004) suggest that another player strategy involves changing the venue of decision making. This tactic was employed by the donors in Bangladesh when confronted with opposition to reform in the MoH – they sought allies in the ministry of finance and parliament who might support their cause. Player strategies aim to alter the balance of players by introducing sympathetic ones and sidelining opposing ones.

Perception strategies

Throughout this book the force of ideas and the role that the framing and perceptions of a problem and its policy solution have on the position and power of different interests have been highlighted. A variety of techniques are used to alter perceptions. Data and arguments can, for example, be questioned as can the relative importance of a problem or the practicality of a policy solution. The appropriateness of public or private action can be attacked using economic theory or philosophy to shift players' perceptions on an issue. Associations can also be altered to give an issue a greater chance of political and social acceptability. For example, those seeking to eliminate congenital syphilis (i.e. syphilis transmitted from mother to infant) may highlight that this is a condition 'inflicted' upon 'innocent' infants, and may not stress the fact that the infection in the mother is sexually transmitted since sexually transmitted infections historically are both low on policy agendas and attract moral opprobrium. Appealing to prevailing values can also work. Advocates for congenital syphilis, for example, stress the principles of fairness and equity – arguing that the elimination of congenital syphilis deserves the same attention as the elimination of mother to child transmission of HIV – an issue that has received much public and policy concern. Invoking symbols can also change perceptions of issues. Thus, reforms can be linked to nationalist sentiments, imperatives or celebrities. Employing celebrities to endorse new reforms and initiatives is becoming common as is the branding of public health interventions.

Feedback

You have now reviewed the range of tools which Roberts et al. (2004) have identified as useful in influencing the position, power, players and perceptions associated with policy change. Some strategies are open to most players, for example, sharing or refusing to share information, changing the perception of an issue, or mobilizing groups. Some strategies may, however, only be available to certain groups. For example, the tactics to increase the political resources of supportive actors require that you have access to resources to distribute to them. Similarly, many strategies which aim to change the position of actors require access to decision making over other issues that can be traded. Even changing the perception of an issue requires communication skills as well as access to the media or social media accounts. Some degree of power is usually necessary to deliver credible threats.

Data for policy analysis

It will come as no surprise to you that the quality of your policy analysis will depend on the accuracy, comprehensiveness and relevance of the information that you are able to access and collect. These, in turn, depend on the time and resources available to you, your official mandate, your contacts in the relevant policy domain and the perceived sensitivity or stakes associated with the policy. The steps describing a stakeholder analysis, above, can be conducted through brainstorming sessions to elicit differing perspectives – but it is also useful for analysts to work independently before comparing their responses. Evidence for policy analysis usually emanates from documents and people – and increasingly from resources available through the Internet, though these need to be interpreted with care.

Policy documents

Policy-relevant documents are those which provide clues as to the likely actors involved in any policy process as well as their interests, positions and commitment to the policy in question. The sources of those documents will depend on specifics of the analysis. Much can be learned about policy actors, process, context and content from academic books and journals. The following journals are likely to have relevant material: *Health Policy and Planning*, *Health Policy*, *International Journal of Health Policy and Management*, *Journal of Health Politics*, *Policy and Law*, *Social Science and Medicine*, *Health Affairs*, *Journal of Health Services Research and Policy*, *Milbank Quarterly*, *Journal of Public Health Policy*, *BMJ Global Health*, *Bulletin of the World Health Organization*, *Global Public Health* and *Global Health Governance*.

A literature search would be likely to start with a topic search on the health problem or policy you are concerned with using a combination of bibliographic services such as the Social Science Citation Index, the US National Library of Medicine's MEDLINE (www.nlm.nih.gov), EMBASE, CINAHL PubMed, PolicyCommons.net, Policy and Society, Scopus or Google Scholar.

'Grey literature', including reports and evaluations produced by interest groups or independent evaluators, think tanks and consultants, government and non-governmental and multilateral organizations, can also be useful. Press releases and editorials in the mass media as well as social media posts provide additional material.

There is likely to be a wealth of information about most policies and many policy contexts available on the Internet. Yet in contrast to journals and most official reports from government and multilateral sources, the information on the Internet is neither necessarily subject to peer review nor is it always obvious which group or individual has published the material (which may have a bearing on its credibility) and whilst some of it may deliberately contain mis-information to sway public or policy maker opinion on an issue, much 'grey' literature can be of great value (Banks 2022).

Indeed, unpublished reports, email messages, minutes of meetings, memoranda and other 'internal' documents can be particularly useful in revealing the true interests and positions of actors as well as their strategies and tactics for influencing policy – but may be generally difficult to access, though some countries have freedom of information legislation allowing citizens to request documents produced by public bodies that can be used by researchers. Internal tobacco industry documents, made public as a result of litigation against companies in the US in 1998, provided a rare and rich account of the industry's aims, interests and activities related to a number of health policies and organizations (e.g. undermining the Framework Convention on Tobacco Control and exerting influence over WHO). Figure 11.2 is a copy of one such internal document which reveals the mechanisms through which Philip Morris sought to influence the policy decisions of legislators in the US.

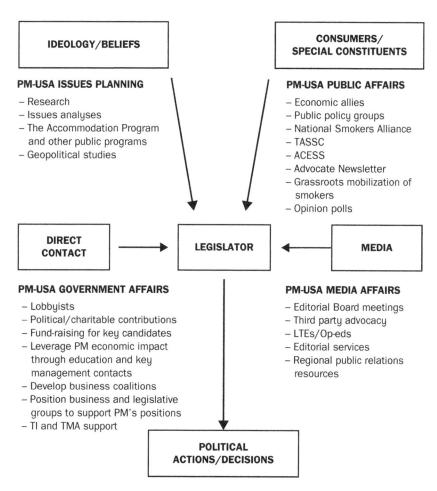

Figure 11.2: Tools to affect legislative decisions

Since this is an internal industry document, not all the acronyms are explained. The following seem likely: PM, Philip Morris; TMA, Tobacco Manufacturing Association; LTE, letter to editor; TASSC, the Advancement of Sound Science Coalition; TI, Tobacco Industry; ACESS, unknown.

Source: Philip Morris (no date)

Depending on the issue, you may also wish to consult statistical data sources, for example, to verify the magnitude of a problem so as to assist in framing a problem or undermining an opponent's argument. International organizations, such as WHO and the World Bank, provide policy relevant data as do most governments and sub-national agencies of government (much of which is available on their websites).

The purpose of documentary analysis is to provide evidence that explains or predicts policy change. Therefore, you might be looking for evidence on relevant contextual variables (situational, structural, cultural and exogenous), actors (their power, interests, positions and commitment), content (policy aims, including target groups, and means), and process (stage, venue and strategies used to influence policy). Although there are a number of approaches to extracting data from documentary sources, most policy analysts will rely on content analysis, of which there are two types. First, quantitative content analysis is a systematic approach that seeks to quantify the content within documents according to pre-determined categories. A policy analyst might, for example, search through a sample of national newspapers to record the number of column inches devoted to different health policy issues, such as planetary health, over a particular time span so as to gauge media and public interest in a policy issue. Here the pre-determined category is planetary health. Alternatively, an analyst may go through a broader range of document types to reveal specific actors' positions with respect to a particular policy over a period of time – in which case the policy (e.g. a specific policy on reducing carbon content in a health food chain), the actors and their positions would be the pre-determined categories.

In contrast, qualitative content analysis aims to uncover underlying themes and structures of argument used in documentary material. The policy analyst searching through newspapers for coverage of planetary health, for example, may examine the editorials to understand whether there is support for the government's above-mentioned policy on carbon in the food chain or to determine whether the press is spreading scientifically inaccurate messages in relation to the issue. Alternatively, an analyst might search documents for evidence of the philosophical arguments used to support or frame a particular policy stance. The themes extracted using qualitative content analysis are often depicted using illustrative quotations from the document.

The utility of documentary analysis rests upon the quality and quantity (i.e. completeness) of the documents used. Bryman (2008) suggests that a number of questions should be posed to assess documentary sources critically, including:

- Who wrote and published the document?
- Why was the document produced?
- Was the author in a position to be authoritative about the subject?
- Is the material authentic?

- What interests did the author have (and did the author declare them)?
- Is the document representative or atypical – and, if so, in what way?
- Is the meaning of the material clear?
- Can the contents be corroborated through other sources?
- Are competing interpretations of the document possible?

Another factor to consider is whether the document has been edited for public release (known as redaction), which can limit the utility of the document but can also reveal the sensitivity of the issue to the actor in question.

Gathering data from people

Interviewing and surveying actors can provide rich information for policy analysis. These methods may be the only way to gather valid information on the political interests and resources of relevant actors or to gather historical and contextual information. Large-scale surveys represent a quantitative method for collection of information often by questionnaire or structured interview. Surveys, which can be administered in person or by post, email or Internet for self-completion, are used by policy analysts to generate basic information in relation to actors' views of a problem or their position in relation to a policy if this information cannot be obtained from documentary sources.

Semi-structured interviews are generally more useful than questionnaire surveys in eliciting information that is often 'richer' and/or of a more sensitive nature. The goal of the semi-structured interview is to obtain in-depth, useful and valid data on actors' perceptions of a given policy issue and how it might affect them and others. Typically, what is called a topic or interview guide will be used to prompt the analyst to cover a given set of issues with each respondent, as opposed to using a pre-determined set of questions as used in surveys. The idea is to allow flexibility and fluidity in the interview so that it resembles a conversation in which the respondent feels sufficiently comfortable to provide a detailed account and to tell their story. Hence, questions should be open (i.e. those which do not invite a 'yes' or 'no' response) and should be sequenced in such a way as to deal with more factual and less contentious issues before tackling more difficult areas and at deeper levels of understanding (Fontana and Frey 1994). Frameworks presented in earlier chapters can help structure and inform question guides.

Health policy interviews undertaken with senior decision makers and representatives of powerful interest groups are of a special nature. These are sometimes called elite interviews. While potentially useful, such interviews pose particular challenges. First, it is often difficult to recruit respondents as they may be wary of how the results might be used, particularly if they are concerned that the analysis may undermine their own policy aims. Second, people in high-status occupations may not have sufficient time for an interview. Third, leaders may simply provide official positions, which may be more efficiently obtained through policy documents. Often it is more productive to interview such officials outside the office (or office hours), which may encourage them to provide 'off the record' comments which are more informative. Fourth, officials may be reluctant to be interviewed on the grounds that it will be difficult to maintain their anonymity.

Relevant individuals to interview can be initially identified through the literature and document review, which should reveal organizations and actors with an interest in the policy issue. These individuals will be likely to be able to identify further informants who may in turn identify others (called 'snowball' sampling). Interviewing retired staff from interested organizations can yield more forthright and analytical perspectives as these individuals will have had time to reflect and may not fear reprisals – and may also have more time available to allow them to participate in an interview. The most knowledgeable informants are likely to be drawn from a sub-group of actors identified in the stakeholder analysis. You may find that it is best to approach first those individuals with rich sources of information and power, and who are supportive of the proposed policy, while those who may be hostile or may block access to other interviewees should be interviewed later in the process.

Thought needs to be given to introducing the purpose of the interview in such a way that is honest and ethical, and yet yields good data. Similarly, it will be necessary to inform respondents how you will use the information and whether they wish to keep their responses anonymous. The pros and cons of using a tape recorder need to be weighed up, but whatever decision is taken, the importance of transcribing the results or writing up notes taken during the interview immediately afterwards cannot be overemphasized. Even if an interview has been recorded, it is helpful for the interviewer to write a few notes covering their impressions of the main findings from the interview and its implications for further data collection.

The central limitation of interview data is that they concern what people say and how they say it, as opposed to what people actually do or think. This problem can be overcome by 'triangulating' their responses with those from other informants, or with data gathered through other means, including observations of meetings or documentary sources (Mays and Pope 2020). It is harder to negotiate access to meetings and other events than to obtain interviews, unless the meetings are held in public.

Social media as a source of data for policy analysis

Social media provides a potentially rich source of material for policy analysis. This type of media is evolving rapidly and takes many different forms, including blogs, microblogs (e.g. Weibo) and vlogs, networking forums (e.g. Facebook, LinkedIn), content sharing sites (e.g. TikTok and Instagram), collaborative knowledge sharing sites (e.g. wikis) podcasts, etc. Social media is increasingly used for communicating, collaborative projects, sharing content within communities, social networking, gaming, influencing and political campaigning. Some have a large user population, which generates a large digital footprint that can serve policy and policy analysis. There is an increasing amount of research on the health impacts of platforms such as WhatsApp or TikTok. From the perspective of policy, however, social media analysis can yield valuable information about participants' positions, interests and commitment from material they post (e.g. Tweets) or the virtual social networks in which they participate around various policy issues. Material can also help identify frames for discourse analysis and reveal how policy actors seek to influence debates and mobilize constituencies in policy processes. Platforms such as WhatsApp could be used to analyse health policy processes, for example in relation to advocacy coalition dynamics or street level bureaucrats engagement in policy implementation. Guides to the analysis of social media data are becoming available (e.g. Powell and van Velthoven 2020).

In summary, documents and people can be important sources of evidence for policy analysis, and both quantitative and qualitative approaches will be required to gather data. Multiple sources and methods can increase understanding and the validity of the results. Once you engage in a real policy analysis, you will be likely to have additional questions on gathering and analysing data and would be well advised to consult a social science research methods guide, such as that by Bryman (2008), or a more in-depth treatment of documentary analysis (Gorsky and Mold 2020).

Data analysis: applying the 'policy triangle'

Many of the frameworks presented in this book provide a structure with which to apply and present policy analysis. You will recall that we gave prominence to the 'policy analysis triangle' in Chapter 1 (Figure 1.1) and will use it illustratively in this section. Although the triangle provides an extremely useful structure to make your exploration of health policy issues and collection of data more systematic, it can be difficult to apply when you come to analysing and presenting your data because the different aspects, such as actors and processes, are so integrally intertwined and the goal of the analysis is generally to draw out their inter-relationships.

Several scholars have presented the finding of policy organized around the policy triangle. Trostle et al. (1999), for example, examined policies on AIDS, cholera, family planning and immunization in Mexico to understand the extent to which researchers influence decision makers. They found a number of common factors enabling or impeding interactions between these two sets of actors and analysed their data by looking at the:

- content of each policy and the factors that promoted (e.g. good quality research) or constrained (e.g. academic jargon, unrealistic recommendations) the relationship;
- actors involved in each policy and the factors that enabled (e.g. networks that agreed on priority issues) or impeded (e.g. lack of technical background among decision makers) the relationship;
- processes, which included communication channels and events that intervened to promote or impede the use of research;
- contextual factors that enabled (e.g. the stability of the state) or constrained the ability of research to influence policy (e.g. centralization of power and information).

Another way of presenting your policy analysis is by applying a different, more explanatory framework. For example, the framework offered by Shiffman and Smith (2007) on priority setting provides more explicit guidance as to what you might include. Whichever framework you use, it is worthwhile consulting a qualitative data analysis textbook. Pope et al. (2020) provide a simple introduction.

There are different ways to organize your analysis and supporting material and it will very much depend on your policy analysis question. On the whole it is usually easier to approach your analysis like a narrative if it is a retrospective policy analysis: a story with a beginning, middle and end. For example, if you arrange your data and analysis chronologically, using the 'stages heuristic' (see Chapter 1), you will start with problem identification and issue recognition (agenda setting), go on to policy formulation and implementation, and end with an evaluation of what happened in this particular policy 'story'. This last part could be an overall discussion of how to understand what happened in this particular issue and consider whether the story did unfold in such a linear fashion in practice.

In gathering your data, you may well have produced a timeline: writing down the dates over a period of time of a series of events such as meetings or conferences, results from research studies, media stories, a change in government or the availability of funding, and decisions which will have informed your analysis of how the issue got on to the policy agenda and was handled. You may start your narrative by describing the background to the issue you are looking at, referring to some or all of Leichter's four contextual factors – situational, structural, cultural or external – that you learned about in Chapter 1. Having done that, you could move on to the problem identification phase, saying how the issue got on to the agenda, whether there was a single focusing event or several, where ideas came from and how they were framed, what role particular actors played in getting attention for the issue, whether the media were involved, and so on.

Having established how and why the issue reached the policy agenda, you might go on to describe who was involved in formulating the policy (see Berlan et al. (2014) for the seven stages of policy formulation): was it largely prepared within a government department, how far did it involve others, such as the finance or social welfare ministries or interest groups? You may refer to the extent to which researchers, non-government organizations or the private sector were consulted or involved directly, or not; or how far they tried to influence the formulation of the policy and go on to describe its content (e.g. the policy mechanism, who was covered by it, or the cost implications).

The third stage in the stages heuristic model is that of implementation. What happened once the policy was formulated? How was it executed? Was there good communication between policy makers and those putting it into practice or was this a top-down instruction, which implementers were expected to carry out without discussion? A good example of this sort of analytical narrative is that by Pelletier and colleagues (2011). They explored the policy process in five LMICs to understand why under-nutrition – a major contributor to the global burden of disease – was neglected in these countries.

Pelletier et al.'s research was undertaken in Bangladesh, Bolivia, Guatemala, Peru and Vietnam, and sought to identify the challenges in the policy process and ways to overcome them. The authors looked specifically at the commitment of governments to under-nutrition policies, and then at the processes of agenda setting, policy formulation and implementation. Among their findings, they suggested that high-level political attention to nutrition could be generated in a number of ways but required sustained efforts from policy entrepreneurs and champions. Further they observed that there were many hurdles in the process of policy formulation, and that mid-level actors from ministries and external partners had difficulty in translating windows of opportunity for nutrition into concrete operational plans. This was often due to capacity constraints, differing professional views of under-nutrition, and disagreements over interventions, ownership, roles and responsibilities. Finally, when it came to implementation, the pace and quality of execution was often constrained by weaknesses in human and organizational capacities from national to front line levels.

In taking such an approach to your narrative, you will be looking very closely at both processes and actors – and having analysed your data from interviews and documents – you will be making a judgement about who exercised their power or influence at each stage of the process. Remember you need to demonstrate that you are presenting your analysis based on your data and not just making a judgement according to your own beliefs – although you should be explicit about your own positionality (see below). You need to support your analysis by giving the sources of your analysis such as: 'Fourteen (out of sixteen) interviewees suggested that the Prime Minister and her commitment to this policy was the single most important factor in getting it on to the policy agenda.'

Ethics of policy analysis

In this book you have learned that policy change is political and, in this chapter, that analysis for policy typically serves political ends. Making policy alternatives and their consequences more explicit and improving the political feasibility of policy are neither value-neutral nor immune to politics. Policy analysis, therefore, will not invariably lead to better policy (e.g. policy which improves efficiency, equity or addresses problems of public health importance), or to better policy processes (e.g. fairer decision making processes in which all those affected are provided opportunities to air their views and influence decisions). The substance and process of policy analysis are influenced by who finances, executes, uses and interprets the analysis.

Ongoing, systematic analysis of a policy can be a resource intensive endeavour. Not all policy actors are equally endowed with resources. Everything else being equal, policy analysis may serve to reinforce the prevailing distribution of political power and economic resources: those with political resources are more likely to be those who can finance analysis, and influence who and how the analysis will be used. Those groups with more political resources are in a better position to develop politically informed strategies to influence the positions, players, power and perceptions surrounding a policy. Although policy analysis can be disruptive and lead to progressive change, it may equally reinforce the status quo.

Policy analysis is influenced not just by interests and power but also by the positionality of the analyst. The policy interests and the choice of questions are affected by individual experiences and social attributes relating to race, caste, gender, class (among others) of the researcher and sometimes for the organization in which the analyst is based. If the analysis is *for* policy, it is almost inevitable that the analyst will have a preferred policy outcome. As no one is value-neutral, it is difficult to produce policy analysis which is entirely unbiased. While there are ways to minimize bias, for example, by triangulating methods and sources of information and testing results with peers, it is probably necessary to accept the fact that the results of policy analysis, especially prospective analysis, will reflect to some degree the perspective of the analyst (e.g. the weight they give to equity versus efficiency in analysing the likely impact of a policy). As part of critical reflexivity, it is the responsibility of the analyst to make clear the values that have shaped their approach to the analysis. As an analyst this can involve asking yourself why you are researching that specific policy issue, who will benefit, for whom (whose interests) you are gathering data and what interests and perspectives will be involved in analysis and writing up of findings (Topp et al. 2021).

Analysis for policy raises other kinds of ethical issues. For example, is it ethical to encourage any group to participate in the policy process so as to develop a more powerful coalition? Is it ethical to undermine the legitimacy of opponents or to withhold information from public discourse for tactical purposes? How far should one compromise on evidence-informed policy content so as to accommodate and win over a policy opponent? Your values will dictate how you answer these questions. In thinking about your response it may be useful to assume that other actors use these and other techniques to manipulate the substance and process of policy to their advantage. This may lead you to decide to join in the process of strategically seeking to influence the policy process to achieve your aims.

Alternatively, you may decide to undertake prospective policy analysis to monitor and describe a policy process and leave it to other actors in the policy arena to use the knowledge in the process of policy debate. You may, however, feel uncomfortable with some of the strategies and decide that the ends do not justify the means. While these means may relate to values and ethics, they may also relate to the time, resources and emotional costs of pursuing, and at times failing to achieve, a particular policy change. There is nothing inherently wrong with abandoning or adopting a political strategy.

Summary

In this chapter you have reviewed the retrospective and prospective uses of policy analysis and been introduced to several methods and tools including policy tracing and discourse analysis. Stakeholder analysis was presented. You used this tool to identify policy actors, assess their power, interests and position with respect to a policy issue of your choice, and developed a position map based on this analysis. A range of strategies to manage the position, power, players and perceptions associated with policy change were reviewed as were sources of information for policy analysis. With these tools in hand, you are now hopefully better equipped to pursue policy change as well as to analyse what happened in the past. The tools call for the systematic and creative collection of evidence and for reflexivity and judgement in their analysis – as all analysis will be infused with values and ethical questions. While analysis may more often serve to reinforce the status quo, without the use of policy analysis tools groups without power will remain at a perpetual disadvantage.

Further reading

Balane, M.A., Palafox, B., Palileo-Villanueva, L.M. et al. (2020) Enhancing the use of stakeholder analysis for policy implementation research: towards a novel framing and operationalised measures, *BMJ Global Health*, 5: e002661.

Browne, J., Coffey, B., Cook, K. et al. (2019) A guide to policy analysis as a research method, *Health Promotion International*, 34: 1032–44. https://doi.org/10.1093/heapro/day052

Kakoti, M., Devaki, N., Bestman, A. et al. (2023) How to do (or not to do)…how to embed equity in health research: lessons from piloting the 8Quity tool, *Health Policy and Planning*, 38(4): 571–8.

Reich, M.R. (1996) Applied political analysis for health policy reform, *Current Issues in Public Health*, 2: 186–91.

Surjadjaja, C. and Mayhew, S.H. (2011) Can policy analysis theories predict and inform policy change? Reflections on the battle for legal abortion in Indonesia, *Health Policy and Planning*, 26(5): 373–84.

References

Balane, M.A., Palafox, B., Palileo-Villanueva, L.M. et al. (2020) Enhancing the use of stakeholder analysis for policy implementation research: towards a novel framing and operationalised measures, *BMJ Global Health* 5: e002661.

Banks, M.A. (2022) Towards a continuum of scholarship: the eventual collapse of the distinction between grey and non-grey literature. Presented at the 7th Grey Literature (GL7) Conference: Open Access to Grey Resources, December 5–6, 2005. Available at: https://bit.ly/3JOklgr (accessed 3 October 2022).

Beach, D. and Pedersen, R.B. (2019) *Process-Tracing Methods: Foundations and Guidelines*. Ann Arbor, MI: University of Michigan Press.

Befani, B. and Stedman-Bryce, G. (2017) Process tracing and Bayesian updating for impact evaluation, *Evaluation*, 23(1): 42–60.

Berlan, D., Buse, K., Shiffman, J. and Tanaka, S. (2014) The bit in the middle: a synthesis of global health literature on policy formulation, *Health Policy and Planning*, 29(suppl 3): iii23–34.

Blanchet, K. and James, P. (2013) The role of social networks in the governance of health systems – the case of eye care systems in Ghana, *Health Policy and Planning*: 28(2): 143–56.

Bryman, A. (2008) *Social Research Methods*, 3rd edn. Oxford: Oxford University Press.

Buse, K. (1998) A policy analysis of aid coordination and management in the health sector in Bangladesh: assessing the instruments, exposing the agendas and considering the prospects for government leadership. PhD Dissertation. London School of Hygiene and Tropical Medicine.

Buse, K., Aftab, W., Akhter, S. et al. (2020) The state of diet-related NCD policies in Afghanistan, Bangladesh, Nepal, Pakistan, Tunisia and Vietnam: a comparative assessment that introduces a 'Policy Cube' approach, *Health Policy and Planning*, 35(5): 503–21.

de Leeuw, E. (2017) Engagement of sectors other than health in integrated health governance, policy, and action, *Annual Review of Public Health*, 38(1): 329–49.

Fontana, A. and Frey, J. (1994) Interviewing: the art of science, in N.K. Denzin (ed.) *The Handbook of Qualitative Research*. Thousand Oaks, CA: SAGE, pp. 361–76.

Gilson, L., Erasmus, E., Borghi, J. et al. (2012) Using stakeholder analysis to support moves towards universal coverage: lessons from the SHIELD project, *Health Policy and Planning*, 27(suppl 1): i64–76.

Glassman, A., Reich, M.R., Laserson, K. and Rojas, F. (1999) Political analysis of health reform in the Dominican Republic, *Health Policy and Planning*, 14: 115–26.

Gorsky, M. and Mold, A. (2020) Documentary analysis, in C. Pope and N. Mays (eds.) *Qualitative Research in Health Care*, 4th edn. Oxford: Wiley Blackwell, pp. 83–96.

Hacker, J.S. (1998) The historical logic of national health insurance: structure and sequence in the development of British, Canadian, and US medical policy, *Studies in American Political Development*, 12(1): 57–130.

Kingdon, J.W. (1995) *Agendas, Alternatives, and Public Policies*, 2nd edn. New York: HarperCollins.

Mays, N. and Pope, C. (2020) Quality in qualitative research, in C. Pope, C. and N. Mays (eds.) *Qualitative Research in Health Care*, 4th edn. Oxford: Wiley Blackwell, pp. 211–33.

Mishra, A. and Nambiar, D. (2018) On the unraveling of 'revitalization of local health traditions' in India: an ethnographic inquiry, *International Journal for Equity in Health*, 17: 175.

Pelletier, D.L, Frongillo, E.A., Gervais, S. et al. (2011) Nutrition agenda setting, policy formulation and implementation: lessons from the Mainstreaming Nutrition Initiative, *Health Policy and Planning*, 27(1): 19–31.

Philip Morris (no date) PM tools to affect legislative decisions. October 2003. Bates No. 204770711. Available at http://legacy.library.ucsf.edu/tid/ (accessed 3 October 2022).

Pope, C., Ziebland, S. and Mays, N. (2020) Analysis, in C. Pope and N. Mays (eds.) *Qualitative Research in Health Care*, 4th edn. Oxford: Wiley Blackwell, pp. 111–34.

Powell, J. and van Velthoven, M.H. (2020) Digital data and online qualitative research, in C. Pope and N. Mays (eds.) *Qualitative Research in Health Care*, 4th edn. Oxford: Wiley Blackwell, pp. 97–110.

Quinn, B. (2012) Jeremy Hunt backs 12-week legal limit on abortions, *The Guardian*, 6 October. Available at: www.theguardian.com/world/2012/oct/06/jeremy-hunt-12-week-abortion-limit (accessed 24 April 2023).

Reich, M.R. (1996) Applied political analysis for health policy reform, *Current Issues in Public Health*, 2: 186–91.

Roberts, M.J., Hsiao, W., Berman, P. and Reich, M.R. (2004) *Getting Health Reform Right: A Guide to Improving Performance and Equity*. Oxford: Oxford University Press.

Scarr, J., Buse, K., Norton, R. et al. (2022) Rising tide: a policy analysis tracing the emergence of drowning prevention on the global health and development agenda, *Lancet Global Health*, 10(7): E1058–66.

Shiffman, J. and Smith, S. (2007) Generation of political priority for global health initiatives: a framework and case study of maternal mortality, *The Lancet*, 370 (9595): 1370–9.

Stedman-Bryce, G. (2013) *Health for All: Towards Free Universal Health Care in Ghana*, End of Campaign Evaluation Report. Oxford: Oxfam.

Topp, S.M., Schaaf, M., Sriram, V. et al. (2021) Power analysis in health policy and systems research: a guide to research conceptualization, *BMJ Global Health*, 6(11): 6:e007268. https://doi.org/10.1136/bmjgh-2021-007268

Trostle, J., Bronfman, M. and Langer, A. (1999) How do researchers influence decision makers? Case studies of Mexican policies, *Health Policy and Planning*, 14(2): 103–14.

Weimer, D.L. and Vining, A.R. (2010) *Policy Analysis: Concepts and Practices*, 5th edn. Englewood Cliffs, NJ: Prentice Hall.

Yazdannik, A., Yousefy, A. and Mohammadi, S. (2017) Discourse analysis: a useful methodology for health-care system researchers, *Journal of Education and Health Promotion*, 6: 111. https://doi.org/10.4103/jehp.jehp_124_15.

Glossary

Accountability The evaluative process by which an individual, group or organization provides an account of its behaviour and/or performance for which they are responsible to another, overseeing person, group or organization, or is held to account on the basis of performance reports provided by an independent body. Poor performance may lead to a range of sanctions of varying degrees of severity.

Actor Shorthand term used to denote any participant in the policy process that affects or has an interest in a policy, including individuals, organizations, groups, governments and international bodies.

Advocacy coalition Grouping of actors within a policy sub-system distinguished by a shared set of norms, beliefs and resources. It can include politicians, civil servants, members of interest groups, journalists and academics who share ideas about policy goals and to a lesser extent about solutions.

Agency The capacity of individuals, groups or organizations to act independently and to make their own free choices.

Agenda setting Process by which certain issues come onto the policy agenda from the much larger number of issues potentially worthy of attention by policy makers.

Audit Examination of the extent to which an activity corresponds with predetermined standards or criteria.

Authority Whereas power concerns the ability to influence others, authority is the right to do so.

Autonomy Self-determination or the state of being or behaving in a self-governing way with the ability to make one's own decisions.

Beneficence Acting for the good of the person or people served with a strong connotation of moral obligation (often applied to clinician behaviour).

Bottom-up approach to understanding policy implementation Approach to explaining policy implementation that focuses on how local actors and contextual factors influence policy implementation.

Bounded rationality Describes the way that people, including policy makers, always operate with imperfect knowledge and thus, at best, can only make decisions that are satisfactory as opposed to optimal.

Bureaucracy This term can refer to: (1) institutions through which government policy is pursued; (2) public officials, often known as civil servants, whose job it is to advise ministers (the executive) on how best to take forward their policy goals and then to manage the process of policy implementation; and (3) a hierarchical and rule-based approach to public administration.

Cause group Civil society group whose main goal is to promote a particular issue or cause such as free speech or prison reform.

Civil society The part of society that is outside the private sphere of the family or household, the market and the state.

Civil society group A non-market (i.e. not-for-profit) interest group or organization which is also not part of the state. These groups are sometimes referred to as the Third Sector.

Cognitive bias A systematic error in reasoning arising from intrinsic limitations in the human brain's ability to process information and its tendency to simplify. For example, because our attention span is limited, we tend to be selective in what we pay attention to and tend to favour evidence that confirms our prior beliefs and values (confirmation bias).

Coloniality The legacy of systems and practices, including particularly 'ways of thinking', resulting from the imposition of the will of one people on another and the use of the resources of the subordinated people for the benefit of the imposer, as in the case of European colonialism.

Colonization The action or process of settling among and establishing control over the indigenous people of an area.

Conflicts of interest A set of circumstances that create a risk that an individual's ability to apply professional judgement is, or could be, or could be perceived to be, impaired or influenced by a secondary interest (such as a financial one).

Content Substance of a particular policy which details its constituent parts (e.g. its specific objectives).

Context Systemic factors – political, economic, social or cultural, local, national and international – which may affect health policy.

Corporation An association of stockholders (shareholders) which is regarded as a legal entity or a 'person' under most national laws. Ownership is marked by ease of transferability and the limited liability of stockholders.

Decentralization The transfer of authority and responsibilities from central government to local levels.

Decolonization The process of undoing colonial dispossession and destruction; for example, through practices that reduce emphasis on Eurocentric knowledge, and emphasize, promote and nurture other indigenous and/or local knowledge production.

Democracy A system of societal governance in which the people elect their representatives to form a time-limited government through periodic elections (indirect democracy) or participate directly in decision making through mechanisms such as referenda.

Dissemination Process by which research findings are made known to audiences, including policy makers.

Donor agency A foreign government or philanthropic organization that provides resources for social welfare, health and social services or development.

Downstream interventions Policies or programmes focused on behaviour change at the individual level, not addressing the structural influences on individual behaviour.

Efficiency A measure of the extent to which (health and health care) resources are being used to produce the greatest possible value. In health policy, efficiency typically focuses on the relationship between resource inputs, outputs (e.g. services delivered or reforms enacted in related policy fields such as education) and outcomes (e.g. health improvements in terms of reductions in mortality, reductions in morbidity or gains in quality-adjusted life years).

Elitism The theory that power is concentrated in the hands of a small minority in society.

Epistemic community Policy community marked by shared political values, and a shared understanding of a problem and its causes.

Epistemicide The destruction of certain forms of knowledge or ways of knowing – most often linked to colonialism in which knowledge practices from the Global North displaced indigenous ones.

Epistemology The theory of knowledge which covers, in particular, the methods used to establish knowledge and the validity of that knowledge; i.e. how to distinguish between knowledge that is justified and mere opinion.

Equity The absence of unfair, avoidable or remediable differences between groups of people defined socially, economically or in other ways (e.g. by gender, ethnicity, disability or sexual orientation).

Evaluation Research designed specifically to assess the operation and/or impact of a programme or policy in order to determine whether the programme or policy is worth pursuing, stopping or amending.

Evidence Any form of data, information or knowledge, including, but not confined to research, that may be used to inform decisions.

Evidence-based medicine Movement within medicine and related professions to base clinical practice on the most rigorous and comprehensive scientific evidence available, ideally from randomized controlled trials of the effectiveness of interventions.

Evidence-based (or evidence-informed) policy Movement within public policy to give evidence greater weight in shaping policy decisions. It is better described as 'evidence-informed' policy than 'evidence-based', since evidence can only ever be one, albeit important, input to decision making.

Executive Leadership of a country (i.e. the president and/or prime minister and other ministers). The prime minister/president and senior ministers are often referred to as the cabinet.

Fairness Fairness is an umbrella term that can refer to equality (equal treatment of all regardless of individual characteristics), equality of opportunity, justice and equity (unequal treatment of unequals, for instance, in relation to their needs). Fairness is one of the most contested but widely sought after features of policy and policy processes. This is because of the many definitions of fairness, and the value many actors accord to these ideas.

Feasibility A characteristic of those issues or policy options or solutions considered practical in a particular political context.

Federal system A government system in which the sub-national (i.e. state or provincial) level of government is not subordinate to the national government but has substantial powers of its own which the national government cannot take away without changing the constitution.

Feminism A range of socio-political movements, ideologies and scholarly theories that aim to define and establish the political, economic, personal and social equality of the sexes.

Formative evaluation Evaluation undertaken in the early or pilot stage of a policy or programme, designed to assess how well it is being implemented with a view to refining it to improve its longer term or full-scale implementation.

Frames Concepts and images by which policy issues are described and understood.

Framing The process by which policy issues are constructed and given particular 'frames' that relate to the values and/or goals of different interests.

Global civil society Civil society groups which are global in their aims, advocacy or organization.

Global constitutionalism Attempts to institutionalize and order governance processes 'above' the level of the state through mechanisms similar to those at state level.

Global public goods Goods which are undersupplied by private markets, inefficiently produced by individual states and have universal benefits.

Global social movements Loose networks of individuals and organizations that collaborate across borders to advance similar policy goals and in doing so have become powerful actors in global governance and policy making.

Globalization The interdependence of the world's economies, cultures and populations, brought about by cross-border trade in goods and services, technology, and flows of investment, people and information.

Governance The process of societal decision making where there are many policy actors involved, and where the relationship between the government of the day and these policy actors is not entirely rules-based or hierarchical.

Government That part of the state comprising the executive ('the government of the day') and the bureaucracy (civil or public service and ministries).

Ideas The values, evidence, anecdote and argument that shape policy, including the way a policy problem or solution is presented or framed.

Implementation Process of turning a policy into practice or action.

Implementation gap Difference between what the policy architect intended and the end-result of a policy.

Implementation science The study of methods and approaches designed to embed evidence-informed policies, programmes and practices in regular use.

Infodemic An excess of information about a health issue that is often invalid, rapidly disseminated and hampers an effective response.

Insider groups Interest groups which pursue a strategy designed to win themselves the status of legitimate participants in the government policy process.

Institutions In political science, the 'rules of the game' determining how organizations, such as governments, operate. These can be formal structures and procedures, but also informal norms of behaviour that may not be written down. Confusingly, the term is also in more general use to refer to 'organizations'.

Interest What an actor or group stands to gain or lose from a policy change.

Interest group Any group outside the state including market-related and civil society groups that attempt to influence government policy to achieve goals that are either directly beneficial to the group's members or advance the societal goal it seeks.

Iron triangle Small, stable and exclusive policy community usually involving executive agencies of government, legislative committees and private market interest groups (e.g. between politicians, policy officials and big pharma).

Issue network Loose extensive, diverse network of policy actors who come together informally to try to draw attention to an issue, address a specific problem or promote a particular solution.

Judiciary Judges and courts responsible for ensuring that the government of the day (the executive) acts according to the laws passed by the legislature and/or in line with the constitution.

Knowledge transfer Information or research dissemination strategy usually incorporating a variety of 'linkage' and 'exchange' activities designed to tighten the links between researchers and policy makers.

Legislature Body that enacts the laws that govern a country and oversees the executive. It is normally democratically elected in order to represent the people of the country and commonly referred to as the parliament or assembly. Many countries have two chambers or 'houses' of parliament.

Legitimacy A characteristic of those issues which public policy makers see as appropriate for government to act on.

Majoritarian A government system in which election results are determined by a simple numerical majority of the votes cast and/or the parliamentary seats won, sometimes referred to as 'first past the post'.

Market-related interest groups Interest groups such as business, professional and employer associations.

Marxism A political theory named after Karl Marx. It asserts that the owners of capital and the means of production inevitably exploit those who only have their labour to offer in the capitalist system. It examines the consequences of this for the position of labour, capitalist productivity and economic development.

Monitoring Routine collection of performance data on an activity usually against a plan or contract.

Multilateral Having members or participation from several groups, especially the governments of different countries.

Multilateralism The practice of co-operation and co-ordination between three or more states to pursue common interests, as well as the more recent phenomenon of formal institutions and organizations (which may or may not include non-state actors) to support such co-operation (e.g. UNICEF or the Global Fund).

Multinational Business which operates in at least one country other than its home country.

Nationalism Identification with one's own nation and support for its interests, especially to the exclusion or detriment of the interests of other nations.

Neoliberalism An ideology and policy model that emphasizes the value of free market competition and reducing, especially through privatization and austerity, state influence in the economy. It has been described as a hyper-form of capitalism and/or a means for wealthy elites to intensify their capital accumulation.

Non-governmental organization (NGO) Any not for-profit organization outside the state (i.e. in civil society), though the term also tends to be used more narrowly to refer to larger, structured organizations providing services rather than all of civil society.

Nonmaleficence The principle of ensuring that no harm is created by an action or omission (often applied to clinician behaviour).

Norms The values accepted in a particular social group (a population or population sub-group) as the correct way to judge specific behaviour or policy decisions.

Outsider groups Interest groups which have either failed to attain insider status or have deliberately chosen a path of confrontation with government.

Parliamentary system A system of government in which the members of the executive (the cabinet) are also members of the legislature and are chosen from the members of the legislature who represent political parties that have a majority in the legislature.

Path dependency The phenomenon in which decisions taken in one period influence the scope and direction of later policy by reinforcing the position of particular interest groups or putting in place specific ways of working that restrict future action.

Pluralism The theory that power is widely distributed in society.

Policy Broad statement of goals, objectives and means that creates the framework for activity leading to implementation with varying degrees of completeness. It often takes the form of explicit written documents, but may also be implicit or unwritten.

Policy agenda List of issues to which an organization, usually the government, is giving serious attention at any one time with a view to taking some sort of action.

Policy community (and sub-system) Relatively stable network of organizations (interest groups and state agencies) and individuals involved in a recognizable field of wider public policy such as health policy. Within each of these fields, there will be identifiable sub-systems, such as for mental health policy, with their own policy communities.

Policy elite Specific group of policy makers who hold senior positions in a policy system, and often have privileged access to other top members of the same, and other, organizations.

Policy instrument One of the range of options at the disposal of the policy maker in order to give effect to a policy goal (e.g. privatization, regulation, subsidy, etc.).

Policy makers Those who influence or make policies in organizations such as central or local government, multinational companies or local businesses, clinics or hospitals.

Policy network Generic term for inter-dependent organizations (e.g. interest groups and state agencies) involved in an area of policy that exchange resources and bargain to varying degrees to attain their specific goals.

Policy process The way in which problems rise to policy makers' attention and policies are initiated, formulated, negotiated, adopted, communicated, implemented and evaluated.

Policy stream The set of possible policy solutions or alternatives developed by experts, politicians, bureaucrats and interest groups, together with the activities of those interested in these options (e.g. debates about the merits of different solutions).

Policy transfer A process in which knowledge and ideas about policies (broadly defined) in one political setting (past or present) are used in the development of policies in another political setting.

Policy windows Points in time when the opportunity arises for an issue to come onto the policy agenda and be taken seriously with a view to action.

Politics stream Political events such as shifts in the national mood or public opinion, elections and changes in government, social uprisings, demonstrations and campaigns by interest groups that influence the likelihood that a problem and its potential solution will be acted on by governments.

Populism An approach to politics that is difficult to define since it is not intellectually coherent but usually includes leaders and potential leaders who define themselves as the champions of the ordinary people, purport to be anti-elitist and who brand opponents as disloyal to the country. Populism particularly appeals to those who are concerned to protect the security and cultural integrity of their country against outsiders ('others') but who are also sceptical of the ability of democratically elected government to do so.

Positionality The stance or positioning of the policy maker or policy researcher, related to their particular identity, in the social, economic and political context of a policy issue. Thought to shape how they think about and tackle the issue.

Positivism A philosophical system that argues that knowledge can only come from observation and experience and rejects metaphysical speculation.

Power The ability to control resources and influence people, leading them to do things that they might otherwise not have done.

Presidential system A system of government in which the president (i.e. the head of the government of the day – the executive) is not a member of the legislature but elected separately. Presidential systems vary in the extent to which the president has directive powers that do not depend on the will of the legislature.

Principal–agent theory Theory of organizational and government behaviour that focuses on the relationship between principals (e.g. purchasers) and their agents (e.g. providers), together with the contracts or agreements that enable the principal to specify what is to be done (e.g. service provision) and check that this has been accomplished.

Private sector The part of the economy that is not under direct government control and operates primarily on a for-profit basis.

Privatization Sale of publicly owned property to the private sector.

Problem stream Indicators of the scale and significance of an issue which give it visibility, together with the activities of those interested in the issue.

Proportional representation Voting system which is designed to ensure as far as possible that the proportion of votes received by each political party equates to their share of the seats in the legislature.

Public choice (theory) The theory that explains government decision making as a result of the actions of self-interested and rational public actors.

Public goods Goods that are available to all and used by the individual but benefit the community as a whole such that the more people avail themselves of the good or service, the greater the social benefit.

Public–private partnership A contract between a private sector organization and a public body (e.g. government agency) to provide a public asset (e.g. a hospital building) or service, in which the private organization bears significant risk and management responsibility, with its remuneration linked to its performance.

Racism The belief that different human groups possess distinct and inherited characteristics, abilities or qualities with some of these groups superior to others as a result.

Regulation The rules and standards made and maintained by an authority – often by government (e.g. in a private market for goods and services to prevent anti-competitive behaviour or false claims).

Research Systematic activity designed to generate rigorous new knowledge and relate it to existing knowledge in order to improve understanding of the physical or social world.

Saviourism A belief in a saviour; also used to describe, critically, a white person or tendency for countries of the Global North to engage in activities that they see as or are as perceived as undertaken with an intention to liberate or rescue non-white people or countries of the Global South.

Social constructivism A sociological theory of knowledge according to which knowledge develops as a result of social interaction, collaboration and language use.

Social contract A theory that concerns the legitimacy of the state's or ruler's authority over the individual. It is based on the idea that individuals have consented, either explicitly or tacitly, to surrender some of their freedoms and submit to the authority of the state or ruler.

Social media Software that uses web-based and mobile technologies for the creation, sharing and exchange of user-generated content in virtual networks and communities.

Social movement Loose grouping of individuals sharing certain views and attempting to influence others (e.g. through use of social media, demonstrations, etc.) but without a formal organizational structure.

Social network analysis Methods used for mapping, measuring and analysing the social relationships between people, groups and organizations.

Social structure The recurrent patterned arrangements that influence or limit the choices and opportunities available to people in society.

Stakeholder analysis Process through which those making policy or affected by it are identified and their likely position and levels of interest and influence are assessed.

State A set of public bodies that enjoy legal sovereignty over a fixed territorial area and extends beyond the government of the day, comprising the executive, legislature, bureaucracy, judiciary, courts and military as well as other public bodies, including the specialized agencies that regulate aspects of health and the health care system.

Stewardship The role of governments in directing and overseeing the health system, improving its performance and ensuring that it is maintained in good order for future generations (e.g. by ensuring a supply of trained health workers).

Stigma The shame, perceived disgrace or social disapproval associated with a particular social status or disease. Policies can amplify or counter stigma through the way they are labelled, designed or implemented (e.g. the 'dole' versus 'social security').

Street-level bureaucrats Frontline staff involved in delivering public services to members of the public who have some discretion and agency in how they apply the objectives of policies handed down to them.

Summative evaluation Evaluation designed to produce an overall verdict on a policy or programme in terms of the balance of costs and benefits.

Technocracy A form of government led by an elite of technical experts.

Top-down approach to understanding policy implementation Sees policy implementation as a linear, rational process in which policy initiated at higher levels of the policy system (e.g. national government) is subsequently executed at subordinate levels.

Transnational advocacy networks Actors, who share common values or policy objectives, collaborate internationally on an issue by sharing complementary resources to highlight specific policy problems and advance solutions (typically more structured than global social movements).

Transnational corporations For-profit enterprises operating across multiple countries comprising parent enterprises and their foreign affiliates.

Transparency A characteristic of a policy process in which the values, evidence, participants, method of deliberation, etc. are visible to those actors not directly involved, especially members of the public.

Unilateral Performed by, or affecting, only one group or country involved in a situation, without the agreement of the other(s).

Unitary system A system of government in which the lower levels of government are constitutionally subordinate to the national government and derive their authority entirely from central government.

Upstream determinants of health Structural features of society (e.g. socio-economic inequalities, urban design, taxation) that shape individuals' exposure to health-harms choices and health-related behaviour.

Upstream interventions Policies involving collective action that focus on structural change in society, with the potential to affect large groups of people, for example, government regulation.

Values The principles or norms people use to decide what, for them, is 'good' and important to pursue in relation to society or their own lives; that is, the basis on which they define 'the good society' or 'the good life' or 'being a good person'.

White supremacy The belief that white people constitute a superior race and should dominate societies, to the exclusion or detriment of other racial and ethnic groups.

Index

Page numbers in italics are figures; with 't' are tables.